Insurance Handbook for the Medical Office

STUDENT WORKBOOK

Insurance Handbook for the Medical Office

STUDENT WORKBOOK

Twelfth Edition

MARILYN TAKAHASHI FORDNEY

CMA-AC (AAMA)

Formerly Instructor of Medical Insurance, Medical Terminology,
Medical Machine Transcription, and Medical Office Procedures
Ventura College
Ventura, California

ELSEVIER
SAUNDERS

ELSEVIER
SAUNDERS

3251 Riverport Lane
St. Louis, Missouri 63043

Workbook for
INSURANCE HANDBOOK FOR THE MEDICAL OFFICE, TWELFTH EDITION

ISBN: 978-1-4377-2255-0

Notices

Knowledge and best practice in this field are constantly changing. As new research and experience broaden our understanding, changes in research methods, professional practices, or medical treatment may become necessary.

Practitioners and researchers must always rely on their own experience and knowledge in evaluating and using any information, methods, compounds, or experiments described herein. In using such information or methods they should be mindful of their own safety and the safety of others, including parties for whom they have a professional responsibility.

With respect to any drug or pharmaceutical products identified, readers are advised to check the most current information provided (i) on procedures featured or (ii) by the manufacturer of each product to be administered, to verify the recommended dose or formula, the method and duration of administration, and contraindications. It is the responsibility of practitioners, relying on their own experience and knowledge of their patients, to make diagnoses, to determine dosages and the best treatment for each individual patient, and to take all appropriate safety precautions.

To the fullest extent of the law, neither the Publisher nor the authors, contributors, or editors, assume any liability for any injury and/or damage to persons or property as a matter of products liability, negligence or otherwise, or from any use or operation of any methods, products, instructions, or ideas contained in the material herein.

Acquisitions Editor: Susan Cole
Developmental Editor: Karen Baer
Publishing Services Manager: Catherine Jackson
Project Manager: Divya Krish
Design Direction: Kim Denando

Printed in the United States

Last digit is the print number: 9 8 7 6 5 4 3 2 1

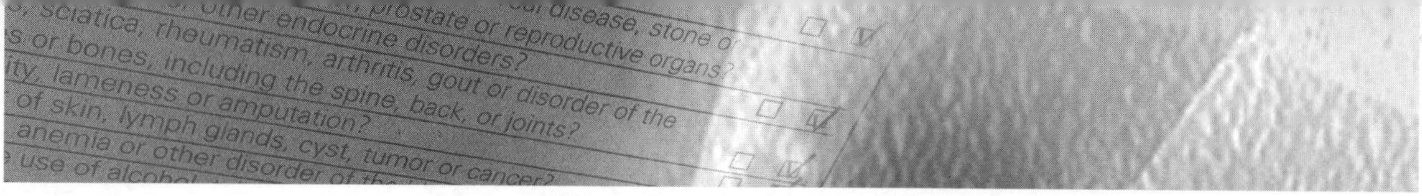

Acknowledgments

This edition of the *Workbook* for *Insurance Handbook for the Medical Office* has had considerable input from many medical professionals. Expert consultation has been necessary because of the complexities of the managed care environment, intricacies of procedural and diagnostic coding, impact of technology on insurance claims processing, and the more sophisticated role the insurance billing specialist has in today's workforce.

I owe an immense debt of gratitude to the reviewers of the *Workbook* assignments and to Karen Levein, instructor at Burbank Adult School, who helped me update the coding data. Also a debt of gratitude is extended to Linda French, CMA-C, NCICS, CPC, and Karen Hawkins, RN, who acted as technical collaborators and helped me update the clinical and coding information of the patient records in the *Workbook* exercises and tests for a previous edition.

Most important, I express overwhelming gratitude to the professional consultants who provided vital information to make this *Workbook* better than previous editions. They are:

Deborah Emmons, CMA
President
S.T.A.T. Transcription Service
Port Hueneme, California

Sandy Gutt
Instructor
Southern California Regional Occupational Center
Torrance, California

Ronna Jurow, MD
Active Staff and Attending Physician in Obstetrics, Gynecology, and Infertility
Community Memorial Hospital
Ventura, California

Lucille M. Loignon, MD, FACS
Diplomate, American Board of Ophthalmology
Oxnard, California

Maria Reyes
Ventura Anesthesia Medical Group
Ventura, California

Lita Starr
Office Manager
Oxnard, California

Paul Wertlake, MD
Formerly Medical Director and Chief Pathologist
Unilab Corporation
Tarzana, California

Shirley Wertlake, CLS
Formerly Technical Specialist
Clinical Laboratories
University of California—Los Angeles Medical Center
Los Angeles, California

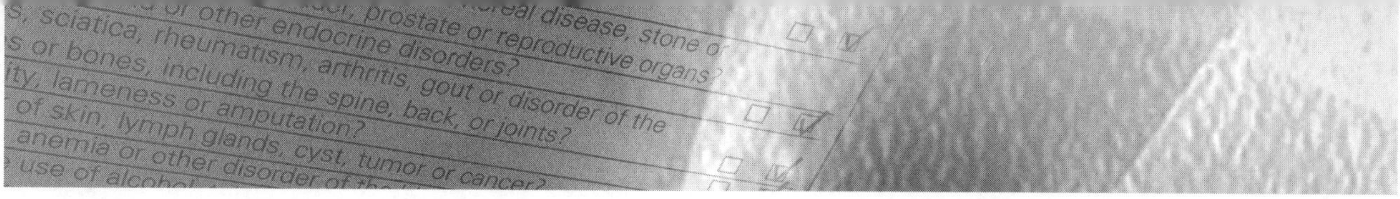

Contents

Instruction Guide to the Workbook, ix

Learning Objectives, ix

- Instructions to the Student, x
- Key Terms and Key Abbreviations, x
- Note Taking, x
- Review Question Assignments, x
- Simulation Assignments, x
- Medical Terminology and Abbreviations, xi
- Patient Records, xi
- Financial Records, xi
- CMS-1500 (08-05) Claim Form, xi
- Performance Evaluation Checklist, xii
- Appendices, xii
- Student Reference Notebook, xii
- Content Suggestions From the Workbook, xii
- Content Suggestions From the Handbook, xii
- Tests, xii
- Reference Material, xii
- Employee Insurance Procedure Manual, xv
- Student Software Challenge, xv

UNIT 1

Career Role and Responsibilities

1 Role of an Insurance Billing Specialist, 1

2 HIPAA Compliance and Privacy in Insurance Billing, 9

UNIT 2

The Claims Process

3 Basics of Health Insurance, 24

4 Medical Documentation and the Electronic Health Record, 41

5 Diagnostic Coding, 63

6 Procedural Coding, 86

7 The Paper Claim: CMS-1500 (08-05), 111

8 Electronic Data Interchange: Transactions and Security, 139

9 Receiving Payments and Insurance Problem Solving, 165

10 Office and Insurance Collection Strategies, 189

UNIT 3

Health Care Payers

11 The Blue Plans, Private Insurance, and Managed Care Plans, 219

12 Medicare, 244

13 Medicaid and Other State Programs, 300

14 TRICARE and CHAMPVA, 325

15 Workers' Compensation, 356

16 Disability Income Insurance and Disability Benefit Programs, 383

UNIT 4

Inpatient and Outpatient Billing

17 Hospital Billing, 415

UNIT 5

Employment

18 Seeking a Job and Attaining Professional Advancement, 447

Tests, 463

Appendix A College Clinic Office Policies and Mock Fee Schedule, 511

Appendix B Medicare Level II HCPCS Codes, 545

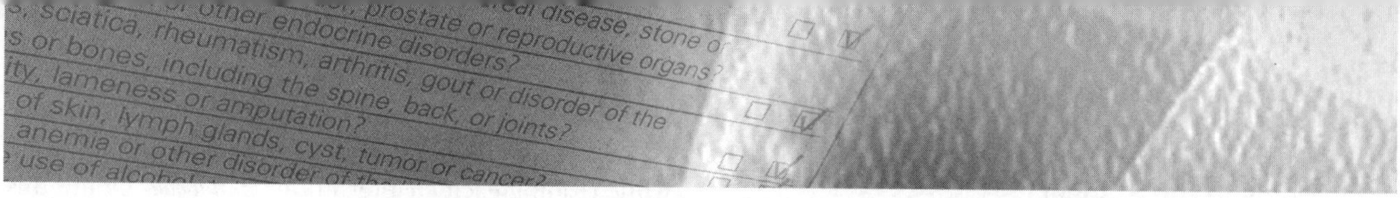

Instruction Guide to the Workbook

LEARNING OBJECTIVES

The student will be able to:

- Define and spell key terms and key abbreviations for each chapter.
- Answer review questions for each chapter of the *Handbook*.
- Complete assignments to enhance and develop better critical thinking skills.
- Define abbreviations as they appear on a patient record.
- Abstract subjective and objective data from patient records.
- Review documentation on patient records.
- Code professional services properly, using the *Current Procedural Terminology* (CPT) Code Book or Appendices A and B.
- Select diagnostic code numbers, using the *International Classification of Diseases, Ninth Revision, Clinical Modification* (ICD-9-CM) and/or the *International Classification of Diseases, Tenth Revision, Clinical Modification* (ICD-10-CM).
- Locate errors on insurance claims before submission to insurance companies.
- Locate errors on returned insurance claims.
- Complete an insurance claim tracer form.
- Carry out collection procedures on delinquent accounts.
- Execute financial management procedures for tracing managed care plans.
- Abstract information necessary to complete insurance claim forms from patient records and billing statement/ledger cards.
- Post payments, adjustments, and balances to patients' statement/ledger cards when submitting insurance claims.
- Compute mathematical calculations for Medicare and TRICARE cases.
- Analyze insurance claims in both hospital inpatient and outpatient settings.
- Prepare a cover letter, résumé, job application, and follow-up letter when searching for employment.
- Access the Internet and visit websites to research and/or obtain data.

Instructions to the Student

The twelfth edition of *Workbook for Insurance Handbook for the Medical Office* has been prepared for those who use the textbook, *Insurance Handbook for the Medical Office* (hereafter referred to as the *Handbook*). It is designed to assist the learner in a practical approach to doing insurance billing and coding. It will also develop a better understanding of the differences among the insurance programs when completing and electronically transmitting the 837 P (Professional) or the paper claim CMS-1500 (08-05).

The key terms and key abbreviations are repeated for quick reference when studying. Each chapter's outline serves as a lecture guide to use for note taking. The review questions in the forms of short answer, true/false, multiple choice, and matching are presented to reinforce learning of key concepts for each topic.

Some assignments give students hands-on experience in typing claim forms for optical character recognition (OCR) scanning equipment, which is used in many states for insurance claims processing and payment. Insurance claim forms and other sample documents that are easily removable are included for keyboarding practice.

Current procedural and diagnostic code exercises for both ICD-9-CM and ICD-10-CM are used throughout to facilitate and enhance coding skills for submitting a claim or making up an itemized billing statement.

Icons appearing throughout the *Workbook* are used to indicate assignment types. An illustration of each icon, along with its description, is outlined below.

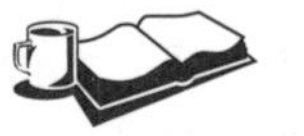

Self-study assignments encompass important points from each chapter and allow you to study at your own pace.

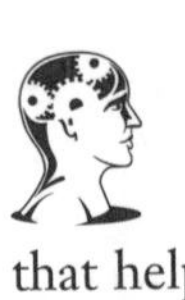

Critical thinking assignments require skills that help prepare you for real-world scenarios encountered in insurance billing.

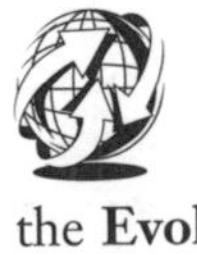

The **Student Software Challenge** located on the **Evolve** website is required for completing selected assignments for several chapters. **Internet** assignments point you to the World Wide Web for resources.

Key Terms and Key Abbreviations

Key terms and key abbreviations are presented for each chapter, and definitions may be located in the glossary at the end of the *Handbook*. It is suggested that you make up 3- by 5-inch index cards for each term or abbreviation and write in the definitions as you encounter them while reading each chapter in the *Handbook*. Doing this will reinforce your knowledge and help you learn the words and abbreviations. Your instructor may wish to select certain words to study for pop quizzes.

Note Taking

Taking notes is an important key to success in studying and learning. Note taking helps an individual pay attention during class and retain information. Each chapter has a study outline for organizational purposes, and the outline may be used as a guide for writing down key points during lectures or when studying or reviewing from the *Handbook* for tests. Use file cards, notepads, or a notebook for taking notes. Underline or highlight important words or phrases. To improve the usefulness of notes, try the following format:

1. On a notepad sheet or file card, draw a margin 3 inches from the left.
2. Use the left side for topic headings and the right side for notes.
3. Skip a few lines when the topic changes.
4. Write numbers or letters to indicate sub-ideas under a heading.
5. Be brief; do not write down every word except when emphasizing a quotation, rule, or law. Write notes in your own words because that is what you will understand.
6. Use abbreviations that you know how to translate.
7. Listen carefully to the lecture.
8. After the lecture, reread your notes. Highlight the word(s) on the left side of the page to identify the topic of the notes on the right.
9. For study purposes, cover the right side and see if you can explain to yourself or someone else the topic or word.
10. Remember: learning is by doing, and doing is up to you. So take notes for better understanding.

Review Question Assignments

Review questions have been designed to encompass important points for each chapter to assist you in studying insurance billing and coding theory. For this edition, crossword puzzles for each chapter and additional quizzes are available on the Evolve website.

Simulation Assignments

Assume that you have been hired as an insurance billing specialist and that you are working in a clinic setting for an incorporated group of medical doctors, other allied health specialists, and a podiatrist. You will be asked to complete various assignments. These doctors will be on the staff of a nearby hospital. Appendix A details this clinic's policies and procedures, which you must read completely before beginning the competency-based assignments. Within each chapter, the simulation assignments progress from easy to more complex. Some assignments are given with critical thinking problems, which the instructor may use for class discussion.

Always read the assignment entirely before beginning it. There are *Workbook* assignments. Table I-1 is a reference guide that lists chapter numbers and titles, along with the corresponding assignment numbers.

Medical Terminology and Abbreviations

A list of abbreviations is provided in Appendix A to help you learn how to abstract and read physicians' notes. Decode any abbreviations that you do not understand or that are unfamiliar to you. To reinforce learning these abbreviations, write their meanings on the assignment pages. If you do not have a background in medical terminology, it may be wise to use a good medical dictionary as a reference or, better yet, enroll in a terminology course to master that skill.

Patient Records

Patient records, financial accounting records (ledgers), and encounter forms are presented as they might appear in a physician's office, so the learner may have the tools needed to extract information to complete claim forms. Patient records have been abbreviated because of space and page constraints. The records contain pertinent data for each type of case, but it was necessary to omit a lengthy physical examination. Because detailed documentation is encouraged in medical practices, the records all appear typewritten rather than in handwritten notes. The physician's signature appears after each dated entry on the record.

All the materials included in the assignments have been altered to prevent identification of the cases or parties involved. The names and addresses are fictitious, and no reference to any person living or dead is intended. No evaluation of medical practice or medical advice is to be inferred from the patient records nor is any recommendation made toward alternative treatment methods or prescribed medications.

Financial Records

Financial accounting record statements (ledgers) are included for practice in posting, totaling fees, and properly recording appropriate information when an insurance claim is submitted. Refer to Appendix A to obtain information about the Mock Fee Schedule and the physicians' fees for posting to the statements.

CMS-1500 (08-05) Claim Form

If you have access to a computer, use the practice management software that accompanies the *Workbook* to complete each assignment and print it out for evaluation. To complete the CMS-1500 (08-05) claim form properly for each type of program, refer to the section in Chapter 7

TABLE I-1

***Workbook* Assignments**

Handbook Chapter	Corresponding *Workbook* Chapter	Assignments
1	Role of an Insurance Billing Specialist	1–1 through 1–3
2	HIPAA Compliance and Privacy in Insurance Billing	2–1 through 2–5
3	Basics of Health Insurance	3–1 through 3–7
4	Medical Documentation and the Electronic Health Record	4–1 through 4–7
5	Diagnostic Coding	5–1 through 5–12
6	Procedural Coding	6–1 through 6–10
7	The Paper Claim: CMS-1500 (08-05)	7–1 through 7–7
8	Electronic Data Interchange: Transactions and Security	8–1 through 8–9
9	Receiving Payments and Insurance Problem Solving	9–1 through 9–9
10	Office and Insurance Collection Strategies	10–1 through 10–7
11	The Blue Plans, Private Insurance, and Managed Care Plans	11–1 through 11–6
12	Medicare	12–1 through 12–11
13	Medicaid and Other State Programs	13–1 through 13–5
14	TRICARE and CHAMPVA	14–1 through 14–7
15	Workers' Compensation	15–1 through 15–6
16	Disability Income Insurance and Disability Benefit Programs	16–1 through 16–6
17	Hospital Billing	17–1 through 17–9
18	Seeking a Job and Attaining Professional Advancement	18–1 through 18–7

of the *Handbook* that describes in detail the correct information to be put in each block. Also view the templates found at the end of Chapter 7 for each insurance type.

Complete all insurance forms in OCR style because this is the format in which insurance carriers process claims most expediently. Chapter 7 gives instructions on OCR do's and don'ts. If you do not have access to a computer, type or neatly write in the information on the insurance form as you abstract it from the patient record.

Performance Evaluation Checklist

The twelfth edition features a competency-based format for each assignment indicating performance objectives to let you know what is to be accomplished. The task (job assignment), conditions (elements needed to perform and complete the task), and standards (time management), as well as directions for the specific task, are included. Use of a checklist with points projected and points earned is available on the Evolve website; the checklist assists in scoring the assignments and helps you develop the skill of speed in completing tasks.

A two-part performance evaluation checklist used when completing a CMS-1500 (08-05) claim form is depicted in Figures I-1 and I-2. Reproduce these sheets only for the assignments that involve completing the CMS-1500 (08-05) claim form. Your instructor will give you the number of points to be assigned for each step.

Appendices

Refer to Table I.2, which shows what is included in each of the appendixes.

Student Reference Notebook

A student reference notebook is recommended so that you can access information quickly to help you complete the *Workbook* assignments. Before beginning the assignments, tear out Appendix A and place it in a three-ring binder with chapter indices. Appendix A includes the clinic policies and guidelines, data about the clinic staff, medical and laboratory abbreviations, and mock fee schedule used while working as an insurance billing specialist for the College Clinic.

Beside these suggestions, you may wish either to tear out or to make photocopies of other sections of the *Handbook* for your personal use. In addition, your instructor may give you handouts from time to time, pertaining to regional insurance program policies and procedures, to place in your notebook.

Content Suggestions From the Workbook

- ✓ Appendix A: College Clinic policies, data about staff physicians, medical and laboratory abbreviations, and mock fee schedule
- ✓ Appendix B: HCPCS codes
- ✓ CMS-1500 (08-05) claim form (photocopy if extra copies are needed for making rough drafts or retyping an assignment)

Content Suggestions From the *Handbook*

- ✓ Evaluation and Management CPT codes: Tables 6.3 and 6.4
- ✓ Insurance form templates from Chapter 7: Figures 7-3 through 7-12
- ✓ Terminology used in coding procedures: Table 4-1
- ✓ CMS-1500 (08-05) block-by-block claim form instructions from Chapter 7
- ✓ Glossary (key terms and key abbreviations)

Tests

Tests are provided at the end of the *Workbook* to provide a complete, competency-based educational program.

Reference Material

To do the assignments in this *Workbook* and gain expertise in coding and insurance claims completion, an individual must have access to the books listed here. Addresses for obtaining these materials are given in parentheses. Additional books and booklets on these topics, as well as Medicaid, Medicare, TRICARE, and more, are listed in the appendix in the *Handbook*.

Dictionary

Dorland's Illustrated Medical Dictionary, 32nd edition, Elsevier, 2011 (6277 Sea Harbor Drive, Orlando, FL 32821-9989; 1-800-545-2522).

Fordney's Medical Insurance Dictionary for Billers and Coders, Elsevier, 2010 (3251 Riverport Lane, St. Louis, Missouri 63043; 1-800-545-2522).

Code Books

Current Procedural Terminology, American Medical Association, published annually (515 North State Street, Chicago, IL 60610; 1-800-621-8335).

International Classification of Diseases, Ninth Revision, Clinical Modification (An inexpensive softcover generic physician version of volumes 1 through 3 is available from Channel Publishing Limited, 4750 Longley Lane, Suite 100, Reno, NV 89502; 1-800-248-2882.)

Rough draft version of *International Classification of Diseases, Tenth Revision, Clinical Modification* available for download from the following website: http://www.cdc.gov/nchs/about/otheract/icd9/icd10cm.htm.

PERFORMANCE EVALUATION CHECKLIST

Assignment No. ____________

Name: ____ Date: ____________________________

Performance Objective

Task: Given access to all necessary equipment and information, the student will complete a CMS-1500 health insurance claim form.

Standards: Claim Productivity Management
Time __________ minutes
Note: Time element may be given by instructor.

Directions: See assignment.

NOTE TIME BEGAN __________ **NOTE TIME COMPLETED** __________

PROCEDURE STEPS	ASSIGNED POINTS	STEP PERFORMED SATISFACTORY	COMMENTS
1. Assembled CMS-1500 claim form, patient record, E/M code slip, ledger card, typewriter or computer, pen or pencil, and code books.	________	________	________
2. Posed ledger card correctly.	________	________	________
3. Proofread form for spelling and typographical errors while form remained in typewriter or on computer screen.	________	________	________
4. Points earned for correct completion of CMS-1500 block-by-block data.	________	________	________

Figure I-1

PERFORMANCE EVALUATION CHECKLIST

BLOCK	INCORRECT	MISSING	NOT NEEDED	REMARKS	BLOCK	INCORRECT	MISSING	NOT NEEDED	REMARKS
					18				
1A					19				
2					20				
3					21				
4									
5					22				
6					23				
7					24A				
8					24B				
					24C				
9					24D				
9A									
9B									
9C					24E				
9D									
					24F				
10A					24G				
10B					24H, 24I				
10C					24J				
10D									
11					25, 26				
11A					27				
11B					28				
11C					29				
11D									
12					30				
13									
14					31				
15									
16					32				
17									
17A					33				
					Reference Initials				

TOTAL POINTS EARNED: ________

TOTAL POINTS POSSIBLE: ________

Evaluator's signature ____________________

NEED TO REPEAT: ________

Figure I-2

TABLE I-2

Appendix	Contents
A	**College Clinic Office Policies and Mock Fee Schedule** College Clinic College Clinic Staff Abbreviations and Symbols Laboratory Abbreviations College Clinic Mock Fee Schedule Index
B	**Medicare Level II HCPCS Codes** Partial List of the Medicare Healthcare Common Procedure Coding System (HCPCS)

Word Book

Medical Abbreviations and Eponyms by Sheila Sloane, Elsevier, 1997 (6277 Sea Harbor Drive, Orlando, FL 32821-9989; 1-800-545-2522).

Pharmaceutical Book

Optional publications for drug names and descriptions might be either drug books used by nurses (e.g., *Mosby's Gen RX*, Elsevier, published annually [3251 Riverport Lane, St. Louis, MO 63043; 1-800-325-4177; www.elsevier.com]) or ones used by physicians (e.g., *Physician's Desk Reference* [PDR], Medical Economics Company, published annually [5 Paragon Drive, Montvale, NJ, 07645; 1-800-432-4570]).

Employee Insurance Procedural Manual

If you currently work in a medical office, you may custom design an insurance manual for your physician's practice as you complete insurance claims in this *Workbook*. Obtain a three-ring binder with indices and label them "Group Plans," "Private Plans," "Medicaid," "Medicare," "Managed Care Plans," "State Disability," "TRICARE," and "Workers' Compensation." If many of your patients have group plans, complete an insurance data or fact sheet for each plan and organize them alphabetically by group plan (Figure I-3). For managed care plans, type a form as shown in Figure 11-6 of the *Handbook*.

An insurance manual with fact sheets listing benefits can keep you up to date on policy changes and ensure maximum reimbursement. Fact sheets can be prepared from information obtained when patients bring in their benefit booklets. Obtain and insert a list of the procedures that must be performed as an outpatient and those that must have second opinions for each of the insurance plans.

As you complete the assignments in this *Workbook*, place them in the insurance manual as examples of completed claims for each particular program.

Student Software Challenge

The Student Software Challenge is another user-friendly software program located on the Evolve website. The software simulates a realistic experience by having students gather necessary documents and extract specific information to complete the CMS-1500 (08-05) insurance claim form. All source documents appear on screen and may be viewed simultaneously or printed for 10 patient cases that escalate in difficulty.

Student Software Challenge exercises are located in Chapters 7, 12, and 14. Some added features on the Evolve site are blank forms that students can fill out and print or save for additional practice or for use in the classroom. Documents available for printing include letterheads, authorization request forms, financial accounting statements (ledgers), and the CMS-1500 (08-05) form.

INSURANCE DATA

1. Employer's name __________
2. Address __________ Telephone Number __________
3. Insurance Company Contact Person __________
4. Insurance Carrier __________
5. Address __________ Telephone Number to Call for Benefits __________
6. Group Policy Number __________
7. Group Account Manager __________ Telephone Number __________
8. **Insurance Coverage:**
   Annual Deductible __________ Patient Copayment Percentage __________
   Noncovered Procedures __________
   Maximum Benefits __________
9. **Diagnostic Coverage:**
   Limited Benefits __________
   Maximum Benefits __________
   Noncovered Procedures __________
10. **Major Medical:**
   Annual Deductible __________ Patient Copayment Percentage __________
   Limited Benefits __________
   Maximum Benefits __________
   Noncovered Procedures __________

Mandatory Outpatient Surgeries __________

Second Surgical Opinions __________

Preadmission Certification Yes _____ No _____ Authorized Labs __________

Payment Plan:

UCR __________ Schedule of Benefits __________ CPT __________ RVS __________

Send claims to: __________

____

Date Entered __________ Date Updated __________

Figure I-3

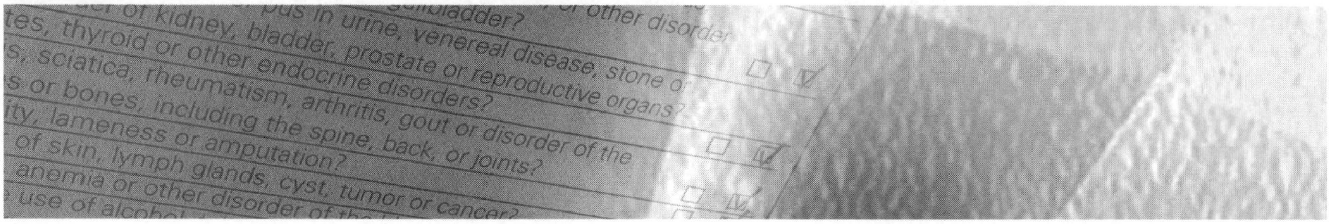

CHAPTER

1

Role of an Insurance Billing Specialist

KEY TERMS

Your instructor may wish to select some specific words pertinent to this chapter for a test. For definitions of the terms, further study, and/or reference, the words, phrases, and abbreviations may be found in the glossary at the end of the Handbook. *Key terms for this chapter follow.*

American Health Information Management Association
American Medical Association
cash flow
claims assistance professional
ethics
etiquette
insurance billing specialist
list service (listserv)
medical billing representative
multiskilled health practitioner
reimbursement specialist
respondeat superior
senior billing representative

KEY ABBREVIATIONS

See how many abbreviations and acronyms you can translate and then use this as a handy reference list. Definitions for the key abbreviations are located near the back of the Handbook *in the glossary.*

AAMA ____________________
ACA ____________________
AHIMA ____________________
AMA ____________________
ASHD ____________________
CAP ____________________
e-mail ____________________
GED ____________________
HIPAA ____________________
listserv ____________________
MSHP ____________________
MSO ____________________
NPP ____________________

PERFORMANCE OBJECTIVES

The student will be able to:

- Define and spell the key terms and key abbreviations for this chapter, given the information from the *Handbook* glossary, within a reasonable time period and with enough accuracy to obtain a satisfactory evaluation.
- Answer the fill-in-the-blank, multiple choice, and true/false review questions after reading the chapter, with enough accuracy to obtain a satisfactory evaluation.
- Use critical thinking to write one or two grammatically correct paragraphs with sufficient information to obtain a satisfactory evaluation.
- Visit websites and site-search information via the Evolve website, with sufficient information to obtain a satisfactory evaluation.

STUDY OUTLINE

Background of Insurance Claims, Coding, and Billing

Role of the Insurance Billing Specialist

- Job Responsibilities
- Educational and Training Requirements
- Career Advantages
- Self-Employment or Independent Contracting
- Flexible Hours
- Disabled Workers
- Qualifications
    - Attributes
    - Skills
    - Personal Image
    - Behavior

Medical Etiquette

Medical Ethics

Employer Liability

Employee Liability

Scope of Practice

Future Challenges

ASSIGNMENT 1-1 ▶ REVIEW QUESTIONS

Part I Fill in the Blank

Review the objectives, key terms, and chapter information before completing the following review questions.

1. Read the job descriptions in Chapter 1 in the *Handbook*. The ability to input data and transmit insurance claims accurately either directly or through a clearinghouse, as well as update and maintain software applications to requirements of third-party payers, is a technical skill required in the job of a/an ______________________.

2. Name some of the facilities where facility billing is used.

    a. ______________________

    b. ______________________

    c. ______________________

    d. ______________________

    e. ______________________

3. Name examples of non-physician practitioners (NPPs).

 a. ______________________________

 b. ______________________________

 c. ______________________________

 d. ______________________________

 e. ______________________________

 f. ______________________________

 g. ______________________________

 h. ______________________________

4. Identify three career opportunities (job titles) available after training in diagnostic and procedural coding and insurance claims completion.

 a. ______________________________

 b. ______________________________

 c. ______________________________

5. List some of the responsibilities and duties an insurance billing specialist might perform generally, as well as when acting as a collection manager. Refer to the section on "Job Responsibilities" on p. 5 in the text.

 a. ______________________________

 b. ______________________________

 c. ______________________________

 d. ______________________________

 e. ______________________________

 f. ______________________________

 g. ______________________________

6. List the duties of a claims assistance professional.

 a. ______________________________

 b. ______________________________

 c. ______________________________

7. Insurance claims must be promptly submitted within ________ business days to ensure continuous cash flow.

8. Define cash flow.

____

9. Reasons for a medical practice's large accounts receivable are

a. ____

b. ____

c. ____

d. ____

10. Skills required for an insurance billing specialist are

a. ____

b. ____

c. ____

d. ____

e. ____

f. ____

g. ____

h. ____

i. ____

j. ____

11. Standards of conduct by which an insurance billing specialist determines the propriety of his or her behavior in a relationship are known as ______________________.

12. Complete these statements with either the word *illegal* or *unethical*.

a. To report incorrect information to the Aetna Casualty Company is ______________________.

b. To report incorrect information to a Medicare fiscal intermediary is ______________________.

c. In certain circumstances, it may be ______________ for two physicians to treat the same patient for the same condition.

13. When a physician is legally responsible for an employee's conduct performed during employment, this is known as ______________________.

14. A claims assistance professional neglects to submit an insurance claim to a Medicare supplemental insurance carrier within the proper time limit. What type of insurance is needed for protection against this loss for the client?

____

Part II Multiple Choice

Choose the best answer.

15. Two billing components are facility billing and professional billing. Professional billing is done for

    a. hospitals

    b. skilled nursing facilities

    c. ambulatory surgical centers

    d. physicians

16. *Physician extenders* are health care personnel trained to provide medical care under the direct or indirect supervision of a physician, such as

    a. multiskilled health practitioners (MSHPs)

    b. claims assistance professionals (CAPs)

    c. non-physician practitioners (NPPs)

    d. insurance billing specialists

17. The individual responsible for documenting the patient's clinical notes and assigning a diagnosis code and a procedure code for medical services rendered is a/an

    a. physician

    b. insurance biller

    c. office manager

    d. financial accounting clerk

18. An individual cross-trained to function in more than one job is known as a/an

    a. administrative medical assistant

    b. receptionist

    c. claims assistance professional

    d. multiskilled health practitioner

19. Third-party payers that require the provider to submit insurance claims for the patient are

    a. federal and state programs

    b. private insurance plans

    c. managed care programs

    d. health care insurance plans

Part III True/False

Write "T" or "F" in the blank to indicate whether you think the statement is true or false.

_______ 20. Physicians are paid according to relative value units that are based on cost of delivering care, malpractice insurance, and the physician's work.

_______ 21. It is not necessary to refer to coding books because medical practices use a fee schedule.

_______ 22. It is the coder's responsibility to inform administration or his or her immediate supervisor if unethical or illegal coding practices are occurring.

_______ 23. When one code is available that includes all of the services, it is permissible to bill using separate codes for the services.

_______ 24. Depending on the circumstances of the case, an insurance billing specialist can be held personally responsible under the law for billing errors.

CRITICAL THINKING

To enhance your critical thinking skills, problems will be interspersed throughout the *Workbook*. Thinking is the goal of instruction and a student's responsibility. When trying to solve a problem by critical thinking, it is desirable to have more than one solution and to take time to think out answers. Remember that an answer may be changed when additional information is provided in a classroom setting.

ASSIGNMENT **1-2 ▶ CRITICAL THINKING**

Performance Objective

Task: Describe why you are training to become an insurance billing specialist.

Conditions: Use one or two sheets of white typing paper and pen or pencil.

Standards: Time: ____________ minutes

Accuracy: ____________

(Note: The time element and accuracy criteria may be given by your instructor.)

Directions: Write one or two paragraphs describing why you are training to become an insurance billing specialist. Or, if enrolled in a class that is part of a medical assisting course, explain why you are motivated to seek a career as a medical assistant. Make sure grammar, punctuation, and spelling are correct.

ASSIGNMENT 1-3 ▶ VISIT WEBSITES

Performance Objective

Task: Access the Internet and visit several websites of the World Wide Web.

Conditions: Use a computer with printer and/or pen or pencil to make notes.

Standards: Time: ____________ minutes

Accuracy: ____________

(Note: The time element and accuracy criteria may be given by your instructor.)

Directions: Access an Internet server and do the following three site searches:

1. Find one of the web search engines (Yahoo, Excite, Google, Alta Vista, Bing). Begin a web search (e.g., key in "insurance billers") to search for information about insurance billers. List three to five websites found. Go to one or more of those resources and list the benefits that those sites might have for a student in locating job opportunities or networking with others for professional growth and knowledge. Bring the website addresses to share with the class.

2. Site-search information on standards of ethical coding by visiting the website of the American Health Information Management Association (AHIMA) and print a hard copy of AHIMA's Code of Ethics. Next, obtain information on the eHealth code of ethics by visiting the website of the Internet Healthcare Coalition (www.iHealthcoalition.org/ehealth-code-of-ethics/). Click on eHealth Code of Ethics, read the article, and respond to the following:

   A. Write a brief definition for each of the following terms: health information, health products, and health services.
   B. State the eight guiding principles of organizations and individuals who provide health information over the Internet.

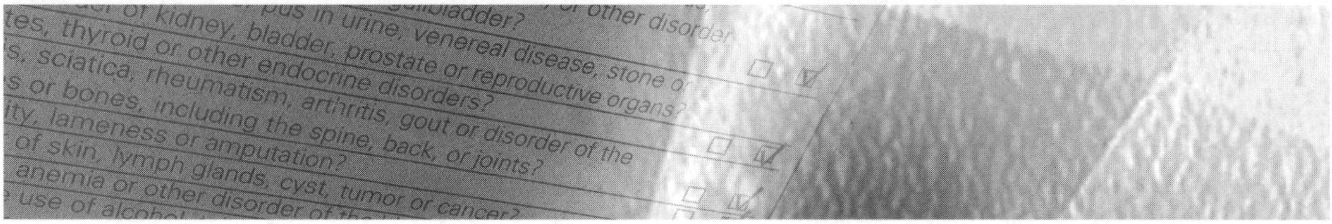

CHAPTER

2

HIPAA Compliance and Privacy in Insurance Billing

KEY TERMS

Your instructor may wish to select some specific words pertinent to this chapter for a test. For definitions of the terms, further study, and/or reference, the words, phrases, and abbreviations may be found in the glossary at the end of the Handbook. *Key terms for this chapter follow.*

abuse
authorization
authorization form
breach of confidential communication
business associate
clearinghouse
code set
compliance
compliance plan
confidential communication
confidentiality
consent
consent form
covered entity
disclosure
e-health information management
electronic media
embezzlement
fraud
health care provider
individually identifiable health information
nonprivileged information
Notice of Privacy Practices
phantom billing
privacy
privacy officer, privacy official
privileged information
protected health information
security officer
Security Rule
standard
state preemption
transaction
use

KEY ABBREVIATIONS

See how many abbreviations and acronyms you can translate and then use this as a handy reference list. Definitions for the key abbreviations are located near the back of the Handbook *in the glossary.*

CCI ____________________
CD ____________________
CDT ____________________
CLIA ____________________
CMS ____________________
CPT ____________________
DHHS ____________________
DOJ ____________________
EDI ____________________
eHIM ____________________
FBI ____________________
FCA ____________________
FDIC ____________________
FTP ____________________
HCFAP ____________________
HIPAA ____________________
HL7 ____________________
IIHI ____________________
MIP ____________________
NCVHS ____________________
NDC ____________________
NHII ____________________
NPP ____________________
OCR ____________________
OIG ____________________
ORT ____________________
OSHA ____________________
P&P ____________________
PHI ____________________
PO ____________________
TCS ____________________
TPO ____________________

PERFORMANCE OBJECTIVES

The student will be able to:

- Define and spell the key terms and key abbreviations for this chapter, given the information from the *Handbook* glossary, within a reasonable time period and with enough accuracy to obtain a satisfactory evaluation.
- Answer the fill-in-the-blank, multiple choice, and true/false review questions after reading the chapter, with enough accuracy to obtain a satisfactory evaluation.
- Make decisions after reading scenarios whether the situations are considered fraud, abuse, or neither, with sufficient information to obtain a satisfactory evaluation.
- Decide when a situation is an incidental disclosure, HIPAA violation, or neither, with sufficient information to obtain a satisfactory evaluation.
- Make a choice after reading scenarios whether to ask for consent or authorization, or perform other office procedures, with sufficient information to obtain a satisfactory evaluation.
- Visit websites and site-search information via the Evolve website, with sufficient information to obtain a satisfactory evaluation.

5. It is 10:30 AM, and you go on a coffee break leaving two patients' charts on the checkout counter.

   ID V N

   Explain ______________________________

6. In the reception room, a patient, Martha Havasi, overhears your telephone conversation even though you spoke quietly and shut the glass window.

   ID V N

   Explain ______________________________

7. You telephone a patient, Alex Massey, to remind him of tomorrow's appointment and leave a voicemail message on his answering machine.

   ID V N

   Explain ______________________________

8. Three patients near the reception area of the office overhear you telling another staff member that Daisy Dotson is scheduled for a Pap smear tomorrow at 4:00 PM.

   ID V N

   Explain ______________________________

9. You telephone a patient, Janet Hudson. She is not home so you leave a message on her answering machine that her breast cancer biopsy results came back negative.

   ID V N

   Explain ______________________________

10. You call out Fran O'Donnell's complete name in the waiting room where other patients are sitting.

    ID V N

    Explain ______________________________

11. You do not close the glass window to the reception room when talking on the telephone with your sister.

    ID V N

    Explain ______________________________

12. The office nurse tells a patient, Hugo Wells, his test results in front of his relatives in a treatment area.

ID V N

Explain ______________________________

13. You leave Katy Zontag's medical chart open at the receptionist's counter.

ID V N

Explain ______________________________

14. You telephone a patient, José Ramirez, and leave your name, the physician's name, and telephone number on his answering machine.

ID V N

Explain ______________________________

15. A patient, Kim Lee, is in the examination room and overhears a conversation concerning blood test results of another patient in an adjoining room.

ID V N

Explain ______________________________

16. While waiting in the reception room, a patient, Xavier Gomez, overhears a receptionist talking with another patient on the telephone about a colonoscopy appointment.

ID V N

Explain ______________________________

17. Betty Burton, a patient who is being weighed on the office scale by the medical assistant, overhears a conversation between an insurance billing specialist and an insurance company representative in which the billing specialist is trying to obtain preauthorization for another patient's medical procedure.

ID V N

Explain ______________________________

18. In a restaurant, a waitress overhears an insurance biller talking to a friend and telling her about a famous actress who visited her physician's office yesterday.

ID V N

Explain ______________________________

ASSIGNMENT 2-3 ▸ CRITICAL THINKING: FRAUD VERSUS ABUSE

Performance Objective

Task: Make a decision after reading each case study, whether it is considered fraud, abuse, or neither.

Conditions: Use pen or pencil.

Standards: Time: ______________________ minutes

Accuracy: ______________________

(Note: The time element and accuracy criteria may be given by your instructor.)

Directions: Read through each scenario and circle whether it is a fraud (F) issue, practice of abuse (A), or neither (N). To distinguish the difference between fraud and abuse situations, remember that under the Medicare program, abuse relates to incidents or practices that are inconsistent with accepted sound business practices, whereas fraud is intentional deception that an individual knows, or should know, to be false, and the individual knows the deception could result in some unauthorized benefit to himself or herself or to some other person(s). Briefly explain the answer you selected.

Scenarios

1. Dr. Pedro Atrics has a friend whose child needs elective surgery. He agrees to perform the surgery and bill it as an "insurance only" case.

   F A N

   Explain ____

2. A patient, Carl Skinner, calls the office repeatedly about his prescriptions. When seen in the office the next time, Dr. Input bills a higher level of evaluation and management service to allow for the additional time.

   F A N

   Explain ____

3. Dr. Skeleton sets a simple fracture and puts a cast on Mr. Davis. He bills for a complex fracture.

   F A N

   Explain ____

4. A patient, Maria Gomez, asks a friendly staff member to change the dates on the insurance claim form. The medical assistant complies with the request.

   F A N

   Explain ____

5. A patient, Roberto Loren, asks the physician to restate a diagnosis so the insurance company will pay, because payment would be denied based on the present statement. The physician complies with the request.

F A N

Explain ______________________________

6. Dr. Rumsey sees a patient twice on the same day but bills as though the patient was seen on two different dates.

F A N

Explain ______________________________

7. A Medicare patient, Joan O'Connor, is seen by Dr. Practon, and the insurance claim shows a charge to the Medicare fiscal intermediary at a fee schedule rate higher than and different from that of non-Medicare patients.

F A N

Explain ______________________________

8. A patient, Hazel Plunkett, receives a service that is not medically necessary to the extent rendered, and an insurance claim is submitted.

F A N

Explain ______________________________

9. A patient, Sun Cho, paid for services that were subsequently declared not medically necessary, and Dr. Cardi failed to refund the payment to the patient.

F A N

Explain ______________________________

10. Dr. Ulibarri tells the insurance biller not to collect the deductible and copayments from Mrs. Gerry Coleman.

F A N

Explain ______________________________

ASSIGNMENT 2-4 ▸ CRITICAL THINKING: CONSENT VERSUS AUTHORIZATION

Performance Objective

Task: Make a decision using your best judgment after reading each scenario and determine whether you should ask for consent or authorization, or do other procedures.

Conditions: Use pen or pencil.

Standards: Time: ____________ minutes

Accuracy: ____________

(Note: The time element and accuracy criteria may be given by your instructor. Class discussion may offer other possible ways of handling the given situations.)

Directions: Read through each case study and determine whether you should ask for consent or authorization, or perform other office procedures.

Scenarios

1. Dr. Practon's patient, Mary Ann Bailey, goes to the College Hospital's emergency department complaining of severe stomach cramps. Subsequently, she is admitted to the hospital for pancreatitis. The floor nurse at the hospital telephones Dr. Practon's office asking for the patient's medical records to be brought over immediately. What should you do?

   Response ____

   ____

   ____

2. Robert Fellow, a patient, telephones the College Clinic and states that he has hired a lawyer and is filing a lawsuit against another driver for an automobile accident that happened about a month ago. The attorney for the other driver needs your patient's medical records to find out what injuries your patient suffered as a result of the accident. The attorney also wants to know if there are any preexisting injuries. Mr. Fellow requests that you send a copy of his medical records to the other attorney. What should you do?

   Response ____

   ____

   ____

3. Consuelo Lopez, the mother of a minor patient, Johnnie Lopez, telephones your office stating that Johnnie is having difficulty staying focused and loses his concentration during classroom activities at school. Mrs. Lopez has made an appointment for him to be seen by a psychologist and has requested that you send his medical records to the psychologist before the date of the appointment. What should you do?

Response ____

____

____

4. Eric Jacobs, a patient, receives psychiatric counseling (not psychotherapy) and treatment for diabetes at the College Clinic. The patient requests a copy of his medical record. (A) Is it necessary to remove the documentation pertaining to the psychiatric counseling sessions before giving the patient a copy of his medical record? (B) Can you disclose to the patient his medical records? Explain.

Response (A) ____

____

Response (B) ____

____

ASSIGNMENT 2-5 ▸ VISIT WEBSITES

Performance Objective

Task: Access the Internet and visit several websites of the World Wide Web.

Conditions: Use a computer with printer and/or pen or pencil to make notes.

Standards: Time: ________________________ minutes

Accuracy: ________________________

(Note: The time element and accuracy criteria may be given by your instructor.)

Directions: Access an Internet server and do the following three site searches.

1. Site-search information on patient confidentiality by visiting the website of the American Medical Association (www.ama-assn.org).

2. Search information on patient confidentiality in health care by using the Google search engine. Key in patient confidentiality in health care. Locate an article and print a hard copy to share and discuss with the class.

3. Site-search for information on fraud and abuse by visiting one or more of the following three federal websites:

   - Centers for Medicare and Medicaid Services - CMS (http://www.cms.hhs.gov/)
   - Federal Bureau of Investigation - FBI (http://www.fbi.gov/)
   - U.S. Department of Health & Human Services Office of Inspector General (http://www.oig.hhs.gov/)

   See what you can discover and either print out or take notes and bring back information to share with the class for discussion.

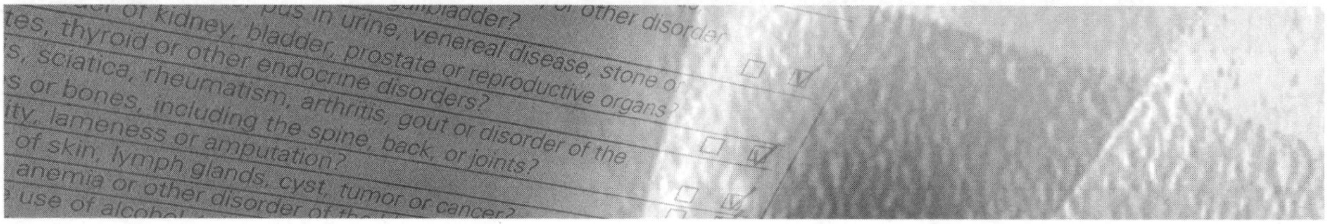

CHAPTER

3

Basics of Health Insurance

KEY TERMS

Your instructor may wish to select some words pertinent to this chapter for a test. For definitions of the terms, further study, and/or reference, the words, phrases, and abbreviations may be found in the glossary at the end of the Handbook. *Key terms for this chapter follow.*

accounts receivable management
applicant
assignment
blanket contract
cancelable
capitation
Civilian Health and Medical Program of the Department of Veterans Affairs
claim
coinsurance
competitive medical plan
conditionally renewable
contract
coordination of benefits
daysheet
deductible
disability income insurance
electronic signature
eligibility
emancipated minor
encounter form
exclusions
exclusive provider organization
expressed contract
extended
financial accounting record
foundation for medical care
guaranteed renewable
guarantor
health insurance
health maintenance organization
high risk
implied contract
indemnity
independent or individual practice association
insured
major medical
Maternal and Child Health Program
Medicaid
Medicare
Medicare/Medicaid
member
noncancelable policy
nonparticipating provider
optionally renewable
participating provider
patient registration form
personal insurance
point-of-service (POS) plan
posted

preauthorization
precertification
predetermination
preexisting conditions
preferred provider organization
premium
running balance
State Disability Insurance
subscriber
TRICARE
Unemployment Compensation Disability
Veterans Affairs outpatient clinic
workers' compensation insurance

KEY ABBREVIATIONS

See how many abbreviations and acronyms you can translate and then use this as a handy reference list. Definitions for the key abbreviations are located near the back of the Handbook *in the glossary.*

AAMB ______
AAPC ______
ADSM ______
A/R ______
CHAMPVA ______
CMP ______
COB ______
COBRA ______
DoD ______
DOS ______
EPO ______
FMC ______
FSA ______
HBMA ______
HDHP ______
HFMA ______
HMO ______
HRA ______
HSA ______
IPA ______
MAB ______
MCD ______
MCHP ______
Medi-Medi ______
MGMA ______
MSA ______
nonpar ______
NPP ______
PAHCOM ______
par ______
PMS ______
POS ______
POS plan ______
PPO ______
ROA ______
SDI ______
SOF ______
UCD ______
VA ______
WC ______

PERFORMANCE OBJECTIVES

The student will be able to:

- Define and spell the key terms and key abbreviations for this chapter, given the information from the *Handbook* glossary, within a reasonable time period and with enough accuracy to obtain a satisfactory evaluation.
- Answer the fill-in-the-blank, multiple choice, and true/false review questions after reading the chapter, with enough accuracy to obtain a satisfactory evaluation.
- Arrange 18 administrative processing steps of an insurance claim in proper sequence, given data from the textbook, within a reasonable time period and with enough accuracy to obtain a satisfactory evaluation.
- Use critical thinking to explain some of the differences in insurance key terms, given data from the textbook, within a reasonable time period and with enough accuracy to obtain a satisfactory evaluation.
- Prepare a financial accounting record, given data from the textbook, within a reasonable time period and with enough accuracy to obtain a satisfactory evaluation.
- Abstract data from some insurance identification cards, given data from the textbook, within a reasonable time period and with enough accuracy to obtain a satisfactory evaluation.

STUDY OUTLINE

History
Insurance in the United States
Health Benefit Exchanges
Legal Principles of Insurance
Insurance Contracts
Physician–Patient Contracts and Financial Obligation
Implied or Expressed Contracts
The Insurance Policy
Policy Application
Policy Renewal Provisions
Policy Terms
Coordination of Benefits
General Policy Limitations
Case Management Requirements
Group Contract
High-Deductible Health Plans
Individual Contract
Prepaid Health Plan
Types of Health Insurance Coverage
CHAMPVA
Competitive Medical Plan
Disability Income Insurance
Exclusive Provider Organization
Foundation for Medical Care
Health Maintenance Organization
Independent or Individual Practice Association
Maternal and Child Health Program
Medicaid
Medicare
Medicare/Medicaid
Point-of-Service Plan
Preferred Provider Organization
TRICARE
Unemployment Compensation Disability
Veterans Affairs Outpatient Clinic
Workers' Compensation Insurance
Examples of Insurance Billing
Procedure: Handling and Processing Insurance Claims
Keeping Up to Date
Procedure: Prepare and Post to a Patient's Financial Accounting Record

ASSIGNMENT 3-3 ▶ CRITICAL THINKING: DIFFERENCES IN INSURANCE KEY TERMS

Performance Objective

Task: Describe and/or explain your responses to five questions.

Conditions: Use one or two sheets of white typing paper and pen or pencil.

Standards: Time: ______________________ minutes

Accuracy: ______________________

(Note: The time element and accuracy criteria may be given by your instructor.)

Directions: Respond verbally or in writing to these questions or statements.

1. Explain the difference between the following:

   Blanket contract ____

   Individual contract ____

2. Explain the difference between a participating provider and a nonparticipating provider for the following:

   Commercial insurance company or managed care plan participating provider:

   ____

   Commercial insurance company or managed care plan nonparticipating provider:

   ____

   Medicare participating provider:

   ____

   Medicare nonparticipating provider:

   ____

3. State the difference between the following:

   Implied contract ____

   Expressed contract ____

4. Explain the birthday law (rule) and when it is used.

   ____

ASSIGNMENT 3-4 ▸ PREPARE A FINANCIAL ACCOUNTING RECORD

Performance Objective

Task: Prepare, insert descriptions, and post fees, payments, credit adjustments, and balances due to a patient's ledger card. If you have access to copy equipment, make a photocopy.

Conditions: Use one patient account or ledger form (Figure 3-1), pen or pencil, and calculator.

Standards: Time: ____________________ minutes

Accuracy: ____________________

(Note: The time element and accuracy criteria may be given by your instructor.)

Directions:

1. Locate a financial accounting record (ledger) (see Figure 3-1) form. Refer to the step-by-step procedures at the end of Chapter 3 in the *Handbook*. In addition, see Figures 3-14 and 10-3 in the *Handbook* for graphic examples of financial accounting records (ledgers).
2. Insert the patient's name and address, including zip code, in the box.
3. Enter the patient's personal data.
4. Ledger lines: Insert date of service (DOS), reference (CPT code number, check number, or dates of service for posting adjustments or when insurance was billed), description of the transaction, charge amounts, payments, adjustments, and running current balance. The posting date is the actual date the transaction is recorded. If the DOS differs from the posting date, list the DOS in the reference or description column.

Note: A good bookkeeping practice is to use a red pen to draw a line across the financial accounting record (ledger) from left to right to indicate the last entry billed to the insurance company.

Account No. 3-3

FINANCIAL STATEMENT

PRACTION MEDICAL GROUP, INC.
4567 Broad Avenue
Woodland Hills, XY 12345-0001
Tel. 555-486-9002
Fax No. 555-487-8976

Phone No. (H) ____________ (W) ____________ Birthdate ____________

Primary Insurance Co. ____________ Policy/Group No. ____________

	REFERENCE	DESCRIPTION	CHARGES	CREDITS		BALANCE
				PYMNTS.	ADJ	
				BALANCE FORWARD →		

PLEASE PAY LAST AMOUNT IN BALANCE COLUMN

THIS IS A COPY OF YOUR FINANCIAL ACCOUNT AS IT APPEARS ON OUR RECORDS

Figure 3-1

Scenario:

A new patient, Miss Carolyn Wachsman, of 4590 Ashton Street, Woodland Hills, XY 12345, was seen by Dr. Practon; her account number is 2-3. Her home telephone number is (555) 340-8876, and her work telephone number is (555) 509-7091. She was born on 5-8-75. She is insured by Blue Cross, and her subscriber number is 540-xx-3209.

Miss Wachsman was seen on March 24 of the current year for a level III evaluation and management office visit ($). She also received an ECG ($). Locate these fees in the Mock Fee Schedule in Appendix A of this *Workbook*.

An insurance claim form was sent to Blue Cross on March 25. On May 15, Blue Cross sent an explanation of benefits stating the patient had previously met her deductible. Check number 433 for $76 was attached to the EOB and $19 was indicated as the adjustment to be made by the provider. On May 25, the patient was billed for the balance.

After the instructor has returned your work to you, either make the necessary corrections and place it in a three-ring notebook for future reference, or, if you received a high score, place it in your portfolio for reference when applying for a job.

ASSIGNMENT 3-5 ▶ ABSTRACT DATA FROM AN INSURANCE IDENTIFICATION CARD

Performance Objective

Task: Answer questions in reference to an insurance identification card for Case A.

Conditions: Use an insurance identification card (Figure 3-2), the questions presented, and pen or pencil.

Standards: Time: ______________ minutes

Accuracy: ______________

(Note: The time element and accuracy criteria may be given by your instructor.)

Directions: An identification card provides much of the information needed to establish a patient's insurance coverage. You have photocopied the front and back sides of three patients' cards and placed copies in their patient records, returning the originals to the patients. Answer the questions by abstracting or obtaining the data from the cards.

CASE A

1. Name of patient covered by the policy. ______________
2. Provide the insurance policy's effective date. ______________
3. List the telephone number for preauthorization. ______________
4. State name and address of insurance company. ______________
5. List the telephone number to call for provider access. ______________
6. Name the type of insurance plan. ______________
7. List the insurance identification number (a.k.a. subscriber, certificate, or member numbers). ______________
8. Furnish the group number. Plan or coverage code. ______________
9. State the copay requirements. ______________
10. Does the card indicate the patient has hospital coverage? ______________

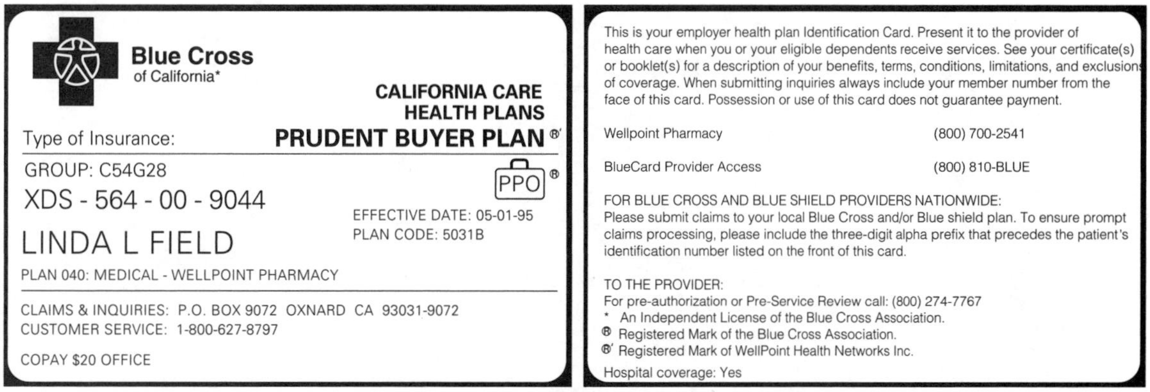

Blue Cross of California*

CALIFORNIA CARE HEALTH PLANS

Type of Insurance: PRUDENT BUYER PLAN ®'

GROUP: C54G28 PPO ®

XDS - 564 - 00 - 9044

EFFECTIVE DATE: 05-01-95
PLAN CODE: 5031B

LINDA L FIELD

PLAN 040: MEDICAL - WELLPOINT PHARMACY

CLAIMS & INQUIRIES: P.O. BOX 9072 OXNARD CA 93031-9072
CUSTOMER SERVICE: 1-800-627-8797

COPAY $20 OFFICE

This is your employer health plan Identification Card. Present it to the provider of health care when you or your eligible dependents receive services. See your certificate(s) or booklet(s) for a description of your benefits, terms, conditions, limitations, and exclusions of coverage. When submitting inquiries always include your member number from the face of this card. Possession or use of this card does not guarantee payment.

Wellpoint Pharmacy (800) 700-2541

BlueCard Provider Access (800) 810-BLUE

FOR BLUE CROSS AND BLUE SHIELD PROVIDERS NATIONWIDE:
Please submit claims to your local Blue Cross and/or Blue shield plan. To ensure prompt claims processing, please include the three-digit alpha prefix that precedes the patient's identification number listed on the front of this card.

TO THE PROVIDER:
For pre-authorization or Pre-Service Review call: (800) 274-7767
* An Independent License of the Blue Cross Association.
® Registered Mark of the Blue Cross Association.
®' Registered Mark of WellPoint Health Networks Inc.
Hospital coverage: Yes

Figure 3-2

ASSIGNMENT 3-6 ▶ ABSTRACT DATA FROM AN INSURANCE IDENTIFICATION CARD

Performance Objective

Task: Answer questions in reference to the insurance identification card for Case B.

Conditions: Use an insurance identification card (Figure 3-3), the questions presented, and pen or pencil.

Standards: Time: ______________________ minutes

Accuracy: ______________________

(Note: The time element and accuracy criteria may be given by your instructor.)

CASE B

1. Name of patient covered by the policy. ______________________
2. Provide the insurance policy's effective date. ______________________
3. List the telephone number for preauthorization. ______________________
4. State name of insurance company. ______________________
5. List the telephone number to call for patient benefits and eligibility. ______________________
6. Name the type of insurance plan. ____________
7. List the insurance identification number (a.k.a. subscriber, certificate, or member numbers).

   ____
8. Furnish the group number. Plan or coverage code. ______________________
9. State the copay requirements, if any. ______________________
10. List the Blue Shield website. ______________________

Blue Shield of California
An Independent Member of the Blue Shield Association

PPO **Preferred Plan**

SUBSCRIBER NAME: M T FORDHAM

EFFECTIVE DATE: 010120XX

SUBSCRIBER ID NUMBER: AJC557469969

GROUP NUMBER: 00P1901

PLAN CODE: 542

CUSTOMER SERVICE: (800) 331-2001

07/16/20XX

Use Blue Shield of California Preferred Physicians and Hospitals to receive maximum benefits.

Carry the Blue Shield Identification Card with you at all times and present it whenever you or one of your covered dependents receives medical services. Read your employee booklet/Health Services Agreement which summarizes the benefits, provisions, limitations and exclusions of your plan. Your health plan may require prior notification of any hospitalization and notification, within one business day, of an emergency admission. Review of selected procedures may be required before some services are performed. To receive hospital pre-admission and pre-service reviews, call 1-800-343-1691. Your failure to call may result in a reduction of benefits.

For questions, including those related to benefits, and eligibility, call the customer service number listed on the front of this card.

The PPO logo on the front of this ID Card identifies you to preferred providers outside the state of California as a member of the Blue Card PPO Program.

When you are outside of California call 1-800-810-2583 to locate the nearest PPO Provider. Remember, any services you receive are subject to the policies and provisions of your group plan.

ID-23200-PPO REVERSE www.blueshieldca.com

Figure 3-3

ASSIGNMENT 3-7 ▶ ABSTRACT DATA FROM AN INSURANCE IDENTIFICATION CARD

Performance Objective

Task: Answer questions in reference to the insurance identification card for Case C.

Conditions: Use an insurance identification card (Figure 3-4), the questions presented, and pen or pencil.

Standards: Time: ______________________ minutes

Accuracy: ______________________

(Note: The time element and accuracy criteria may be given by your instructor.)

CASE C

1. Name of patient covered by the policy. ______________________
2. Provide the insurance policy's effective date, if there is one. ______________________
3. List the number to call for out-of-network preauthorization. ______________________
4. State name and address of insurance company. ______________________
5. List the telephone number to call for member inquiries. ______________________
6. Name the type of insurance plan. ______________________
7. List the insurance identification number (a.k.a. subscriber, certificate, or member numbers).

   ____

8. Furnish the group number. ______________________
9. State the copay requirements, if any. ______________________
10. Who is the patient's primary care physician? ______________________

UNITEDhealthcare

LINDA L. FLORES
Member # 52170-5172

CALMAT

Group # 176422
COPAY: Office Visit $10 ER $50
Urgent $35

Electronic Claims Payor ID 87726

Call 800-842-5751 for Member Inquiries

POS PCP Plan
WITH RX D - UHC
and MH/CD
PCP: G. LOMAN
805-643-9973

MTH

This identification card is not proof of membership nor does it guarantee coverage. Persons with coverage that remains in force are entitled to benefits under the terms and conditions of this group health benefit plan as detailed in your benefit description.

IMPORTANT MEMBER INFORMATION
In non-emergencies, call your Primary Care Physician to receive the highest level of benefits. If you have an emergency and are admitted to a hospital, you are required to call your Primary Care Physician within two working days.
For out of network services that require authorization, call the Member Inquiries 800 number on the front of this card.

Claim Address: P.O. Box 30990, Salt Lake City, UT 84130-0990

Figure 3-4

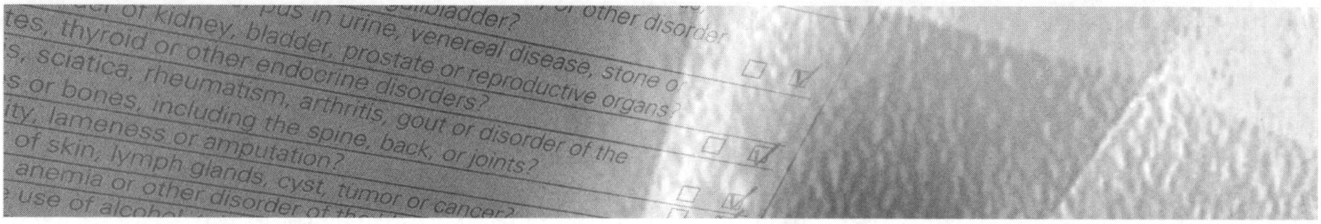

CHAPTER

4

Medical Documentation and the Electronic Health Record

KEY TERMS

Your instructor may wish to select some words pertinent to this chapter for a test. For definitions of the terms, further study, and/or reference, the words, phrases, and abbreviations may be found in the glossary at the end of the Handbook. *Key terms for this chapter follow.*

acute
attending physician
chief complaint
chronic
comorbidity
comprehensive
concurrent care
consultation
consulting physician
continuity of care
counseling
critical care
detailed
documentation
electronic health record
emergency care
eponym
established patient
expanded problem focused
external audit
facsimile
family history
health record/medical record
high complexity
history of present illness
internal review
low complexity
medical decision making
medical necessity
medical report
moderate complexity
new patient
non-physician practitioner
ordering physician
past history
physical examination
primary care physician
problem focused
prospective review
referral
referring physician
resident physician

retrospective review
review of systems
social history
straightforward
subpoena
subpoena duces tecum
teaching physician
treating or performing physician

KEY ABBREVIATIONS

See how many abbreviations and acronyms you can translate and then use this as a handy reference list. Definitions for the key abbreviations are located near the back of the Handbook *in the glossary.*

AARA ______
C ______
CC ______
CCU ______
CHEDDAR ______
D ______
dx, Dx ______
ED or ER ______
EHR ______
E/M service ______
EMR ______
EPF level of history or examination ______
ESI ______
fax ______
FH ______
HC medical decision making ______
HIM ______
HIV ______
HPI ______
ICU ______
imp ______
LC medical decision making ______
LLQ ______
LUQ ______
MC medical decision making ______
MDM ______
NLP ______
NP ______
NPP ______
PCP ______
PE or PX ______
PF level of history or examination ______
PFSH ______
PH ______
PO ______
POR system ______
RCU ______
RLQ ______
R/O ______
ROS ______
RUQ ______
SF medical decision making ______
SH ______
SOAP style ______
SOR system ______
WNL ______

c. symptoms, objective findings, and professional services

d. subjective, opinions, assistance, and present illness

21. A physical examination of a patient performed by a physician is

a. descriptive

b. comprehensive

c. subjective

d. objective

22. A health care management process after doing a history and physical examination on a patient that result in a plan of treatment is called

a. selecting a treatment option

b. medical decision making

c. establishing a diagnosis

d. choosing a management option

23. When there is an underlying disease or other conditions are present at the time of the patient's office visit, this is termed

a. mortality

b. continuity

c. comorbidity

d. complexity

Part IV True/False

Write "T" or "F" in the blank line to indicate whether you think the statement is true or false.

_______ 24. A patient's hospital discharge summary contains the discharge diagnosis but not the admitting diagnosis.

_______ 25. An eponym should not be used when a comparable anatomic term can be used in its place.

_______ 26. If the phrase "rule out" appears in a patient's health record in connection with a disease, then code the condition as if it existed.

_______ 27. During a prospective review or prebilling audit, all procedures or services and diagnoses listed on the encounter form must match the data on the insurance claim form.

_______ 28. Assigned insurance claims for Medicaid and Medicare cases must be kept for a period of 7 years.

ASSIGNMENT 4-2 ▸ REVIEW DIAGNOSTIC TERMINOLOGY AND ABBREVIATIONS

In the *Handbook*, review Table 4-1 and anatomic figures, as well as Appendix A in the *Workbook*, which has a list of abbreviations and symbols.

1. Match the following terms in the right column with the descriptions and fill in the blank line with the appropriate letter.

_______	Pertaining to both sides	a. acute
_______	Act of cutting out	b. chronic
_______	Condition that runs a short but severe course	c. percutaneous
_______	Localized or in one specific location	d. bilateral
_______	Through the skin	e. excision
_______	Condition persisting over a long period of time	f. in situ

2. Write in the meaning for these abbreviations and/or symbols commonly encountered in a patient's medical record.

RLQ ____

DC ____

WNL ____

R/O ____

URI ____

$\bar{c}$ ____

3. When documenting incisions, the unit of measure length should be listed in

____.

Multiple Choice Questions

Circle the letter that gives the best answer to each question.

4. If a physician called and asked for a patient's medical record STAT, what would he or she mean?

   a. The physician wants a statistic from a patient's record

   b. The physician wants the record delivered on Tuesday

   c. The physician wants the record delivered immediately

5. If a physician asks you to locate the results of the last UA, what would you be searching for?

   a. a urinalysis report

   b. an x-ray report of the ulna

   c. uric acid test results

6. If a physician telephoned and asked for a copy of the last H&P to be faxed, what is being requested?

   a. heart and pulmonary findings

   b. H_2 antagonist test results

   c. a history and physical

7. If a hospital nurse telephoned and asked you to read the results of the patient's last CBC, what would you be searching for?

   a. carcinoma basal cell report

   b. complete blood count

   c. congenital blindness, complete report

8. If you were asked to make a photocopy of the patient's last CT, what would you be searching for?

   a. chemotherapy record

   b. connective tissue report

   c. computed tomography scan

ASSIGNMENT 4-3 ▶ CRITICAL THINKING: SOLVE AN OFFICE PROBLEM

Performance Objective

Task: Answer questions after reviewing the case study using critical thinking skills.

Conditions: Use a case study and a pen or pencil.

Standards: Time: ____________________ minutes

Accuracy: ____________________

Directions: Answer questions after reviewing the case study using your critical thinking skills. Record your answer on the blank lines.

1. A patient comes into the office for treatment. He does not return, because he is dissatisfied with Dr. Practon's treatment. Is it necessary to keep his records when he obviously will not return? __________ Why?

____

____

ASSIGNMENT 4-4 ▶ ABSTRACT SUBJECTIVE OBSERVATIONS AND OBJECTIVE FINDINGS FROM PATIENT RECORDS

Performance Objective

Task: List subjective observations and objective findings after reading each of the case studies.

Conditions: Use a pencil and four case studies.

Standards: Time: ____________________ minutes

Accuracy: ____________________

(Note: The time element and accuracy criteria may be given by your instructor.)

Case Study 1 Mrs. Smith is 25 years old and was brought into the emergency department of College Hospital with complaints of difficulty breathing and chest pain. Her vital signs show an elevated temperature of 101° F and pulse rate of 90. Respirations are labored at 30/min. BP is 140/80. Her skin is warm and diaphoretic (perspiring). She states, "This condition has been going on for the past 3 days."

Subjective observations: ____________________

Objective findings: ____________________

Case Study 2 Mr. Jones is 56 years old and was admitted to the hospital with chest pain and elevated pulse and blood pressure. His skin is cold and clammy.

Subjective observations: ____________________

Objective findings: ____________________

Case Study 3 You are assisting the radiology technician with Sally Salazar, a 6-year-old Hispanic girl who was brought into the pediatrician's office with a suspected fracture of the right arm. Sally states she was "running at school, tripped on my shoelace, and fell." She tells you her "arm hurts," points out how "funny my arm looks," and starts to cry. You notice her arm looks disfigured and is covered with dirt. Sally is cradling her arm against her body and is unwilling to let go because "it's going to fall off."

Subjective observations: ____________________

Objective findings: ____________________

Case Study 4 You are working in the business office of College Hospital. A former patient in your hospital comes in complaining of his billing. He states he was never catheterized, never had any of the medications listed on his itemized bill, and has "never been in this hospital for that length of time." His face is red, his voice is gradually getting louder, and you notice he is standing with the aid of crutches because his left leg is in a full cast.

Subjective observations: ____________________

Objective findings: ____________________

ASSIGNMENT 4-5 ▶ REVIEW OF A PATIENT RECORD

Performance Objective

Task: Answer questions after reviewing a patient's record.

Conditions: Use a pencil, internal record review sheet, medical dictionary, abbreviation reference list, drug reference book (e.g., *Mosby's MD Consult*), and laboratory reference book.

Standards: Time: ______________________ minutes

Accuracy: ______________________

(Note: The time element and accuracy criteria may be given by your instructor.)

Directions: In many instances, when developing the skill of reviewing a patient record, you may need critical thinking in addition to efficient use of reference books. Answer only those questions you think can be justified by the documentation presented in the patient's record. Because the content of each record is variable, you may or may not have answers to all eight questions.

Answer the questions by recording on the blank lines the documentation found identifying the components from the patient's record.

If your answers vary, perhaps you have a reason for them that may or may not be valid. List your reasons in the response section. Differences may be reviewed with your instructor privately or via class discussion.

Patient Record

10-21-20xx HPI This new pt is an 80-year-old white male who has had problems with voiding since 9-5-20xx.

During the night the pt had only 50 cc output and was catheterized this morning because of his poor urinary output (200 cc). He was thought to have a distended bladder; he complains of pressure in the suprapubic region. He has not had any gross hematuria. He has voiding difficulty especially lying down and voiding in the supine position. His voiding pattern is improved while standing and sitting.

Gene Ulibarri, MD

mtf

1. Location: In what body system is the sign or symptom occurring?

   Response: ______________________________________

2. Quality: Is the symptom or pain burning, gnawing, stabbing, pressure-like, squeezing, fullness?

   Response: ______________________________________

3. Severity: In this case, how would you rank the symptom (how was distress relieved) or pain (slight, mild, severe, persistent)?

   Response: ______________________________________

4. Duration: How long has the symptom been present or how long does it last?

   Response: ______________________________

5. Timing: When does(do) a sign(s) or symptom(s) occur (AM, PM, after or before meals)?

   Response: ______________________________

6. Context: Is the pain/symptom associated with big meals, dairy products, etc.?

   Response: ______________________________

7. Modifying factors: What actions make symptoms worse or better?

   Response: ______________________________

8. Associated signs and symptoms: What other system or body area produces complaints when the presenting problem occurs? (Example: chest pain leads to shortness of breath.)

   Response: ______________________________

ASSIGNMENT 4-6 ▶ KEY A LETTER OF WITHDRAWAL

Performance Objective

Task: Key letter for physician's signature with envelope, prepare U.S. Postal Service forms, and complete an authorization form.

Conditions: Use one sheet of letterhead (print from Evolve website), U.S. Postal Service forms for certified mail with return receipt requested (Figure 4-1), Authorization for Release of Information form (Figure 4-2), a number 10 envelope, thesaurus, English dictionary, medical dictionary, computer, printer, and pen or pencil.

Standards: Time: ______________________ minutes

Accuracy: ______________________

(Note: The time element and accuracy criteria may be given by your instructor.)

Directions: Mrs. McLean is negligent about following Dr. Ulibarri's advice after she received surgery. Refer to *Workbook* Assignment 7-2 for information from the patient record of Mrs. Merry M. McLean. Use a letterhead and type in modified block style an appropriate letter to Mrs. McLean advising her of the doctor's withdrawal from the case (see *Handbook* Figure 4-21). Date the letter June 30 of the current year. Dr. Ulibarri will be available to this patient for 30 days after receipt of this letter.

This letter must be prepared for Dr. Ulibarri's signature because it is a legal document. Type Mrs. McLean's address on a number 10 envelope, referring to *Workbook* Figure 4-3. Send the letter by certified mail with return receipt requested, referring to *Handbook* Figure 4-22 and enclose a completed Authorization for Release of Information form (see Figure 4-2).

After the instructor has returned your work to you, either make the necessary corrections and place it in a three-ring notebook for future reference, or, if you receive a high score, place it in your portfolio for reference when applying for a job.

UNITED STATES POSTAL SERVICE

First-Class Mail
Postage & Fees Paid
USPS
Permit No. G-10

• Sender: Please print your name, address, and ZIP+4 in this box •

SENDER: *COMPLETE THIS SECTION*

- Complete items 1, 2, and 3. Also complete item 4 if Restricted Delivery is desired.
- Print your name and address on the reverse so that we can return the card to you.
- Attach this card to the back of the mailpiece, or on the front if space permits.

1. Article Addressed to:

COMPLETE THIS SECTION ON DELIVERY

A. Signature
X
☐ Agent
☐ Addressee

B. Received by (*Printed Name*)

C. Date of Delivery

D. Is delivery address different from item 1? ☐ Yes
If YES, enter delivery address below: ☐ No

3. Service Type
☐ Certified Mail ☐ Express Mail
☐ Registered ☐ Return Receipt for Merchandise
☐ Insured Mail ☐ C.O.D.

4. Restricted Delivery? (*Extra Fee*) ☐ Yes

2. Article Number
(*Transfer from service label*)

PS Form 3811, February 2004 Domestic Return Receipt 102595-02-M-1540

7006 0810 0001 6207 8857

PLACE STICKER AT TOP OF ENVELOPE TO THE RIGHT
OF THE RETURN ADDRESS, FOLD AT DOTTED LINE

CERTIFIED MAIL™

7006 0810 0001 6207 8857
7006 0810 0001 6207 8857

U.S. Postal Service™
CERTIFIED MAIL™ RECEIPT
(Domestic Mail Only; No Insurance Coverage Provided)

For delivery information visit our website at www.usps.com®

OFFICIAL USE

Postage	$
Certified Fee	
Return Receipt Fee (Endorsement Required)	
Restricted Delivery Fee (Endorsement Required)	
Total Postage & Fees	**$**

Postmark
Here

Sent To

Street, Apt. No.; or PO Box No.

City, State, ZIP+4

PS Form 3800, June 2002 **See Reverse for Instructions**

Figure 4-1

AUTHORIZATION FOR RELEASE OF INFORMATION

Section A: Must be completed for all authorizations.

I hereby authorize the use or disclosure of my individually identifiable health information as described below.
I understand that this authorization is voluntary. I understand that if the organization to receive the information is not a health plan or health care provider, the released information may no longer be protected by federal privacy regulations.

Patient name: ______________________ **ID Number:** ______________

Persons/organizations providing information: ______________________

Persons/organizations receiving information: ______________________

Specific description of information [including date(s)]: ______________________

Section B: Must be completed only if a health plan or a health care provider has requested the authorization.

1. The health plan or health care provider must complete the following:
   a. What is the purpose of the use or disclosure? ______________________
   b. Will the health plan or health care provider requesting the authorization receive financial or in-kind compensation in exchange for using or disclosing the health information described above? Yes ____ No ____
2. The patient or the patient's representative must read and initial the following statements:
   a. I understand that my health care and the payment of my health care will not be affected if I do not sign this form.
   Initials: ____________
   b. I understand that I may see and copy the information described on this form if I ask for it, and that I get a copy of this form after I sign it.
   Initials: ____________

Section C: Must be completed for all authorizations.

The patient or the patient's representative must read and initial the following statements:

1. I understand that this authorization will expire on ____/____/____(DD/MM/YR).
   Initials: ____________
2. I understand that I may revoke this authorization at any time by notifying the providing organization in writing, but if I do not it will not have any effect on actions they took before they received the revocation.
   Initials: ____________

______________________ ______________

Signature of patient or patient's representative **Date**
(Form MUST be completed before signing)

Printed name of patient's representative: ______________________

Relationship to patient: ______________________

YOU MAY REFUSE TO SIGN THIS AUTHORIZATION
You may not use this form to release information for treatment or payment except when the information to be released is psychotherapy notes or certain research information.

Figure 4-2

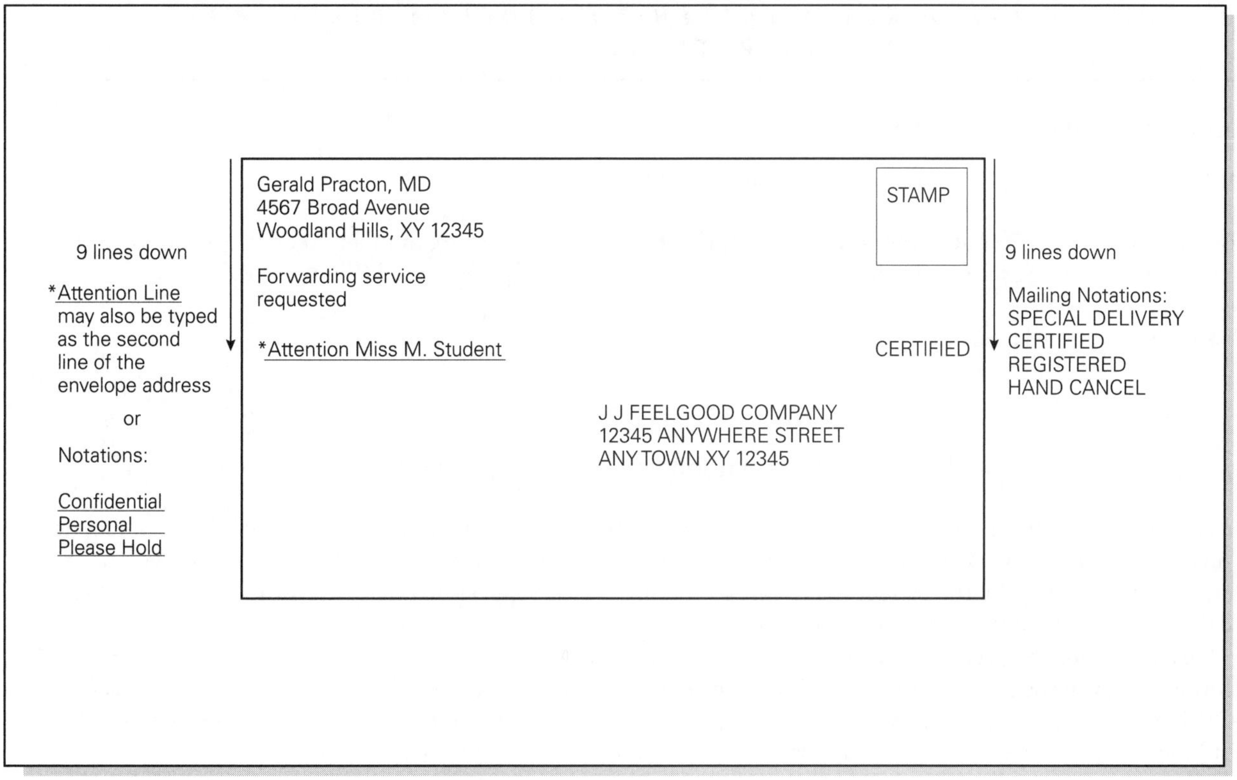
9 lines down
*Attention Line may also be typed as the second line of the envelope address
or
Notations:
Confidential
Personal
Please Hold
Gerald Practon, MD
4567 Broad Avenue
Woodland Hills, XY 12345
Forwarding service requested
*Attention Miss M. Student
STAMP
CERTIFIED
J J FEELGOOD COMPANY
12345 ANYWHERE STREET
ANY TOWN XY 12345
9 lines down
Mailing Notations:
SPECIAL DELIVERY
CERTIFIED
REGISTERED
HAND CANCEL

Figure 4-3

ASSIGNMENT 4-7 ▶ KEY A LETTER TO CONFIRM DISCHARGE BY THE PATIENT

Performance Objective

Task: Key letter for the physician's signature.

Conditions: Use one sheet of letterhead (print from Evolve website), number 10 envelope, and U.S. Postal Service forms for certified mail with return receipt requested (Figure 4-4).

Standards: Time: ______________________ minutes

Accuracy: ______________________

(Note: The time element and accuracy criteria may be given by your instructor.)

Directions: Mr. Walter J. Stone telephones on June 3, sounding extremely upset and irrational. He says that he is unable to return to work on June 22 and that he does not want to be seen by Dr. Input again. Type a letter to confirm this discharge by the patient (see *Handbook* Figure 4-23). Suggest that he contact the local medical society for the names of three internists for further care.

This letter must be prepared for Dr. Input's signature because it is a legal document. Refer to Assignment 7-4 for information from the patient record. Use a letterhead and key in modified block style as shown in *Handbook* Figure 4-21. Use the current date. Key Mr. Stone's address on a number 10 envelope, referring to *Workbook* Figure 4-3. Send the letter by certified mail with return receipt requested, referring to *Handbook* Figure 4-22.

After the instructor has returned your work to you, either make the necessary corrections and place it in a three-ring notebook for future reference, or, if you receive a high score, place it in your portfolio for reference when applying for a job.

UNITED STATES POSTAL SERVICE

First-Class Mail
Postage & Fees Paid
USPS
Permit No. G-10

• Sender: Please print your name, address, and ZIP+4 in this box •

SENDER: ***COMPLETE THIS SECTION***

- Complete items 1, 2, and 3. Also complete item 4 if Restricted Delivery is desired.
- Print your name and address on the reverse so that we can return the card to you.
- Attach this card to the back of the mailpiece, or on the front if space permits.

1. Article Addressed to:

COMPLETE THIS SECTION ON DELIVERY

A. Signature
☐ Agent
x ☐ Addressee

B. Received by (*Printed Name*) C. Date of Delivery

D. Is delivery address different from item 1? ☐ Yes
If YES, enter delivery address below: ☐ No

3. Service Type
☐ Certified Mail ☐ Express Mail
☐ Registered ☐ Return Receipt for Merchandise
☐ Insured Mail ☐ C.O.D.

4. Restricted Delivery? *(Extra Fee)* ☐ Yes

2. Article Number
(Transfer from service label)

PS Form 3811, February 2004 Domestic Return Receipt 102595-02-M-1540

7006 0810 0001 6207 8857

PLACE STICKER AT TOP OF ENVELOPE TO THE RIGHT OF THE RETURN ADDRESS, FOLD AT DOTTED LINE

CERTIFIED MAIL™

7006 0810 0001 6207 8857
7006 0810 0001 6207 8857

U.S. Postal Service™
CERTIFIED MAIL™ RECEIPT
(Domestic Mail Only; No Insurance Coverage Provided)

For delivery information visit our website at www.usps.com®

OFFICIAL USE

Postage	$
Certified Fee	
Return Receipt Fee (Endorsement Required)	
Restricted Delivery Fee (Endorsement Required)	
Total Postage & Fees	**$**

Postmark Here

Sent To

Street, Apt. No.; or PO Box No.

City, State, ZIP+4

PS Form 3800, June 2002 **See Reverse for Instructions**

Figure 4-4

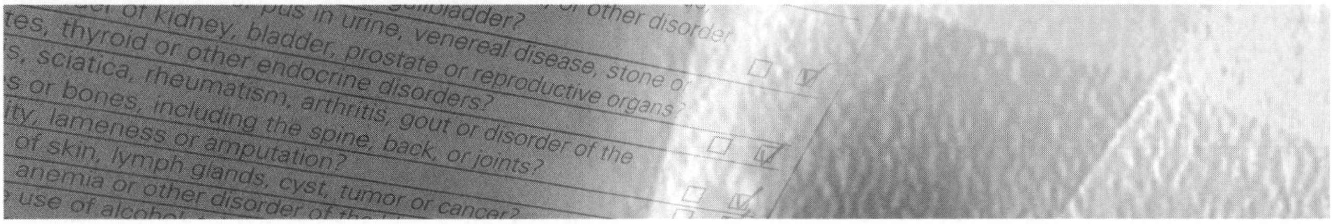

CHAPTER

5

Diagnostic Coding

KEY TERMS

Your instructor may wish to select some words pertinent to this chapter for a test. For definitions of the terms, further study, and/or reference, the words, phrases, and abbreviations may be found in the glossary at the end of the Handbook. *Key terms for this chapter follow.*

adverse effect
benign tumor
chief complaint
combination code
complication
computer-assisted coding
conventions
E codes
eponym
etiology
in situ
International Classification of Diseases, Ninth Revision, Clinical Modification
International Classification of Diseases, Tenth Revision, Clinical Modification
International Classification of Diseases, Tenth Revision, Procedural Coding System
intoxication
italicized code
late effect
malignant tumor
metastasis
neoplasm
not elsewhere classifiable
not otherwise specified
physician's fee profile
poisoning
primary diagnosis
principal diagnosis
secondary diagnosis
slanted brackets
syndrome
V codes

KEY ABBREVIATIONS

AHA ______

AHIMA ______

ASCVD ______

ASHD ______

CAC ______

CC ______

CM ______

CPT ______

DRG ______

DSM-IV ______

E codes ______

ICD-9-CM ______

ICD-10-CM ______

ICD-10-PCS ______

IDDM (type I diabetes) ______

MRI ______

NCHS ______

NEC ______

NIDDM ______

NOS ______

SNOMED ______

V codes ______

PERFORMANCE OBJECTIVES

The student will be able to:

- Define and spell the key terms and key abbreviations for this chapter, given the information from the *Handbook* glossary, within a reasonable time period and with enough accuracy to obtain a satisfactory evaluation.
- Answer the fill-in-the-blank, multiple choice, and true/false review questions after reading the chapter, with enough accuracy to obtain a satisfactory evaluation.
- Assignment 5-2: Indicate main terms, subterms, subterms to subterms, and carryover lines, given a section of a page from the ICD-9-CM code book, with enough accuracy to obtain a satisfactory evaluation.
- Assignment 5-3: Answer questions given a section of a page from the ICD-9-CM code book, with enough accuracy to obtain a satisfactory evaluation.
- Assignment 5-4: Select the correct diagnostic code numbers, given diagnoses, and locate the conditions using Volumes 1 and 2 of the ICD-9-CM code book, with enough accuracy to obtain a satisfactory evaluation.
- Assignments 5-5 through 5-12: Select the correct diagnostic code numbers, given a series of scenarios and diagnoses using Volumes 1 and 2 of the ICD-9-CM code book, with enough accuracy to obtain a satisfactory evaluation.

STUDY OUTLINE

The Diagnostic Coding System
- Sequencing of Diagnostic Codes
- Reasons for the Development and Use of Diagnostic Codes
- Physician's Fee Profile

History of Coding Diseases
- Computer-Assisted Coding

International Classification of Diseases
- History
- Organization and Format
- Contents

Diagnostic Code Book Conventions
- General Coding Guidelines

Rules for Coding
- Signs, Symptoms, and Ill-Defined Conditions
- Sterilization
- Neoplasms
- Circulatory System Conditions
- Diabetes Mellitus
- Pregnancy, Delivery, or Abortion
- Admitting Diagnoses
- Burns
- Injuries and Late Effects

ICD-10-CM Diagnosis and Procedure Codes
- ICD-10-CM Versus ICD-9-CM
- Format and Structure
- ICD-10-CM Coding Conventions
- Other and Unspecified Codes
- Gender and Age Codes

Procedure: Basic Steps in Selecting Diagnostic Codes from ICD-9-CM

Procedure: Basic Steps in Selecting Diagnostic Codes from ICD-10-CM

ASSIGNMENT 5-3 ▸ LOCATING INFORMATION IN ICD-9-CM, VOLUME 2

Performance Objective

Task: Answer questions pertaining to categories 320 and 321 of ICD-9-CM, Volume 2.

Conditions: Use the abstracted section from ICD-9-CM, Volume 2 (Figure 5-1) and pen or pencil.

Standards: Time: ____________________ minutes

Accuracy: ____________________

(Note: The time element and accuracy criteria may be given by your instructor.)

Directions: Refer to a section from a page of ICD-9-CM, Volume 2 (see Figure 5-1), and answer questions pertaining to categories 320 and 321.

1. Locate the section title ____

2. Refer to the INCLUSION TERMS listed under category code 320, titled "Bacterial meningitis." Place an "X" in front of each of the following diagnostic statements that are included in category 320.

____________ purulent meningitis

____________ bacterial meningomyelitis

____________ meningitis

____________ meningoencephalitis

____________ pyogenic meningitis

____________ meningococcal

3. Refer to the EXCLUSION TERMS located under code 320.7, titled "Meningitis in other bacterial diseases classified elsewhere." Place an "X" in front of the following code number(s) that are excluded.

____________ secondary syphilis 091.81

____________ acquired syphilis 097.9

____________ gonococcal meningitis 098.82

____________ congenital syphilis 090.42

____________ primary syphilis 091.2

____________ gram-negative anaerobes 320.81

6. NERVOUS SYSTEM AND SENSE ORGANS (320-389)

INFLAMMATORY DISEASES OF THE CENTRAL NERVOUS SYSTEM (320-326)

320 Bacterial meningitis
Includes: arachnoiditis, leptomeningitis, meningitis, meningoencephalitis, meningomyelitis, pachymeningitis } bacterial

320.0 *Haemophilus* meningitis
Meningitis due to *Haemophilus influenzae* [*H. Influenzae*]

320.1 Pneumococcal meningitis

320.2 Streptococcal meningitis

320.3 Staphylococcal meningitis

320.7 Meningitis in other bacterial diseases classified elsewhere

Code first underlying diseases as:
actinomycosis (039.8)
listeriosis (027.0)
typhoid fever (002.0)
whooping cough (033.0-033.9)

Excludes: meningitis (in):
epidemic (036.0)
gonococcal (098.82)
meningococcal (036.0)
salmonellosis (003.21)
syphilis:
NOS (094.2)
congenital (090.42)
meningovascular (094.2)
secondary (091.81)
tuberculous (013.0)

320.8 Meningitis due to other specified bacteria

320.81 Anaerobic meningitis
Bacteroides (fragilis)
Gram-negative anaerobes

320.82 Meningitis due to gram-negative bacteria, not elsewhere classified
Aerobacter aerogenes | *Klebsiella pneumoniae*
Escherichia coli [E. coli] | *Proteus morganii*
Friedländer bacillus | *Pseudomonas*

Excludes: gram-negative anaerobes (320.81)

320.89 Meningitis due to other specified bacteria
Bacillus pyocyaneus

320.9 Meningitis due to unspecified bacterium
Meningitis:
bacterial NOS
purulent NOS
pyogenic NOS
suppurative NOS

321 Meningitis due to other organisms
Includes: arachnoiditis, leptomeningitis, meningitis, pachymeningitis } due to organisms other than bacteria

321.0 Cryptococcal meningitis
Code first underlying disease (117.5)

Figure 5-1

4. Place an "X" in front of each of the following diagnostic statements included in category code 320 and its subcategories.

_______________ leptomeningitis

_______________ meningitis resulting from *E. coli*

_______________ pyogenic meningitis

_______________ epidemic meningitis

_______________ tuberculous meningitis

5. Write the code numbers for category 320 that require fifth digits.

____

DIAGNOSTIC CODING ASSIGNMENTS

In this chapter, the point awarded for assignments that require diagnostic codes is 1 point for each correct digit.

ASSIGNMENT 5-4 ▶ OBTAIN GENERAL DIAGNOSTIC CODES FOR CONDITIONS

Performance Objective

Task:	Locate the correct diagnostic code for each diagnosis listed.
Conditions:	Use pen or pencil and ICD-9-CM diagnostic code book.
Standards:	Time: ________________ minutes
	Accuracy: ________________
	(Note: The time element and accuracy criteria may be given by your instructor.)

Directions: Using the *International Classification of Diseases, Ninth Revision, Clinical Modification* (ICD-9-CM) code book, read each diagnosis and locate the condition in Volume 2, the Alphabetic Index. Then go to Volume 1, to the Tabular List of Diseases. Match the definition as closely as possible to the written description and assign the correct code, entering it on the blank line. If your instructor tells you to also find the ICD-10-CM codes, a draft version may be downloaded from the following website: http://www.cdc.gov/nchs/icd/icd10cm.htm11update. This website address changes each year to present a current version. As you can read, 11 relates to the year 2011.

Problems	**ICD-9-CM Codes**	**ICD-10-CM Codes**
1. Breast mass	____________	____________
2. *Klebsiella* pneumonia	____________	____________
3. Acute lateral wall myocardial infarction; initial episode	____________	____________
4. Acute cerebrovascular accident	____________	____________
5. Arteriosclerotic cardiovascular disease	____________	____________
6. Dyspnea, R/O cystic fibrosis	____________	____________
7. Ileitis	____________	____________
8. Arthritis of elbow	____________	____________
9. Ringing in the ears	____________	____________
10. Acute exacerbation of chronic asthmatic bronchitis	____________	____________

ASSIGNMENT 5-5 ▶ CODE DIAGNOSES FROM MEDICAL RECORDS

Performance Objective

Task: Locate the correct diagnostic code for each case scenario.

Conditions: Use pen or pencil and ICD-9-CM diagnostic code book.

Standards: Time: ________________ minutes

Accuracy: ________________

(Note: The time element and accuracy criteria may be given by your instructor.)

Directions: This exercise will give you experience in basic diagnostic coding for physicians' insurance claims. First list the ICD-9-CM code for the diagnosis, condition, problem, or other reason for the admission and/or encounter (visit) shown in the medical record to be chiefly responsible for the services provided. Then list additional diagnostic codes that describe any coexisting conditions that affect patient care. Always assign codes to their highest level of specificity—the more digits, the more specific. Do not code probable, rule out, suspected, or questionable conditions. Assign the correct code(s), entering it (them) on the blank line. If your instructor tells you to also find the ICD-10-CM codes, a draft version may be downloaded from the following website: http://www.cdc.gov/nchs/icd/icd10cm.html1update. This website address changes each year to present a current version. As you can read, 11 relates to the year 2011.

Problems	ICD-9-CM Codes	ICD-10-CM Codes
Problem 1. A patient, Mrs. Jennifer Hanson, calls Dr. Input's office stating she has blood in her stool. Dr. Input suspects a GI bleed and tells Mrs. Hanson to come in immediately. It is discovered that the reason for the blood in the stool is a bleeding duodenal ulcer. Code the diagnosis to be listed on the insurance claim for the office visit.	________________	________________
Problem 2. a. Jason Belmen comes in with a fractured humerus. He also has chronic obstructive pulmonary disease (COPD), which is not treated. Code the diagnosis.	a. ________________	a. ________________
b. Assume Mr. Belmen needs general anesthesia for open reduction of the fractured humerus. The COPD could now be considered a risk factor. List the diagnostic code in the second part of this scenario.	b. ________________	b. ________________
Problem 3. Margarita Sanchez came into the office for removal of sutures. Code the diagnosis.	________________	________________

Problem 4. A patient, George Martin, has benign prostatic hypertrophy (BPH). He is seen for catheterization because of urinary retention. Code the primary and secondary diagnoses for the office visit. (Note: BPH is an enlargement of the prostate gland, due to overgrowth of androgen-sensitive glandular elements, which occurs naturally with aging.)

a. ____________________ a. ____________________

b. ____________________ b. ____________________

Problem 5. Mia Bartholomew is seen in the office complaining of a sore throat. A throat culture is done and the specimen is sent to an outside laboratory for a culture and sensitivity study to determine the presence of *Streptococcus*. List the diagnostic code the physician would use if the insurance claim is submitted before the results are known. List the diagnostic code used if the physician submits the insurance claim after the laboratory report is received indicating *Streptococcus* is present.

a. ____________________ a. ____________________

b. ____________________ b. ____________________

ASSIGNMENT 5-6 ▶ CODE DIAGNOSES USING V CODES

Performance Objective

Task: Locate the correct diagnostic code for each case scenario.

Conditions: Use pen or pencil and ICD-9-CM diagnostic code book.

Standards: Time: ________________________ minutes

Accuracy: ________________________

(Note: The time element and accuracy criteria may be given by your instructor.)

Directions: In this exercise you will be reviewing V codes in the ICD-9-CM code book. Assign the correct code, entering it on the blank line. These are some key words under which V codes may be located in Volume 2:

admission	checking/checkup	donor	insertion of	status post
aftercare	conflict	evaluation	maintenance	vaccination
attention to	contact	examination	observation	
border	contraception	fitting of	person with	
care of	counseling	follow-up	problem with	
carrier	dialysis	history of	screening	

If your instructor tells you to also find the ICD-10-CM codes, a draft version may be downloaded from the following website: http://www.cdc.gov/nchs/icd/icd10cm.htm11update. This website address changes each year to present a current version. As you can read, 11 relates to the year 2011.

Problems	ICD-9-CM Codes	ICD-10-CM Codes
1. Kathy Osborn, a patient, is seen in the office for an annual checkup.	________________	________________
2. Daniel Matsui is seen in the office for adjustment of a lumbosacral corset.	________________	________________
3. Philip O'Brien comes into the office to receive a prophylactic flu shot.	________________	________________
4. Bernadette Murphy is seen in the office for a pregnancy test.	________________	________________
5. Michiko Fujita is seen in the office for a fractured rib. No x-rays are taken because Mrs. Fujita thinks she is pregnant.	a. ________________ b. ________________	a. ________________ b. ________________

6. Dr. Perry Cardi sees Kenneth Pickford in the office for cardiac pacemaker adjustment. The pacemaker was implanted because of sick sinus syndrome. ____________ ____________

7. Frank Meadows returns for follow-up, postoperative transurethral prostatic resection (TURP) for prostate cancer after treatment has been completed.

a. ____________ a. ____________

b. ____________ b. ____________

ASSIGNMENT 5-7 ▸ CODE NEOPLASTIC DIAGNOSES

Performance Objective

Task: Locate the correct diagnostic code for each diagnosis listed.

Conditions: Use pen or pencil and ICD-9-CM diagnostic code book.

Standards: Time: ________________ minutes

Accuracy: ________________

(Note: The time element and accuracy criteria may be given by your instructor.)

Directions: In this exercise, you will be reviewing diagnostic codes in the ICD-9-CM code book involving neoplasms. The morphology of neoplasm is found in Appendix A of Volume 1. Neoplasms are classified according to their histology. Morphology (M) codes are sometimes used to supplement a diagnostic code. M codes are not used on insurance forms when submitting claims by physicians; therefore, they will not be used in this assignment. M codes are never used as a primary diagnostic code. Assign the correct code, entering it on the blank line.

If your instructor tells you to also find the ICD-10-CM codes, a draft version may be downloaded from the following website: http://www.cdc.gov/nchs/icd/icd10cm.htm11update. This website address changes each year to present a current version. As you can read, 11 relates to the year 2011.

Problems	ICD-9-CM Codes	ICD-10-CM Codes
1. Leiomyoma, uterus	________	________
2. Ewing's sarcoma, forearm	________	________
3. Adenocarcinoma, right breast, central portion, female	________	________
4. Dyspnea resulting from carcinoma of the breast, female with metastasis to the upper lobe, right lung	a. ________ b. ________	a. ________ b. ________
5. Patient is seen for a yearly examination 1 year after a mastectomy for breast cancer; she is disease-free at this time	a. ________ b. ________	a. ________ b. ________
6. Patient comes in for chemotherapy because of lymphosarcoma of the intrathoracic lymph nodes	a. ________ b. ________	a. ________ b. ________

ASSIGNMENT 5-8 ▶ CODE DIAGNOSES FOR PATIENTS WITH DIABETES

Performance Objective

Task: Locate the correct diagnostic code for each diagnosis listed.

Conditions: Use pen or pencil and ICD-9-CM diagnostic code book.

Standards: Time: ________________ minutes

Accuracy: ________________

(Note: The time element and accuracy criteria may be given by your instructor.)

Directions: In this exercise, you will review diagnostic codes in the ICD-9-CM code book involving cases of patients with diabetes. When coding diabetes, first find out the type of diabetes being treated, type I or type II. Then look to see whether the diabetes is under control. These two answers determine the assignment of the fifth digit.

For diabetic complications, determine whether the complication is due to the diabetes and whether the diabetes is out of control. These points need to be regarded as two distinctly different issues. A patient can have controlled diabetes but still have a complication caused by diabetes. Complications arising from diabetes must be coded. The code for the complication is listed after the subterm in brackets.

Example: If a patient with type II uncontrolled diabetes is treated for a skin ulcer on the lower extremity, look up "diabetes" in Volume 2 and find the subterm "ulcer." The diabetes code listed is 250.8 and under the subterm "ulcer" is a sub-subterm of "lower extremity" with the code 707.1 in brackets. Go to Volume 1 and verify the diabetes code and assign a fifth digit. The correct code is 250.82 (2 for type II, uncontrolled). Now verify the ulcer code in Volume 1. You will see that code 707.1 does not mention diabetes. If diabetes is the cause of the ulcer, code the diabetes first and the ulcer second. If the patient's diabetes is under control and is not being treated at the visit, code the ulcer first and diabetes second as an underlying disease. Other complications, such as bone changes (731.8), may tell you to code the underlying disease first. Therefore, always verify all codes in Volume 1 before assigning them.

Assign the correct code(s) for each case involving diabetes, entering it (them) on the blank line.

If your instructor tells you to also find the ICD-10-CM codes, a draft version may be downloaded from the following website: http://www.cdc.gov/nchs/icd/icd10cm.htm11update. This website address changes each year to present a current version. As you can read, 11 relates to the year 2011.

Problems	ICD-9-CM Codes	ICD-10-CM Codes
1. Diabetes mellitus	________	________
2. Type II, uncontrolled non–insulin-dependent diabetes mellitus with ketoacidosis	________	________
3. Diabetic gangrene (type I diabetes, out of control)	a. ________	a. ________
	b. ________	b. ________
4. Controlled type II diabetes with cataract	a. ________	a. ________
	b. ________	b. ________
5. Type I diabetes with diabetic polyneuropathy and retinopathy	a. ________	a. ________
	b. ________	b. ________
	c. ________	c. ________
	d. ________	d. ________

ASSIGNMENT 5-9 ▶ CODE DIAGNOSES FOR PATIENTS WITH HYPERTENSION

Performance Objective

Task: Locate the correct diagnostic code for each diagnosis listed.

Conditions: Use pen or pencil and ICD-9-CM diagnostic code book.

Standards: Time: ______________________ minutes

Accuracy: ______________________

(Note: The time element and accuracy criteria may be given by your instructor.)

Directions: In this exercise, you will review diagnostic codes in the ICD-9-CM code book involving patients who have hypertension. To begin coding, look in Volume 2 under "hypertension" and find the Hypertension Table. This is designed to simplify coding conditions caused by, or associated with, hypertension or hypertensive disease. At the beginning of the table, many terms are listed in parentheses. These terms are nonessential modifiers, which means that the absence or presence of one of these terms does not change the meaning of the code. From the table, the codes relating to hypertension begin with 401. Go to this number in Volume 1 and look through this section to become familiar with it.

Assign the correct code(s) for each case, entering it (them) on the blank line.

If your instructor tells you to also find the ICD-10-CM codes, a draft version may be downloaded from the following website: http://www.cdc.gov/nchs/icd/icd10cm.htm11update. This website address changes each year to present a current version. As you can read, 11 relates to the year 2011.

Problems	ICD-9-CM Codes	ICD-10-CM Codes
1. High blood pressure	______________	______________
2. Malignant hypertension	______________	______________
3. Antepartum hypertension complicating pregnancy	______________	______________
4. Hypertension with kidney disease	______________	______________
5. Hypertension due to arteriosclerotic cardiovascular disease (ASCVD) and systolic congestive heart failure (CHF)	______________	______________
6. Myocarditis and CHF due to malignant hypertension	a. ______________	a. ______________
	b. ______________	b. ______________

ASSIGNMENT 5-10 ▶ CODE DIAGNOSES FOR INJURIES, FRACTURES, BURNS, LATE EFFECTS, AND COMPLICATIONS

Performance Objective

Task: Locate the correct diagnostic code for each diagnosis listed.

Conditions: Use pen or pencil and ICD-9-CM diagnostic code book.

Standards: Time: ________________________ minutes

Accuracy: ________________________

(Note: The time element and accuracy criteria may be given by your instructor.)

Directions: In this exercise, you will review diagnostic codes from the ICD-9-CM code book involving patients who have suffered injuries, burns, fractures, and late effects. If your instructor tells you to also find the ICD-10-CM codes, a draft version may be downloaded from the following website: http://www.cdc.gov/nchs/icd/icd10cm.htm11update. This website address changes each year to present a current version. As you can read, 11 relates to the year 2011. Some guidelines for coding injuries, fractures, burns, late effects, and complications are:

Injuries

✓ Code injuries separately according to their general type and then by anatomic site. Fifth digits are commonly used in the injury section to specify anatomic sites and severity.
✓ Code injuries separately if they are classifiable to more than one subcategory unless the diagnosis does not support separate injuries or the Alphabetic Index provides instructions to use combination code.

Fractures

✓ Fractures are presumed to be closed unless otherwise specified.
✓ Fracture/dislocations are coded as fractures.
✓ Pathologic fractures are coded first and the cause (disease process) coded second.

Burns

✓ Multiple burns at the same site, but of different degrees, are coded to the most severe degree.
✓ Code the extent of body surface involved (percentage of body surface), when specified, as an additional code.

Late Effects

✓ A residual, late effect is defined as the current condition resulting from a previous acute illness or injury that is no longer the current problem. Late effects are coded using the residual or late effect as the primary diagnosis. The cause of the residual or late effect is coded second.

Complications

✓ For conditions resulting from the malfunction of internal devices, use the subterm “mechanical” found under the main term “complication.”
✓ Postoperative complications are sometimes found under the subterm “postoperative,” which appears under the main term identifying the condition. If not found there, look for a subterm identifying the type of procedure, type of complication, or surgical procedure under the main term “complication.”

Assign the correct code(s) for each case, entering it (them) on the blank line.

Problems	ICD-9-CM Codes	ICD-10-CM Codes
1. Supracondylar fracture of right femur with intracondylar extension of lower end	________________	________________
2. Fracture of left humerus and left foot	a. ________________	a. ________________
	b. ________________	b. ________________
3. Comminuted fracture of left radius and ulna, not displaced.	________________	________________
4. Pathologic fracture of right hip due to drug-induced osteoporosis	a. ________________	a. ________________
	b. ________________	b. ________________
5. Lacerations of the upper arm with embedded glass	________________	________________
6. Burns on the face and neck	________________	________________
7. Second- and third-degree burns on chest wall; 20% of body involved, 10% third-degree burns	a. ________________	a. ________________
	b. ________________	b. ________________
8. Bursitis of the knee resulting from crushing injury to the knee 1 year ago	a. ________________	a. ________________
	b. ________________	b. ________________

ASSIGNMENT 5-11 ▸ CODE DIAGNOSES FOR PREGNANCY, DELIVERY, AND NEWBORN CARE

Performance Objective

Task: Locate the correct diagnostic code for each case scenario.

Conditions: Use pen or pencil and ICD-9-CM diagnostic code book.

Standards: Time: ________________________ minutes

Accuracy: ________________________

(Note: The time element and accuracy criteria may be given by your instructor.)

Directions: In this exercise, you will review diagnostic codes from the ICD-9-CM code book involving patients who have conditions involving pregnancy and delivery, and newborn infants.

For the supervision of a normal pregnancy, turn to Volume 2 and look up "pregnancy." This is a long category. Look up the subterm "supervision" and find the sub-subterm "normal" (NEC V22.1) and "first" (V22.0). Check Volume 1 to verify these codes. Also see code V22.2 "pregnancy state, incidental." This code is used in the second position to tell the insurance carrier that the patient is pregnant in addition to any other diagnosis.

If a patient has complications, turn to Volume 2 and look under the main term "pregnancy." Find the subterm "complicated by" and find the sub-subterm stating the complication. These are codes from ICD-9-CM Chapter 11: "Complications of Pregnancy, Childbirth, and Puerperium" (630-677).

Delivery in a completely normal case is coded 650 and is listed under the main term "delivery, uncomplicated." Normal is described as "delivery without abnormality or complication and with spontaneous cephalic delivery, without mention of fetal manipulation or instrumentation." A different code must be used to describe any complication or deviation from this description of normal.

When coding deliveries, always include a code for the status of the infant. Look up "outcome of delivery" in Volume 2 and you will find various V27 codes listing possible outcomes. These codes would be listed as secondary codes on the insurance claim form for the delivery.

On the insurance claim form for the newborn, turn to "newborn" in Volume 2. You will find V codes from V30.X to V39.X describing the birth of the newborn. Use these codes in the first position when billing for services for the newborn infant.

Assign the correct code(s) for each case entering it (them) on the blank line.

If your instructor tells you to also find the ICD-10-CM codes, a draft version may be downloaded from the following website: http://www.cdc.gov/nchs/icd/icd10cm.htm11update. This website address changes each year to present a current version. As you can read, 11 relates to the year 2011.

Problems	ICD-9-CM Codes	ICD-10-CM Codes
1. A pregnant patient who is due to deliver in 6 weeks presents in the office with preeclampsia.	______	______
2. A patient presents with a chief complaint of severe episodes of pain and vaginal hemorrhage. The physician determines that the patient has an incomplete spontaneous abortion complicated by excessive hemorrhage; she was 6 weeks' pregnant.	______	______
3. A patient comes in who is diagnosed with a kidney stone; the patient is also pregnant.	a. ______ b. ______	a. ______ b. ______
4. A patient is delivered of twins both live born by cesarean section because of cephalopelvic disproportion, which caused an obstruction.	a. ______ b. ______ c. ______ d. ______	a. ______ b. ______ c. ______ d. ______

ASSIGNMENT 5-12 ▶ CODE DIAGNOSES USING E CODES

Performance Objective

Task: Locate the correct diagnostic code for each diagnosis listed.

Conditions: Use pen or pencil and the ICD-9-CM diagnostic code book.

Standards: Time: ________________ minutes

Accuracy: ________________

(Note: The time element and accuracy criteria may be given by your instructor.)

Directions: In this exercise you will be reviewing diagnostic codes from the ICD-9-CM code book involving patients who may have been in an accident, had an adverse effect from ingesting a toxic substance, or suffered an injury. Read the definitions for poisoning and drug intoxication in the *Handbook*.

✓ E codes are not used to describe the primary reason for a patient's visit but identify external environmental events, circumstances, and conditions as the cause of injury, poisoning, and other adverse effects (unfavorable results).

✓ E codes that identify external environmental events, such as an injury, are used only as supplemental codes to describe how an injury occurred. These codes are listed in the back of Volume 2 and provide a more descriptive clinical picture for the insurance carrier. They may or may not be required and in some cases may speed up the payment of the claim.

✓ E codes are used for coding adverse effects of drugs and chemicals but are not required when coding a poisoning. Use the Table of Drugs and Chemicals at the back of Volume 2 and go to the column titled "Therapeutic Use." In addition, it is necessary to use a code to describe the adverse effect of using a particular drug or medicine. Find this in Volume 2 and verify it in Volume 1.

Assign the correct code(s) for each case and enter it (them) on the blank line.

If your instructor tells you to also find the ICD-10-CM codes, a draft version may be downloaded from the following website: http://www.cdc.gov/nchs/icd/icd10cm.htm11update. This website address changes each year to present a current version. As you can read, 11 relates to the year 2011.

Problems	ICD-9-CM Codes	ICD-10-CM Codes
1. Light-headedness caused by digitalis intoxication.	a. ________	a. ________
	b. ________	b. ________
2. Treatment of a rash after an initial dose of penicillin is given.	a. ________	a. ________
	b. ________	b. ________
3. Accidental overdose of meperidine (Demerol).	a. ________	a. ________
	b. ________	b. ________

4. A 20-month-old baby accidentally ingests approximately 15 aspirin and is severely nauseated.

a. ______________ a. ______________

b. ______________ b. ______________

c. ______________ c. ______________

5. A patient presents in the physician's office with a vague complaint of not feeling well. The physician notices that the patient has ataxia (a staggering gait). After reviewing the patient's history, the physician determines the ataxia is due to the meprobamate the patient is taking.

a. ______________ a. ______________

b. ______________ b. ______________

6. Internal bleeding: abnormal reaction to a combination of chloramphenicol and warfarin (Coumadin).

a. ______________ a. ______________

b. ______________ b. ______________

c. ______________ c. ______________

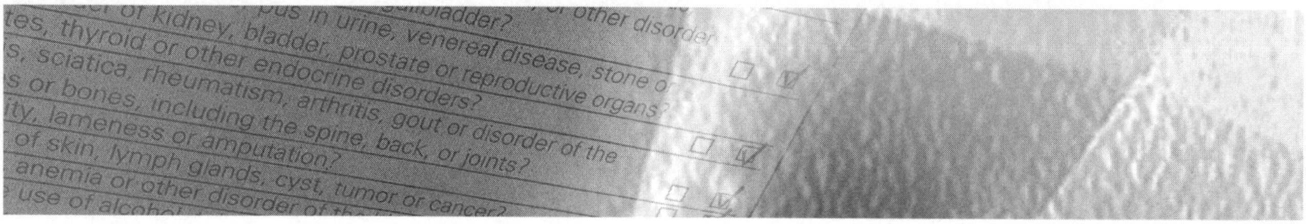

CHAPTER

6

Procedural Coding

KEY TERMS

Your instructor may wish to select some words pertinent to this chapter for a test. For definitions of the terms, further study, and/or reference, the words, phrases, and abbreviations may be found in the glossary at the end of the Handbook. *Key terms for this chapter follow.*

alternative billing codes
bilateral
bundled codes
comprehensive code
conversion factor
Current Procedural Terminology
customary fee
downcoding
fee schedule
global surgery policy
Healthcare Common Procedure Coding System
modifiers
never event
procedure code numbers
professional component
reasonable fee
relative value studies
relative value unit
resource-based relative value scale
surgical package
technical component
unbundling
upcoding
usual, customary, and reasonable

3. Evaluation and Management (E/M) codes are used by physicians to report a significant portion of their services. Remember, it is the physician's responsibility to assign E/M codes, and the exercises presented here are only for familiarization. The problems will acquaint you with terminology for this section of the CPT code book. Select the appropriate **new patient** office visit codes using the key components:

   a. This is a Level 3 case: Detailed history

      Detailed examination

      Low-complexity decision-making ________________

   b. This is a Level 1 case: Problem-focused history

      Problem-focused examination

      Straightforward decision-making ________________

   c. This is a Level 5 case: Comprehensive history

      Comprehensive examination

      High-complexity decision-making ________________

4. Select the appropriate **established patient** office visit codes using the key components. Coding these cases illustrates consideration of two of three components.

   a. This is a Level 4 case: Detailed history

      Detailed examination

      Low-complexity decision-making ________________

   b. This is a Level 5 case: Comprehensive history

      Comprehensive examination

      Moderate-complexity decision-making ________________

   c. This is a Level 5 case: Detailed history

      Comprehensive examination

      High-complexity decision-making ________________

5. Evaluation and Management (E/M) codes **99201** to **99239** are used for services provided in the physician's office or in an outpatient or hospital facility. Read the brief statement and then locate the code number in the *Current Procedural Terminology* code book.

   a. Office visit of a 20-year-old patient seen within the past 3 years for instruction in diabetes injection sites by RN (minimal problem). Patient not seen by physician at this brief visit. ________________

   b. Office visit of a 30-year-old new patient with allergic rhinitis. This case had an expanded problem-focused hx & exam and straightforward decision-making. ________________

   c. Discussion of medication with the son of an 80-year-old patient with dementia on discharge from the observation unit. ________________

   d. Admission to hospital of 60-year-old established patient in acute respiratory distress with bronchitis. Comprehensive hx & exam and medical decision making of moderate complexity. ________________

   e. Hospital visit of a 4-year-old boy, now stable, who will be discharged the next day. This is a problem-focused interval hx & exam and medical decision making of low complexity. ________________

   f. New patient seen in the office for chest pain, congestive heart failure, and hypertension. Comprehensive hx & exam and highly complex decision-making. ________________

6. Evaluation and Management codes **99241** to **99255** are used for consultations provided in the physician's office or in an outpatient or inpatient hospital facility. A consultation is a service provided by a physician whose opinion about a case is requested by another physician. Read the brief statement and then locate the code number in the *Current Procedural Terminology* code book.

   a. Office consultation for a 30-year-old woman complaining of palpitations and chest pains. Her family physician described a mild systolic click. This is an expanded problem-focused hx & exam and straightforward decision-making. ________________

   b. Follow-up inpatient consultation for a 54-year-old woman, who is now stable, admitted 2 days ago for a bleeding ulcer. This case is a detailed hx & exam and low-complexity decision-making. ________________

   c. Office consultation for a 14-year-old boy with poor grades in school and suspected alcohol abuse. This is a comprehensive hx & exam and medical decision making of moderate complexity. ________________

   d. Follow-up inpatient consultation for a 50-year-old man who is diabetic and is suffering with fever, chills, gangrenous heel ulcer, rhonchi, and dyspnea (difficulty breathing), an unstable condition. The patient appears lethargic and tachypneic (rapid breathing). This case is comprehensive hx & exam with highly complex medical decision making. ________________

   e. Initial emergency department consultation for a senior who presents with thyrotoxicosis, exophthalmos, cardiac arrhythmia, and congestive heart failure. This case is a comprehensive hx & exam with highly complex medical decision making. ________________

   f. Initial hospital consultation for a 30-year-old woman, postabdominal surgery, who is exhibiting a fever. This case is an expanded problem-focused hx & exam and straightforward medical decision making. ________________

7. Evaluation and Management codes **99281** to **99499** are used for emergency department, critical care, nursing facility, rest home, custodial care, home, prolonged, physician standby, and preventive medicine services. Read the brief statement and then locate the code number in the *Current Procedural Terminology* code book.

   a. First hour of critical care of a senior who, following major surgery, suffers a cardiac arrest from a pulmonary embolus. ________________

   b. A 40-year-old woman is admitted to the OB unit, and the primary care physician has requested the neonatologist to stand by for possible cesarean section and neonatal resuscitation. Code for a 1-hour standby. ________________

   c. A child is seen in the emergency department with a fever, diarrhea, abdominal cramps, and vomiting. This case had an expanded problem-focused hx & exam and a moderately complex medical decision was made. ________________

   d. A patient is seen for an annual visit at a nursing facility for a detailed hx & comprehensive exam and low-complexity medical decision making. ________________

   e. An initial visit is made to a domiciliary care facility for a developmentally disabled individual with a mild rash on the hands and face. This case had an expanded problem-focused hx & exam and low-complexity medical decision making. ________________

   f. A 50-year-old man with a history of asthma comes into the office with acute bronchospasm and moderate respiratory distress. Office treatment is initiated. The case requires intermittent physician face-to-face time with the patient for 2 hours and prolonged services. Assume the appropriate E/M code has been assigned for this case. ________________

ASSIGNMENT 6-4 ▸ CODE ANESTHESIA PROBLEMS

Performance Objective

Task: Locate the correct procedure and modifier, if necessary, for each question and/or case scenario.

Conditions: Use pen or pencil and *Current Procedural Terminology* code book.

Standards: Time: ________________________ minutes

Accuracy: ________________________

(Note: The time element and accuracy criteria may be given by your instructor.)

Directions: Anesthesia codes **00100** to **01999** may be used by anesthesiologists and physicians. Some plastic surgeons, other medical specialists, and large clinics may have a room set aside to perform surgical procedures that might be performed in a hospital outpatient surgical department. For Medicare claims, some regions do not use the Anesthesia Section of CPT for billing but use a surgical code with an HCPCS modifier appended. Read the brief statement and then locate the code number in the *Current Procedural Terminology* code book. Special modifiers **P1** through **P6** may be needed when coding for this section, as well as code numbers for cases that have difficult circumstances. Definitions for abbreviations may be found in Appendix A of this *Workbook*.

a. Cesarean delivery following neuraxial labor anesthesia, normal healthy patient ________________ _____
________________ _____

b. Reduction mammoplasty of a woman with mild systemic disease ________________ _____

c. Total right hip replacement, 71-year-old patient, normal healthy patient ________________ _____
____

d. Repair of cleft palate, newborn infant, normal healthy patient ________________ _____
____

e. TURP, normal healthy male ________________ _____

ASSIGNMENT 6-5 ▶ CODE SURGICAL PROBLEMS

Performance Objective

Task: Locate the correct procedure code and modifier, if necessary, for each question and/or case scenario.

Conditions: Use pen or pencil and *Current Procedural Terminology* code book.

Standards: Time: ________________ minutes

Accuracy: ________________

(Note: The time element and accuracy criteria may be given by your instructor.)

Directions: Surgery codes **10040** to **69979** are used for each anatomic part of the body. Read over each case carefully. It is preferable to use the *Current Procedural Terminology* code book, but if you do not have one, then refer to the Mock Fee Schedule found in Appendix A of this *Workbook* to obtain the correct code number for each descriptor given. Full descriptors for services rendered have been omitted in some instances to give you practice in abstracting the correct descriptor from the available information. Indicate the correct two-digit modifier if necessary. The skill of critical thinking enters this section of the assignment, in that you may have to use your own judgment to code because the cases do not contain full details. Definitions for abbreviations may be found in Appendix A of this *Workbook*. Remember to use the index at the back of the CPT code book.

a. Suppose you work in an office that has an encounter form listing code 36540. Check your edition of CPT and see whether you can locate this code number. If the code does not appear, what code number are you directed to use? ________________

Integumentary System 10040-19499

b. Removal of benign lesion from the back (1.0 cm) and left foot (0.5 cm) ________________

____

c. Drainage of deep breast abscess ________________

d. Laser destruction of two benign facial lesions ________________

____

Musculoskeletal System 20000-29909

Reminder: Be sure to read the "Application of casts and strapping" guidelines in your CPT code book that appears before the 29000 codes. ________________

e. Aspiration of fluid (arthrocentesis) from right knee joint; not infectious ________________

f. Deep tissue biopsy of left upper arm ________________

g. Fracture of the left tibia, closed treatment ________________

Does the procedural code include application and removal of the first cast? ________________

If done as an office procedure, may supplies be coded? ________________

If so, what is the code number from the Medicine section? ____________

Does the procedural code include subsequent replacement of a cast for follow-up care? ____________

If not, list the code number for application of a walking short leg cast. ____________

Respiratory System 30000-32999

h. Parietal pleurectomy ____________

i. Removal of two nasal polyps, simple ____________

j. Diagnostic bronchoscopy with bronchial biopsy ____________

Cardiovascular System 33010-37799

k. Pacemaker insertion with transvenous electrode, atrial ____________

l. Thromboendarterectomy with patch graft ____________

m. Introduction of intracatheter and injection procedure for contrast venography ____________

Hemic/Lymphatic/Diaphragm 38100-39599

n. Repair, esophageal/diaphragmatic hernia transthoracic ____________

o. Partial splenectomy ____________

p. Excision, two deep cervical nodes ____________

Digestive System 40490-49999

q. T & A, 12-year-old boy ____________

r. Balloon dilation of esophagus ____________

Urinary System/Male and Female Genital 50010-55980

s. Removal of urethral diverticulum from female patient ____________

t. Anastomosis of single ureter to bladder ____________

Laparoscopy/Peritoneoscopy/Hysteroscopy/Female Genital/Maternity 56300-59899

u. Routine OB care, antepartum and postpartum care ____________

v. Therapeutic D & C, nonobstetric ____________

ASSIGNMENT 6-6 ▶ CODE PROBLEMS FOR RADIOLOGY AND PATHOLOGY

Performance Objective

Task: Locate the correct procedure code and modifier, if necessary, for each question and/or case scenario.

Conditions: Use pen or pencil and *Current Procedural Terminology* code book.

Standards: Time: ______________________ minutes

Accuracy: ______________________

(Note: The time element and accuracy criteria may be given by your instructor.)

Radiologists, as well as other physicians in many specialties, perform these studies. A physician who interprets, dictates, and signs a report may not bill for the report separately because it is considered part of the radiology procedure.

Some medical practices perform basic laboratory tests under a waived test certificate that complies with the rules of the Clinical Laboratory Improvement Amendments (CLIA) of 1988, implemented in September 1992.

a. Upper GI x-ray study with films and KUB ________________

b. Ultrasound, pregnant uterus after first trimester, two gestations ________________

____

c. Routine urinalysis with microscopy, nonautomated ________________

d. Hemoglobin (Hgb), electrophoretic method ________________

ASSIGNMENT 6-7 ▸ PROCEDURE CODE AND MODIFIER PROBLEMS

Performance Objective

Task: Locate the correct procedure code and modifiers, if necessary, for each case scenario.

Conditions: Use pen or pencil and *Current Procedural Terminology* code book.

Standards: Time: ________________________ minutes

Accuracy: ________________________

(Note: The time element and accuracy criteria may be given by your instructor.)

Directions: Find the correct procedure codes and modifiers, if necessary. This assignment will reinforce what you have already learned about procedural coding because code numbers for the case scenarios presented are located in all the sections of the CPT code book. Also search for codes in the Medicine Section, if necessary. The CPT list of modifiers may be found in the *Handbook*.

1. A new patient had five benign skin lesions on the right arm destroyed with surgical curettement. Complete the coding for the surgery.

Code Number	*Description*
a. ________________	Level 3, detailed history and exam with low-complexity decision-making, initial new pt office visit
b. ________________	Destruction of 5 benign skin lesions rt arm

2. Mrs. Stayman had four moles on her back. Dr. Davis excised the multiple nevi in one office visit. The information on the pathology report stated nonmalignant lesions measuring 2.2 cm, 1.5 cm, 1 cm, and 0.75 cm.

Code Number		*Description*
a. ______________	_______	Initial OV
b. ______________	_______	Excision, benign lesion 2.2 cm
c. ______________	_______	Excision, benign lesion 1.5 cm
d. ______________	_______	Excision, benign lesion 1 cm
e. ______________	_______	Excision, benign lesion 0.75 cm

In another case, if a patient required removal of a 1-cm lesion on the back and a 0.5-cm lesion on the neck, the procedural codes would be ________________________ for the back lesion and ________________ for the neck lesion.

3. Dr. Davis stated on his operative report that Mr. Allen was suffering from a complex, complicated nasal fracture. Dr. Davis débrided the wound because it was contaminated and performed an open reduction with internal fixation in a complex and complicated procedure.

Code Number		*Description*
a. ______________	_______	Initial OV, complex hx & exam, moderate-complexity decision-making
b. ______________		Open tx nasal fracture complicated
c. ______________	_______	Débridement, skin, subcutaneous tissue, muscle, and bone

4. An RN, an established patient (est pt), age 40 years, sees the doctor for an annual physical. A Pap (Papanicolaou) smear is obtained and sent to an outside laboratory. The patient also has a furuncle on the right axilla at the time of the visit, which the doctor incises and drains (I & D).

Code Number	*Description*
a. ______________	Periodic physical examination
b. ______________	Handling of specimen
c. ______________	I & D, furuncle, right axilla
d. ______________	5-mL penicillin inj IM

5. While making his rounds in the hospital during the noon hour, Dr. James sees a new patient in the ED (emergency department) for a laceration of the forehead, 5 cm long. The doctor does a workup for a possible concussion.

Code Number		*Description*
a. ______________	_______	ED care, expanded problem-focused history, expanded problem-focused examination, low-complexity decision-making
b. ______________		Repair of laceration, simple, face

6. The physician sees a new patient in the office with the same condition as the patient in Problem 5; however, an infection has developed, and the patient is seen for daily dressing changes. On day 11, the sutures are removed, and on day 12 a final dressing change is made, and the patient is discharged.

Code Number		*Description*
a. ______________	_______	Level 3, detailed history and exam with low-complexity decision-making, initial new patient office visit
b. ______________		Repair of laceration
c. ______________		Tet tox (tetanus toxoid) 0.5 cc
d. ______________		Administration intramuscular injection
e. ______________		Minimal service, OV (suture removal)
f. ______________		Minimal service, OV (dressing change)

Note: Some fee schedules allow no follow-up days; Medicare fee schedule allows 10 follow-up days for the procedural code number for repair of laceration.

7. The physician sees 13-year-old Bobby Jones (est pt) for a Boy Scout physical. Bobby is in good health and well groomed. His troop is going for a 1-week camping trip in 12 days. The physician reviewed safety issues with Bobby, talked to him about school, and counseled him about not getting into drugs or alcohol. Bobby denied any problems with that or of being sexually active. He said that he plays baseball. He has no allergies. The physician performed a detailed examination. The physician completed information for scouting papers and cleared him for camping activity.

Code Number	*Description*
a. ________________	Periodic preventive evaluation and management

8. A new patient, David Ramsey, age 15 years, was seen by Dr. Menter for lapses of memory and frequent headaches. The doctor performed an EEG (electroencephalogram) and some psychological tests (including psychodiagnostic assessment of personality and psychopathology tests [Rorschach and MMPI]). Dr. Astro Parkinson was called in as a consultant. All the test results were negative, and the patient was advised to come in for weekly psychotherapy.

Code Number	*Description*
Dr. Menter's bill:	
a. ________________	OV, comp hx & exam, moderate-complexity decision-making
b. ________________	EEG, extended monitoring (1 hour)
c. ________________	Psychological tests (Rorschach and MMPI)
d. ________________	Psychotherapy (50 minutes)
Dr. Parkinson's bill:	
e. ________________	Consultation, expanded problem-focused hx and exam, straightforward decision-making

9. An est pt, age 70 years, requires repair of a bilateral initial inguinal hernia (reducible). The code for this initial procedure is

a. ____________________ ____________________

ASSIGNMENT 6-8 ▶ HCPCS/MODIFIER CODE MATCH

Performance Objective

Task: Locate the correct HCPCS code and modifier, if necessary, for each medical drug, supply item, or service presented.

Conditions: Use pen or pencil and HCPCS code reference list in Appendix B of this *Workbook*.

Standards: Time: ______________ minutes

Accuracy: ______________

(Note: The time element and accuracy criteria may be given by your instructor.)

Directions: Match the HCPCS code in the first or second column with the description of the drug, supply item, or service presented in the third or fourth column. Write the correct letters in the blanks.

E1280	______	J0760	______	a. Vitamin B_{12}, 1000 mg	k. Blood (whole) for transfusion/unit
E0141	______	A9150	______	b. Injection, insulin per 5 units	l. Heavy duty wheelchair with detachable arms
J0290	______	J2001	______	c. Rigid walker, wheeled, without seat	m. Ampicillin inj, up to 500 mg
J3420	______	L0160	______	d. Waiver of liability statement on file	n. Dimethyl sulfoxide (DMSO) inj
J1815	______	L3100-RT	______	e. Nonemergency transportation, taxi	o. Urine strips
P9010	______	A4250	______	f. Inj of colchicine	p. Vancomycin (Vancocin) inj
J1212	______	J2590	______	g. Cervical occipital/ mandibular support	q. Oxytocin (Pitocin) inj
J3370	______	A4927	______	h. Inj of lidocaine (Xylocaine)	r. Wide, heavy-duty wheelchair with detachable arms and leg rests
E1092	______	A0100	______	i. Gloves, nonsterile	s. Rt hallux valgus night splint
A4211	______	-GA	______	j. Supplies for self-administered drug injections	t. Aspirin, nonprescription

ASSIGNMENT 6-9 ▶ PROCEDURAL CODING CASE SCENARIOS

Performance Objective

Task: Locate the correct procedure code and modifier, if necessary, for each case scenario.

Conditions: Use pen or pencil and *Current Procedural Terminology* code book.

Standards: Time: ________________________ minutes

Accuracy: ________________________

(Note: The time element and accuracy criteria may be given by your instructor.)

Directions: Find the correct procedure codes and modifiers, if necessary, for each case scenario.

1. The physician sees Horace Hart, a 60-year-old new patient, in the office for bronchial asthma, ASHD (arteriosclerotic heart disease), and hypertension. He performs an ECG (electrocardiogram) and UA (urinalysis) without microscopy, and obtains x-rays. Comprehensive metabolic and lipid panels and a CBC (complete blood count) are done by an outside laboratory.

Code Number — *Description*

Physician's bill:

a. ________________ Initial OV, comp hx & exam, high-complexity decision-making

b. ________________ ECG with interpret and report

c. ________________ UA, routine, nonautomated

d. ________________ Chest x-ray, two views

e. ________________ Routine venipuncture for handling of specimen

Laboratory's bill:

f. ________________ Comprehensive metabolic panel: albumin, bilirubin, calcium, carbon dioxide, chloride, creatinine, glucose, phosphatase (alkaline), potassium, protein, sodium, ALT, AST, and urea nitrogen

g. ________________ Lipid panel

h. ________________ CBC, completely automated with complete differential

If the doctor decides to have the chest x-rays interpreted by a radiologist, the procedural code billed by the radiologist would be ________________ ________________.

2. Mr. Hart is seen again in the office on May 12. On May 25 he is seen at home at 2 AM with asthma exacerbation, possible myocardial infarct, and congestive heart failure. The doctor consulted with a thoracic cardiovascular surgeon by telephone. He also called to make arrangements for hospitalization. To complete the patient care, these services required 2 hours and 40 minutes of non–face-to-face time in addition to the time spent examining the patient during the house call.

Code Number	*Description*
a. ______________	OV, problem-focused hx & exam, straightforward decision-making
b. ______________	Home visit, detailed interval hx & exam, high-complexity decision-making
c. ______________	Detention time, prolonged (list time required)

3. On June 9, Horace Hart is seen again in the hospital. The thoracic cardiovascular surgeon who was telephoned the previous day was called in for consultation to formally examine him and says that surgery is necessary, which is scheduled the following day. The patient's physician sees the patient for his asthmatic condition and acts as assistant surgeon. The surgeon does the follow-up care and assumes care in the case.

Code Number *Description*

Primary care physician/assistant surgeon's bill:

a. ______________	Hospital visit, problem-focused hx & exam, low-complexity decision-making
b. ______________	Pericardiotomy

Thoracic cardiovascular surgeon's bill:

c. ______________	Consultation, comp hx & exam, moderate-complexity decision-making
d. ______________	Pericardiotomy

ASSIGNMENT 6-10 ▶ CASE SCENARIO FOR CRITICAL THINKING

Performance Objective

Task: Locate the correct procedure codes and modifiers, if necessary, for a case scenario.

Conditions: Use pen or pencil and *Current Procedural Terminology* code book.

Standards: Time: ______________________ minutes

Accuracy: ______________________

(Note: The time element and accuracy criteria may be given by your instructor.)

Directions: Read through this progress note on Roy A. Takashima. Abstract information from the note about the subjective symptoms, objective findings, and diagnoses. List the diagnostic and procedure codes you think this case would warrant. If your instructor tells you to also find the ICD-10-CM codes, a draft version may be downloaded from the following web site: http://www.cdc.gov/nchs/icd/icd10cm.htm11update. This website address changes each year to present a current version. As you can read, 11 relates to the year 2011.

Takashima, Roy A.
October 5, 20xx

Pt. has many things going on. First, he's had no difficulties following the feral cat bite, and the cat was normal on quarantine.

He seemed to be recovering from the flu but is plagued with a persistent cough and pain down the center of his chest without fever or grossly discolored phlegm.

Physical exam shows expiratory rhonchi and gross exacerbation of his cough on forced expiration. Spirometry before and after bronchodilator was remarkably good; nonetheless, it is improved and he is symptomatically improved with a Proventil inhaler, which he is given as a sample. I don't think other antibiotics would help.

His reflux is under good control with proprietary antacids with a clear exam.

He has several areas of seborrheic keratoses on his face and head that need attention.

Finally, in follow-up of all the above, he needs a complete physical exam.

Ting Cho, MD

Diagnosis: Influenza and acute bronchitis.

Subjective symptoms ____

____

Objective findings ____

____

____

Diagnosis and Dx code ______________________________ __________

______________________________ __________

______________________________ __________

______________________________ __________

E/M code __________

Spirometry code ______________________________ __________

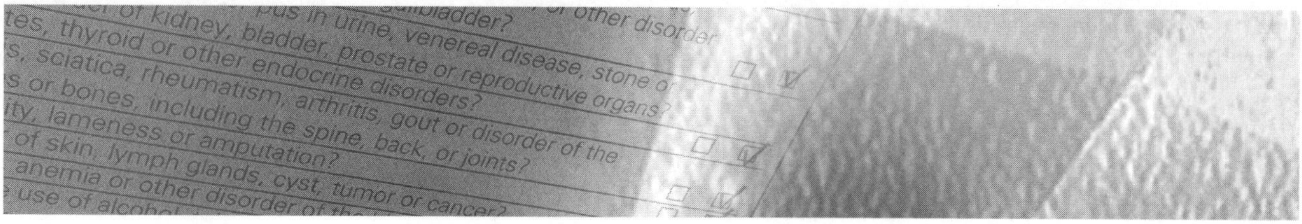

CHAPTER

7

The Paper Claim: CMS-1500 (08-05)

KEY TERMS

Your instructor may wish to select some words pertinent to this chapter for a test. For definitions of the terms, further study, and/or reference, the words, phrases, and abbreviations may be found in the glossary at the end of the Handbook. Key terms for this chapter follow.

clean claim
deleted claim
dirty claim
durable medical equipment number
electronic claim
employer identification number
facility provider number
group National Provider Identifier
Health Insurance Claim Form (CMS-1500 [08-05])
incomplete claim
intelligent character recognition
invalid claim
National Provider Identifier
optical character recognition
"other" claims
paper claim
pending claim
physically clean claim
rejected claim
Social Security number
state license number

KEY ABBREVIATIONS

See how many abbreviations and acronyms you can translate and then use this as a handy reference list. Definitions for the key abbreviations are located near the back of the Handbook in the glossary.

CMS-1500 ____________________
DME ____________________
DNA ____________________
EIN ____________________
EMG ____________________
EPSDT ____________________
FDA ____________________
HHA ____________________
ICR ____________________
IDE ____________________
LMP ____________________
MG ____________________

MSP ______________________________

NA, N/A ______________________________

NOC ______________________________

NPI ______________________________

OCNA key ______________________________

OCR ______________________________

PAYERID ______________________________

PRO ______________________________

SOF ______________________________

SSN ______________________________

TMA ______________________________

PERFORMANCE OBJECTIVES

The student will be able to:

- Define and spell the key terms and key abbreviations for this chapter, given the information from the *Handbook* glossary, within a reasonable time period and with enough accuracy to obtain a satisfactory evaluation.
- After reading the chapter, answer the fill-in-the-blank, mix and match, multiple choice, and true/false review questions, with enough accuracy to obtain a satisfactory evaluation.
- Given a handwritten CMS-1500 (08-05) form, type a CMS-1500 (08-05) Health Insurance Claim Form and list the reasons why the claim was either rejected or delayed, within a reasonable time period and with enough accuracy to obtain a satisfactory evaluation.
- Given the patients' medical chart notes, ledger cards, encounter forms, and blank insurance claim forms, complete each CMS-1500 (08-05) Health Insurance Claim Form for billing, within a reasonable time period and with enough accuracy to obtain a satisfactory evaluation.
- Using the Mock Fee Schedule in Appendix A in this *Workbook*, correctly post payments, adjustments, and balances to the patients' ledger cards, within a reasonable time period and with enough accuracy to obtain a satisfactory evaluation.
- Given a list of common medical abbreviations and symbols that appear in chart notes, fill in the correct meaning of each abbreviation, within a reasonable time period and with enough accuracy to obtain a satisfactory evaluation.

STUDY OUTLINE

History

Compliance Issues Related to Insurance Claim Forms

Types of Submitted Claims

- Claim Status

Abstracting from Medical Records

- Cover Letter Accompanying Insurance Claims
- Life or Health Insurance Applications

Health Insurance Claim Form (CMS-1500 [08-05])

- Basic Guidelines for Submitting a Claim
- Completion of Insurance Claim Forms

Common Reasons Why Claim Forms Are Delayed or Rejected

Additional Claim Submission Errors

Optical Scanning Format Guidelines

- Optical Character Recognition
- Do's and Don'ts for Optical Character Recognition

Procedure: Instructions for the Health Insurance Claim Form (CMS-1500 [08-05])

- Insurance Program Templates

14. The insurance claim form required when submitting Medicare claims is

    a. CMS-1500 (08-05) claim form

    b. Attending Physicians Statement

    c. COMB-1

    d. HIPAA form

15. The maximum number of diagnostic codes in the ANSI 837P claim format for transmitting electronic health insurance claims is

    a. four

    b. six

    c. eight

    d. ten

16. If a patient's gender is not indicated in the CMS-1500 (08-05) claim form, the gender block defaults to

    a. male

    b. female

    c. denies the claim

    d. there is no default; it will appear blank

17. If a provider of medical services does not have an NPI number, the characters or digits that must be entered in Block 24I is/are

    a. leave blank

    b. IC

    c. ID

    d. NPI

Part IV True/False

Write "T" or "F" in the blank to indicate whether you think the statement is true or false.

________ 18. A photocopy of a claim form may be optically scanned.

________ 19. Handwriting is permitted on optically scanned paper claims.

________ 20. A CMS-assigned National Provider Identifier (NPI) number consists of 10 characters.

________ 21. When listing a diagnostic code on an insurance claim, insert the decimal points.

________ 22. A diagnosis reference pointer should be entered in Block 24E and not an ICD-9-CM diagnostic code.

General Directions for Claim Form Completion

Assume that the Health Insurance Claim Form* CMS-1500 (08-05) is printed in red ink for processing by OCR or ICR. Complete the form using OCR/ICR guidelines pertinent to the type of carrier that you are billing (e.g., private, Medicare, TRICARE) and send it to the proper insurance carrier. Refer to Chapter 7 in the *Handbook* for block instructions for each major type of insurance carrier. All blocks are clearly labeled, and each major carrier has an icon that is color coded for easy reference. Claim form templates have been completed to use as visual examples for placement of data; they may be found at the end of Chapter 7 in the *Handbook*. Screened areas on each form do not apply to the insurance program example shown and should be left blank.

Many physicians complete an evaluation and management (E/M) code slip for each patient encounter. Chapter 7 assignments feature this form as a reference for part of each exercise and are used to assist you with E/M CPT code selection. In future assignments, you will identify key components for E/M services in the medical record. All physicians in College Clinic accept assignment of benefits for all types of insurance that you will be billing for; indicate this by checking "yes" in Block 27. For each claim completed, be sure to insert your initials in the lower left-hand corner of the claim form. When coding services from the Surgery Section of CPT, be sure to check the Mock Fee Schedule in Appendix A in this *Workbook* to determine how many follow-up days are included in the surgical or global package. Services provided during the surgical/global package time frame should not be included on the claim form; however, such services should be documented on the financial accounting record, referenced with code 99024 (postoperative follow-up visit; included in global service), and listed as no charge (N/C). Refer to the *Handbook* for detailed information about surgical/global package and follow-up days.

A list of abbreviations pertinent to the medical record has been provided as an exercise to reinforce learning. Not all medical offices use abbreviations in medical record documentation. In the College Clinic scenario, abbreviations are used in patient progress notes to give you an opportunity to practice reading and interpreting them.

ASSIGNMENT 7-2 ▶ COMPLETE A HEALTH INSURANCE CLAIM FORM FOR A PRIVATE CASE

Performance Objective

Task: Complete a health insurance claim form and post the information to the patient's financial account record/statement.

Conditions: Use Merry M. McLean's E/M code slip (Figure 7-1), patient record (Figure 7-2), and financial account record/statement (Figure 7-3); one health insurance claim form (print from Evolve website); a computer or pen; procedural and diagnostic code books; and Appendices A and B in the *Workbook*.

Standards: Claim Productivity Measurement

Time: ________ minutes

Accuracy: ________

(Note: The time element and accuracy criteria may be given by your instructor.)

E/M Code Slip

Patient *McLean, Merry M.* Date *5-6-XX*

CPT Code ________

Dx Code ________

HISTORY

- [ ] Problem Focused
  Chief complaint; Brief history of present illness
- [ ] Expanded Problem Focused
  Chief complaint; Brief history of present illness; Problem pertinent system review
- [x] Detailed
  Chief complaint: Extended history of present illness; Extended system review; Pertinent past family, social history
- [ ] Comprehensive
  Chief complaint; Extended history of present illness; Complete system review; Complete past family, social history

EXAMINATION

- [ ] Problem Focused
  Exam limited to affected body area or organ system
- [ ] Expanded Problem Focused
  Exam extended to other symptomatic or related organ systems
- [x] Detailed
  Extended exam of affected area(s) and other symptomatic or related systems
- [ ] Comprehensive
  Complete single system specialty exam or complete multi-system exam

MEDICAL DECISION MAKING

	Medical Decision	Number of Dx Options	Amount of Data	Risk M and M
[ ]	Straightforward	minimal 1 dx	minimal	minimal
[x]	Low Complexity	limited 1-2 dx	limited	low
[ ]	Moderate Complexity	multiple 1-2 dx	moderate	moderate
[ ]	High Complexity	extensive 2-3 dx	extensive	high

- [ ] Counseling [ ] Time ________
- [ ] Consult [ ] Referring Dr. *Emdee Fine*

Diagnosis *See Pt record*

NP ✓ Est pt ____

Figure 7-1

Directions: Complete the Health Insurance Claim Form,* using OCR or ICR guidelines, and send the form to the Prudential Insurance Company for Mrs. Merry M. McLean by referring to her E/M code slip, patient record, and financial account record/statement. Date the claim June 15. Refer to Appendix A in this *Workbook* to fill in the fees on the financial account record/statement.

1. Use your CPT code book or Appendix A in this *Workbook* to determine the correct 5-digit code number and modifiers for each professional service rendered. To determine diagnostic codes, refer to ICD-9-CM and/or ICD-10-CM code books.

2. Record on the financial account record/statement when you have billed the insurance company.

3. A Performance Evaluation Checklist may be reproduced from the "Instruction Guide to the Workbook" chapter if your instructor wishes you to submit it to assist with scoring and comments.

4. After the instructor has returned your work to you, either make the necessary corrections and place your work in a three-ring notebook for future reference or, if you received a high score, place it in your portfolio for reference when applying for a job.

Abbreviations pertinent to this record:

NP	______	LC	______
UA	______	MDM	______
Dx	______	HV	______
ptr	______	PF	______
Cysto	______	SF	______
Pt	______	RTO	______
Cont	______	postop	______
adm	______	OV	______
hosp	______	lb	______
C	______	adv	______
Hx	______	retn	______
exam	______	est	______

*See Chapter 7 in the *Handbook* for help in completing the form.

PATIENT RECORD NO. 7-2

LAST NAME	FIRST NAME	MIDDLE NAME	BIRTH DATE	SEX	HOME PHONE
McLean	Merry	M.	02-02-48	F	555-486-1859

ADDRESS	CITY	STATE	ZIP CODE
4919 Dolphin Way	Woodland Hills,	XY	12345

CELL PHONE	PAGER NO.	FAX NO.	E-MAIL ADDRESS
555-430-7709	555-098-3456	555-486-1859	McLean@WB.net

PATIENT'S SOC. SEC. NO.	DRIVER'S LICENSE
459-XX-9989	M0039857

PATIENT'S OCCUPATION	NAME OF COMPANY
Secretary	Porter Company

ADDRESS OF EMPLOYER	PHONE
5490 Wilshire Blvd., Merck, XY 12346	555-446-7781

SPOUSE OR PARENT	OCCUPATION
Harry L. McLean	Computer programmer

EMPLOYER	ADDRESS	PHONE
IBM Corporation	5616 Wilshire Blvd., Merck, XY 12346	555-664-9023

NAME OF INSURANCE	INSURED OR SUBSCRIBER
Prudential Insurance Co., 5621 Wilshire Blvd., Merck, XY 12346	Harry L. McLean

POLICY/CERTIFICATE NO.	GROUP NO.
459-XX-9989	8832

REFERRED BY: Emdee Fine, MD, 5000 Wilshire Blvd., Merck, XY 12346 NPI # 73027175XX

DATE	PROGRESS NOTES No. 7-2
5-6-xx	NP presents in office with constant dribbling and wetting at night; uses 15 pads/day.
	Began March 10, 20xx. Pelvic exam done—normal findings. No bladder or uterine
	prolapse noted. UA dipstick performed (nonautomated with microscopy); few bacteria,
	few urates. Dx: urinary incontinence. ptr 4 days for cystourethroscopy.
	GU/llf Gene Ulibarri, MD
5-10-xx	Cysto performed—revealed vesico-vaginal fistula of bladder with an opening into urinary bladder
	and copious leakage into vagina. Schedule surgery to repair fistula. Pt cont to work.
	GU/llf Gene Ulibarri, MD
5-16-xx	Adm to College hosp. C hx/exam LC MDM. Dx: vesicovaginal fistula.
	GU/llf Gene Ulibarri, MD
5-17-xx	Closure of vesicovaginal fistula; abdominal approach.
	GU/llf Gene Ulibarri, MD
5-18-xx thru	Saw patient in hospital (HV) PF hx/exam SF MDM.
5-21-xx	GU/llf Gene Ulibarri, MD
5-22-xx	Discharge from hospital. RTO 2 weeks.
	GU/llf Gene Ulibarri, MD
6-5-xx	Post-op OV. Patient has no pain near operative site. Pt reports she has
	been walking daily and lifting more than 5 lb objects. Pt adv no excessive walking,
	no lifting, stooping, or bending until surgical site is completely healed. Retn to clinic in
	1 wk. Est return to work 7-1-xx. PF hx/exam SF MDM.
	GU/llf Gene Ulibarri, MD

Figure 7-2

Acct No. 7-2

STATEMENT
Financial Account
COLLEGE CLINIC
4567 Broad Avenue
Woodland Hills, XY 12345-0001
Tel. 555-486-9002
Fax No. 555-487-8976

Merry McLean
4919 Dolphin Way
Woodland Hills, XY 12345

Phone No. (H) (555) 486-1859 (W) (555) 446-7781 Birthdate 02-02-48

Primary Insurance Co. Prudential Insurance Co. Policy/Group No. 459-XX-9989/8832

	REFERENCE	DESCRIPTION	CHARGES	CREDITS PYMNTS.	CREDITS ADJ.	BALANCE
20XX		BALANCE FORWARD →				
05-06-xx		OV NP				
05-06-xx		UA				
05-10-xx		Cystourethroscopy				
5-16-xx		Initial hosp care				
05-17-xx		Repair vesicovaginal fistula				
05-18 to 05-22-xx		HV				
05-22-xx		Discharge				
06-05-xx		PO-OV				

PLEASE PAY LAST AMOUNT IN BALANCE COLUMN

THIS IS A COPY OF YOUR FINANCIAL ACCOUNT AS IT APPEARS ON OUR RECORDS

Figure 7-3

ASSIGNMENT 7-3 ▶ COMPLETE A HEALTH INSURANCE CLAIM FORM FOR A PRIVATE CASE

Performance Objective

Task: Complete a health insurance claim form and post the information to the patient's financial account record/statement.

Conditions: Use Billy S. Rubin's E/M code slip (Figure 7-4), patient record (Figure 7-5), and financial account record/statement (Figure 7-6); one health insurance claim form (print from Evolve website); a computer or pen; procedural and diagnostic code books; and Appendices A and B in this *Workbook*.

Standards: Claim Productivity Measurement

Time: ______________ minutes

Accuracy: ______________

(Note: The time element and accuracy criteria may be given by your instructor.)

E/M Code Slip

Patient *Rubin, Billy S.*

Date *
CPT Code
Dx code

HISTORY

- [x] Problem Focused
  Chief complaint; Brief history of present illness
- [ ] Expanded Problem Focused
  Chief complaint; Brief history of present illness; Problem pertinent system review
- [ ] Detailed
  Chief complaint; Extended history of present illness; Extended system review; Pertinent past family, social history
- [ ] Comprehensive
  Chief complaint; Extended history of present illness; Complete system review; Complete past family, social history

EXAMINATION

- [x] Problem Focused
  Exam limited to affected body area or organ system
- [ ] Expanded Problem Focused
  Exam extended to other symptomatic or related organ systems
- [ ] Detailed
  Extended exam of affected area(s) and other symptomatic or related symptoms
- [ ] Comprehensive
  Complete single system specialty exam or complete multi-system exam

MEDICAL DECISION MAKING

Medical Decision	Number of Dx Options	Amount of Data	Risk M and M
[ ] Straightforward	minimal 1 dx	minimal	minimal
[x] Low Complexity	limited 1-2 dx	limited	low
[ ] Moderate Complexity	multiple 1-2 dx	moderate	moderate
[ ] High Complexity	extensive 2-3 dx	extensive	high

[ ] Counseling [ ] Time
[ ] Consult [x] Referring Dr. *U.R. Wright*
Diagnosis *see pt. record*

NP____ Est pt ✓

* For space constraints, this E/M code slip is being used for 8-7-00, 8-14-00, and 8-16-00

Figure 7-4

Directions: Complete the Health Insurance Claim Form* on Mr. Billy S. Rubin for processing and send it to Aetna Life and Casualty Company by referring to Mr. Rubin's E/M code slip, patient record, and financial account record/statement. Date the claim August 30. Refer to Appendix A in this *Workbook* to fill in the fees on the financial statement. Use OCR guidelines.

1. Use your CPT code book or Appendix A in this *Workbook* to determine the correct 5-digit code number and modifiers for each professional service rendered. Do not include no-charge entries on the claim form. To determine diagnostic codes, refer to ICD-9-CM and/or ICD-10-CM code books.

2. Record when you have billed the insurance company on the financial account record/statement.

3. On September 1, Mr. Rubin sends you check No. 421 in the amount of $200 to apply to his account. Post this entry and calculate the balance due.

4. A Performance Evaluation Checklist may be reproduced from the "Instruction Guide to the Workbook" chapter if your instructor wishes you to submit it to assist with scoring and comments.

5. After the instructor has returned your work to you, either make the necessary corrections and place your work in a three-ring notebook for future reference, or, if you received a high score, place it in your portfolio for reference when applying for a job.

Abbreviations pertinent to this record:

est	______	TURP	______
pt	______	wks	______
CBC	______	HV	______
CC	______	PF	______
diff	______	hx	______
PSA	______	exam	______
bx	______	SF	______
STAT	______	MDM	______
PTR	______	Disch	______
CA	______	hosp	______
adm	______	postop	______
surg	______		

*See Chapter 7 in the *Handbook* for help in completing the form.

Additional Coding

1. Determine CPT codes that you would use to bill for College Hospital from the following services mentioned in the patient's progress notes.

	CPT code
A. Blood draw (venipuncture)	____________
B. Complete blood cell (CBC) count (automated) with differential	____________
C. Prostate-specific antigen (PSA) (total)	____________
D. Ultrasonography with guided fine-needle biopsy	____________

PATIENT RECORD NO. 7-3

LAST NAME	FIRST NAME	MIDDLE NAME	BIRTH DATE	SEX	HOME PHONE
Rubin	Billy	S.	11-09-53	M	555-893-5770

ADDRESS	CITY	STATE	ZIP CODE
547 North Oliver Rd.	Woodland Hills	XY	12345

CELL PHONE	PAGER NO.	FAX NO.	E-MAIL ADDRESS
555-430-9080	555-987-7790	555-893-5770	Rubin@WB.net

PATIENT'S SOC. SEC. NO.	DRIVER'S LICENSE
505-XX-1159	R0398056

PATIENT'S OCCUPATION	NAME OF COMPANY
salesman	Nate's Clothier's

ADDRESS OF EMPLOYER	PHONE
7786 East Chabner Blvd., Dorland, XY 12347	555-449-6605

SPOUSE OR PARENT: Lydia B. Rubin (wife)

EMPLOYER	ADDRESS	PHONE

NAME OF INSURANCE	INSURED OR SUBSCRIBER
Aetna Life and Casualty Co., 3055 Wilshire Blvd., Merck, XY 12345	Billy S. Rubin

POLICY/CERTIFICATE NO.	GROUP NO.
42107	2641

REFERRED BY: U. R. Wright, MD, 5010 Wrong Road, Torres, XY 12349 555-907-5440 NPI # 271385554XX

DATE	PROGRESS NOTES No. 7-3
8-7-xx	Office exam est pt. CC: urinary hesitancy, frequency and posturinary dribbling since
	July 15 of this year. Exam revealed hard nodule in prostate. Sent pt to College Hospital for
	laboratory work; CBC (automated with diff) and PSA (total). PTR in 1 wk.
	GU/llf Gene Ulibarri, MD
8-14-xx	Office exam. PSA elevated (5.6), CBC normal. Explained to pt that biopsy is needed at this
	point; may be done as outpatient at College Hospital. Pt elected to have immediate
	bx; arrangements made for stat. Ultrasound with guided fine needle bx. PTR in 2 days for
	results.
	GU/llf Gene Ulibarri, MD
8-16-xx	Pt returns for bx report; positive for CA in situ of prostate. Advised patient that an
	operation is necessary and explained surgical procedure, risks, and complications.
	Arranged for adm to College Hospital on 8/22/xx.
	GU/llf Gene Ulibarri, MD
8-22-xx	Admit to College Hospital. Surg: TURP, complete. Pt tolerated surg well and is comfortable
	in the recovery room. Pt last worked 8/21/xx; est disability 6 to 8 wks. Est return to work
	on 10/22/xx.
	GU/llf Gene Ulibarri, MD
8-23-xx thru	HV (PF hx/exam SF MDM)
8-26-xx	GU/llf Gene Ulibarri, MD
8-27-xx	Disch from hosp. Pt confined at home for 1 week at which time patient will return to
	office for postop check.
	GU/llf Gene Ulibarri, MD

Figure 7-5

Acct No. 7-3

STATEMENT
Financial Account
COLLEGE CLINIC
4567 Broad Avenue
Woodland Hills, XY 12345-0001
Tel. 555-486-9002
Fax No. 555-487-8976

Billy S. Rubin
547 North Oliver Road
Woodland Hills, XY 12345

Phone No. (H) (555) 893-5770 (W) (555) 449-6605 Birthdate 11-09-53

Primary Insurance Co. Aetna Life and Casualty Co. Policy/Group No. 421074/2641

	REFERENCE	DESCRIPTION	CHARGES	CREDITS PYMNTS.	CREDITS ADJ.	BALANCE
20XX		**BALANCE FORWARD** →				
08-07-xx		OV Est Pt				
08-14-xx		OV Est Pt				
08-16-xx		OV Est Pt				
08-22-xx		TURP				
08-23 to 08-26-xx		HV				
08-27-xx		Discharge				

PLEASE PAY LAST AMOUNT IN BALANCE COLUMN

THIS IS A COPY OF YOUR FINANCIAL ACCOUNT AS IT APPEARS ON OUR RECORDS

Figure 7-6

ASSIGNMENT 7-4 ▸ COMPLETE ONE HEALTH INSURANCE CLAIM FORM FOR A PRIVATE CASE

Performance Objective

Task: Complete one health insurance claim form and post the information to the patient's financial account record/statement.

Conditions: Use Walter J. Stone's E/M code slip (Figure 7-7), patient record (Figure 7-8), and financial account record/statement (Figure 7-9); one health insurance claim form (print from Evolve website); a computer or pen; procedural and diagnostic code books; and Appendices A and B in this *Workbook*.

Standards: Claim Productivity Measurement

Time: ______________ minutes

Accuracy: ______________

(Note: The time element and accuracy criteria may be given by your instructor.)

E/M Code Slip

Patient *Stone, Walter J.*

Date *5/12/XX*
CPT Code ________
Dx Code ________

HISTORY

- [ ] Problem Focused
  Chief complaint; Brief history of present illness
- [x] Expanded Problem Focused
  Chief complaint; Brief history of present illness; Problem pertinent system review
- [ ] Detailed
  Chief complaint; Extended history of present illness; Extended system review; Pertinent past family, social history
- [ ] Comprehensive
  Chief complaint; Extended history of present illness; Complete system review; Complete past family, social history

EXAMINATION

- [ ] Problem Focused
  Exam limited to affected body area or organ system
- [x] Expanded Problem Focused
  Exam extended to other symptomatic or related organ systems
- [ ] Detailed
  Extended exam of affected area(s) and other symptomatic or related systems
- [ ] Comprehensive
  Complete single system specialty exam or complete multi-system exam

MEDICAL DECISION MAKING

	Medical Decision	Number of Dx Options	Amount of Data	Risk M and M
[ ]	Straightforward	minimal 1 dx	minimal	minimal
[x]	Low Complexity	limited 1-2 dx	limited	low
[ ]	Moderate Complexity	multiple 1-2 dx	moderate	moderate
[ ]	High Complexity	extensive 2-3 dx	extensive	high

[ ] Counseling [ ] Time ____________
[ ] Consult [ ] Referring Dr. ____________
Diagnosis *see pt. record*

NP ____ Est pt ✓

Figure 7-7

Directions: You will be billing for all services listed on the patient's progress notes for Dr. Clarence Cutler. Complete one Health Insurance Claim Form,* addressing it to Travelers Insurance Company for Mr. Walter J. Stone by referring to his E/M code slip, patient record, and financial account record/statement. Date the claim May 5. Refer to Appendix A in this *Workbook* to fill in the fees on the financial account record/statement. Use OCR guidelines.

1. Use your CPT code book or Appendix A in this *Workbook* to determine the correct 5-digit code number and modifiers for each professional service rendered. To determine diagnostic codes, refer to ICD-9-CM and/or ICD-10-CM code books.

2. On May 14, the insurance company sends the physician a check, number 48572, for $25. Post this entry.

3. Record on the financial account record/statement when you have billed the insurance company.

4. A Performance Evaluation Checklist may be reproduced from the "Instruction Guide to the Workbook" chapter if your instructor wishes you to submit it to assist with scoring and comments.

5. After the instructor has returned your work to you, either make the necessary corrections and place your work in a three-ring notebook for future reference or, if you received a high score, place it in your portfolio for reference when applying for a job.

Abbreviations pertinent to this record:

est	______________________	exam	______________________
pt	______________________	LC	______________________
ER	______________________	MDM	______________________
BP	______________________	EGD	______________________
Dx	______________________	bx	______________________
GI	______________________	ofc	______________________
HV	______________________	wk	______________________
PF	______________________	OV	______________________
hx	______________________	adv	______________________

Additional Coding

1. Refer to Mr. Stone's patient record, abstract information, and code the procedures for services that would be billed by the hospital.

Description of Service	*Code*
a. ______________________	______________________
b. ______________________	______________________
c. ______________________	______________________

*See Chapter 7 in the *Handbook* for help in completing the form.

PATIENT RECORD NO. 7-4

LAST NAME	FIRST NAME	MIDDLE NAME	BIRTH DATE	SEX	HOME PHONE
Stone	Walter	J.	03-14-49	M	555-345-0776

ADDRESS	CITY	STATE	ZIP CODE
2008 Converse Street	Woodland Hills	XY	12345

CELL PHONE	PAGER NO.	FAX NO.	E-MAIL ADDRESS
555-980-7750	555-930-5674	555-345-0776	Stone@WB.net

PATIENT'S SOC. SEC. NO.	DRIVER'S LICENSE
456-XX-9989	H9834706

PATIENT'S OCCUPATION	NAME OF COMPANY
advertising agent	R. V. Black and Associates

ADDRESS OF EMPLOYER	PHONE
1267 Broad Street, Woodland Hills, XY 12345	555-345-6012

SPOUSE OR PARENT
widower

EMPLOYER	ADDRESS	PHONE

NAME OF INSURANCE	INSURED OR SUBSCRIBER
Travelers Insurance Co., 5460 Olympic Blvd., Woodland Hills, XY 12345	Walter J. Stone

POLICY/CERTIFICATE NO.	GROUP NO.
456-XX-9989	6754

REFERRED BY: John B. Stone (brother), former patient of Dr. Input

DATE	PROGRESS NOTES
5-3-xx	Est pt presented in ER after experiencing sudden onset of profuse rectal bleeding with nausea and severe abdominal pain. BP 130/80. Dr. Cutler called to ER by Dr. Input who recommended pt be admitted for further evaluation and diagnostic workup. Dr. Cutler performed a comprehensive history and examination with moderate complexity decision making and admitted the pt to College Hospital. Dx: Unspecified GI hemorrhage. Pt disabled from work.
	CC/llf Clarence Cutler, MD
5-4-xx	Pt underwent upper GI endoscopy to control bleeding. Endoscopy procedure was performed by Dr. Cutler. In the radiology department, the pt had a cholecystography with oral contrast and complete abdominal ultrasound that confirmed inflammatory gallbladder with stones. EGD with bx confirmed prepyloric gastric ulcer with hemorrhage. BP of 135/80. Dr. Cutler performed a laparoscopic cholecystectomy. DX: Cholecystitis with cholelithiasis.
	CC/llf Clarence Cutler, MD
5-5-xx	Pt discharged to home. Pt placed on amoxicillin t.i.d. for 2 wks to prevent infection and Prilosec in A.M. for 2 weeks to control stomach acid. Pt to be seen in ofc in 1 wk. It is estimated pt will resume work on 6/22/xx.
	CC/llf
	Clarence Cutler, MD

Figure 7-8

Acct No. 7-4

STATEMENT
Financial Account
COLLEGE CLINIC
4567 Broad Avenue
Woodland Hills, XY 12345-001
Tel. 555-486-9002
Fax No. 555-487-8976

Walter J. Stone
2008 Converse Street
Woodland Hills, XY 12345

Phone No. (H) (555) 345-0776 (W) (555) 345-6012 Birthdate 03-14-49

Primary Insurance Co. Travelers Insurance Co. Policy/Group No. 456-XX9989/6754

	REFERENCE	DESCRIPTION	CHARGES		CREDITS PYMNTS.		CREDITS ADJ.		BALANCE	
20XX		BALANCE FORWARD →								
01-03-xx	99214	OV	61	51					61	51
01-15-xx	01-03-xx	Billed Travelers Ins.							61	51
03-02-xx	Ck 95268	ROA Travlers Ins.			49	21			12	30
03-03-xx	99213	OV	40	20					52	50
04-03-xx	3-3-xx	Billed Travelers Ins.							52	50
05-03-xx		Initial hosp care								
05-04-xx		Endoscopy								
05-04-xx		Cholecystectomy								

PLEASE PAY LAST AMOUNT IN BALANCE COLUMN

THIS IS A COPY OF YOUR FINANCIAL ACCOUNT AS IT APPEARS ON OUR RECORDS

Figure 7-9

ASSIGNMENT 7-5 ▶ LOCATE ERRORS ON A COMPLETED HEALTH INSURANCE CLAIM FORM

Performance Objective

Task:	Locate errors on a completed health insurance claim form and post the information to the patient's ledger card.
Conditions:	Use Tom N. Parkinson's completed insurance claim (Figure 7-10), one health insurance claim form (print from Evolve website), and a computer or a pen.
Standards:	Time: ________________________ minutes
	Accuracy:
	(Note: The time element and accuracy criteria may be given by your instructor.)

Guidance: To alleviate frustration and ease the process of completing a claim form for the first time, you will be editing a claim and then taking the correct information and inserting it on a blank CMS-1500 (08-05) form. Refer to Chapter 7 in the *Handbook* for block-by-block private payer instructions for completing the CMS-1500 (08-05) insurance claim form. Refer to Figure 7-3 in the *Handbook* for visual placement of data. Refer to Appendix A in this *Workbook* for the physician/clinic information and the clinic's mock fee schedule. The billing physician is Gerald Practon. The name of the insurance carrier is ABC Insurance Company at 111 Main Street in Denver, CO 80210.

Directions: Study the completed claim form (see Figure 7-10) and search for missing or incorrect information. If possible, verify all information. Highlight or circle in red all incorrect or missing information. Insert the correct information on the claim form. Now transfer all the data to a blank CMS-1500 (08-05) claim form. If mandatory information is missing, insert the word "NEED" in the corresponding block of the claim form.

A Performance Evaluation Checklist may be reproduced from the "Instruction Guide to the Workbook" chapter if your instructor wishes you to submit it to assist with scoring and comments.

Optional: List, in block-by-block order, the reasons why the claim may be either rejected or delayed according to the errors found.

---

*See Chapter 7 in the *Handbook* for help in completing the form.

1500

HEALTH INSURANCE CLAIM FORM

APPROVED BY NATIONAL UNIFORM CLAIM COMMITTEE 08/05

PICA — CARRIER — PICA

1. MEDICARE (Medicare #) ☐ MEDICAID (Medicaid #) ☐ TRICARE CHAMPUS (Sponsor's SSN) ☐ CHAMPVA (Member ID#) ☐ GROUP HEALTH PLAN (SSN or ID) ☐ FECA BLK LUNG (SSN) ☐ OTHER (ID) ☐

1a. INSURED'S I.D. NUMBER (For Program in Item 1): PX4278A

2. PATIENT'S NAME (Last Name, First Name, Middle Initial): PARKINSON TOM N

3. PATIENT'S BIRTH DATE MM DD YY: 04 06 1993 SEX M [X] F ☐

4. INSURED'S NAME (Last Name, First Name, Middle Initial): PARKINSON JAMIE B

5. PATIENT'S ADDRESS (No., Street): 4510 SOUTH A STREET

6. PATIENT RELATIONSHIP TO INSURED: Self ☐ Spouse ☐ Child [X] Other ☐

7. INSURED'S ADDRESS (No., Street): 4510 SOUTH A STREET

CITY: WOODLAND HILLS STATE: XY

8. PATIENT STATUS: Single [X] Married ☐ Other ☐; Employed ☐ Full-Time Student [X] Part-Time Student ☐

CITY: WOODLAND HILLS STATE: XY

ZIP CODE: 12345 TELEPHONE (Include Area Code): (555) 74221580

ZIP CODE: 12345 TELEPHONE (INCLUDE AREA CODE): (555) 742 1560

9. OTHER INSURED'S NAME (Last Name, First Name, Middle Initial)

10. IS PATIENT'S CONDITION RELATED TO:

11. INSURED'S POLICY GROUP OR FECA NUMBER

a. OTHER INSURED'S POLICY OR GROUP NUMBER

a. EMPLOYMENT? (CURRENT OR PREVIOUS) ☐ YES [X] NO

a. INSURED'S DATE OF BIRTH MM DD YY — SEX M ☐ F ☐

b. OTHER INSURED'S DATE OF BIRTH MM DD YY — SEX M ☐ F ☐

b. AUTO ACCIDENT? ☐ YES [X] NO PLACE (State)

b. EMPLOYER'S NAME OR SCHOOL NAME

c. EMPLOYER'S NAME OR SCHOOL NAME

c. OTHER ACCIDENT? ☐ YES [X] NO

c. INSURANCE PLAN NAME OR PROGRAM NAME

d. INSURANCE PLAN NAME OR PROGRAM NAME

10d. RESERVED FOR LOCAL USE

d. IS THERE ANOTHER HEALTH BENEFIT PLAN? ☐ YES [X] NO *If yes,* return to and complete item 9 a-d.

READ BACK OF FORM BEFORE COMPLETING & SIGNING THIS FORM.

12. PATIENT'S OR AUTHORIZED PERSON'S SIGNATURE I authorize the release of any medical or other information necessary to process this claim. I also request payment of government benefits either to myself or to the party who accepts assignment below.

SIGNED SOF DATE

13. INSURED'S OR AUTHORIZED PERSON'S SIGNATURE I authorize payment of medical benefits to the undersigned physician or supplier for services described below.

SIGNED SOF

PATIENT AND INSURED INFORMATION

14. DATE OF CURRENT: MM DD YY ILLNESS (First symptom) OR INJURY (Accident) OR PREGNANCY(LMP)

15. IF PATIENT HAS HAD SAME OR SIMILAR ILLNESS. GIVE FIRST DATE MM DD YY

16. DATES PATIENT UNABLE TO WORK IN CURRENT OCCUPATION MM DD YY FROM TO

17. NAME OF REFERRING PHYSICIAN OR OTHER SOURCE 17a. 17b. NPI

18. HOSPITALIZATION DATES RELATED TO CURRENT SERVICES MM DD YY FROM TO

19. RESERVED FOR LOCAL USE

20. OUTSIDE LAB? ☐ YES [X] NO $ CHARGES

21. DIAGNOSIS OR NATURE OF ILLNESS OR INJURY. (RELATE ITEMS 1,2,3 OR 4 TO ITEM 24E BY LINE)

1. ___ . ___ 3. ___ . ___

2. ___ . ___ 4. ___ . ___

22. MEDICAID RESUBMISSION CODE ORIGINAL REF. NO.

23. PRIOR AUTHORIZATION NUMBER

	24. A. DATE(S) OF SERVICE From MM DD YY	To MM DD YY	B. PLACE OF SERVICE	C. EMG	D. PROCEDURES, SERVICES, OR SUPPLIES (Explain Unusual Circumstances) CPT/HCPCS	MODIFIER	E. DIAGNOSIS POINTER	F. $ CHARGES	G. DAYS OR UNITS	H. EPSDT Family Plan	I. ID. QUAL.	J. RENDERING PROVIDER ID. #
1	07 14 20XX				99242			80 24	1		NPI	
2	07 14 20XX				71020		1	38 96	1		NPI	4627889700
3											NPI	
4											NPI	
5											NPI	
6											NPI	

PHYSICIAN OR SUPPLIER INFORMATION

25. FEDERAL TAX I.D. NUMBER SSN EIN: 7034597 ☐ ☐

26. PATIENT'S ACCOUNT NO.

27. ACCEPT ASSIGNMENT? (For govt. claims, see back) [X] YES ☐ NO

28. TOTAL CHARGE $ 119 20

29. AMOUNT PAID $

30. BALANCE DUE $

31. SIGNATURE OF PHYSICIAN OR SUPPLIER INCLUDING DEGREES OR CREDENTIALS (I certify that the statements on the reverse apply to this bill and are made a part thereof.)

GERALD PRACTON 07/14/20XX

SIGNED DATE

32. SERVICE FACILITY LOCATION INFORMATION

a. NPI b.

33. BILLING PROVIDER INFO & PH # (555) 486 9002

COLLEGE CLINIC
4567 BROAD AVENUE
WOODLAND HILLS XY 12345 0001

a. 3664021CC NPI b.

NUCC Instruction Manual available at: www.nucc.org **PLEASE PRINT OR TYPE** APPROVED OMB-0938-0999 FORM CMS-1500 (08-05)

Figure 7-10

ASSIGNMENT 7-6 ▶ REVIEW PATIENT RECORD ABBREVIATIONS

Performance Objective

Task: Insert meanings of abbreviations.

Conditions: Use a pencil or pen.

Standards: Time: ____________________ minutes

Accuracy: ____________________

(Note: The time element and accuracy criteria may be given by your instructor.)

Directions: After completing all the patient records in the *Workbook* that are pertinent to this chapter, you will be able to answer the next two questions.

1. What do these abbreviations mean?

a. PTR ____________________

b. TURP ____________________

c. HX ____________________

d. IVP ____________________

e. c̄ ____________________

f. Dx ____________________

g. BP ____________________

h. CC ____________________

i. UA ____________________

j. PE ____________________

2. Give the abbreviations for the following terms.

a. return ____________________

b. cancer, carcinoma ____________________

c. patient ____________________

d. established ____________________

e. discharged ____________________

f. gallbladder ____________________

g. initial ____________________

ASSIGNMENT 7-7 ▶ STUDENT SOFTWARE CHALLENGE: ASSIGNMENTS FOR CASES 1 THROUGH 6 ONSCREEN COMPLETION OF CMS-1500 (08-05) INSURANCE CLAIM FORMS FOR PRIVATE INSURANCE

Performance Objective

Task: Enter transactions from patients' onscreen encounter forms (superbills) and complete block-by-block onscreen health insurance claim forms

Conditions: Onscreen encounter forms (superbills), patient records, and health insurance claim forms, and computer; procedural and diagnostic code books.

Standards: Time: ________________________ minutes

Accuracy: ________________________

(Note: The time element and accuracy criteria may be given by your instructor.)

Directions: Log on to your Evolve account at *http://evolve.elsevier.com* and access the student resources for Fordney: *Insurance Handbook for the Medical Office*, 12th edition. Then choose Student Software Challenge.

1. For these assignments, follow the instructions for entering data into the onscreen CMS-1500 (08-05) health insurance claim form completing blocks 1 through 33 for Cases 1 through 6.

2. Use your CPT code book or Appendix A in this *Workbook* to determine the correct five-digit code number and modifiers for each professional service rendered. To determine diagnostic codes, refer to ICD-9-CM and/or ICD-10-CM code books.

3. Print a hard copy of the completed health insurance claim form for each case.

4. After the instructor has returned your work to you, either make the necessary corrections and place your work in a three-ring notebook for future reference, or, if you received a high score, place it in your portfolio for reference when applying for a job.

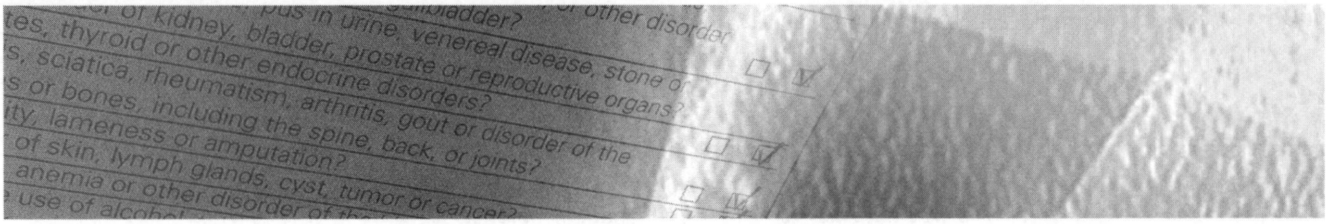

CHAPTER

8

Electronic Data Interchange: Transactions and Security

KEY TERMS

Your instructor may wish to select some words pertinent to this chapter for a test. For definitions of the terms, further study, and/or reference, the words, phrases, and abbreviations may be found in the glossary at the end of the Handbook. *Key terms for this chapter follow.*

Accredited Standards Committee X12
Accredited Standards Committee X12 Version 5010
application service provider
back up
batch
business associate agreement
cable modem
clearinghouse
code sets
covered entity
data elements
digital subscriber line
direct data entry
electronic data interchange
electronic funds transfer
electronic remittance advice
encoder
encryption
HIPAA Transaction and Code Set Rule
National Standard Format
password
real time
standard transactions
T-1
taxonomy codes
trading partner agreement

KEY ABBREVIATIONS

See how many abbreviations and acronyms you can translate and then use this as a handy reference list. Definitions for the key abbreviations are located near the back of the Handbook *in the glossary.*

ANSI ____________________
ASC X12 ____________________
ASET ____________________
ASP ____________________
ATM ____________________
DDE ____________________
DSL ____________________
EDI ____________________
EFT ____________________
EHR ____________________
EMC ____________________
EOMB ____________________
ePHI ____________________
ERA ____________________
HHS ____________________
IRS ____________________
MTS ____________________
NSF ____________________
PMS ____________________
TCS rule ____________________
UPS ____________________

PERFORMANCE OBJECTIVES

The student will be able to:

- Define and spell the key terms and key abbreviations for this chapter, given the information from the *Handbook* glossary, within a reasonable time period and with enough accuracy to obtain a satisfactory evaluation.
- After reading the chapter, answer the fill-in-the-blank, multiple choice, and true/false review questions with enough accuracy to obtain a satisfactory evaluation.
- Decide whether keyed medical and nonmedical data elements are required, situational, or not used when electronically submitting the 837P health care claim.
- State which medical and nonmedical code sets for 837P electronic claims are required, situational, or not used.
- Input data into the element for place of service codes for 837P electronic claims submission.
- Indicate the patient's relationship to the insured by using the individual relationship code numbers for 837P electronic claims submission.
- Select the correct individual relationship code number for 837P electronic claims submission.
- Select the correct taxonomy codes for the specialists for submission of 837P electronic claims submission.
- Locate errors, given computer-generated insurance forms, within a reasonable time period and with enough accuracy to obtain a satisfactory evaluation.
- Fill in the correct meaning of each abbreviation, given a list of common medical abbreviations and symbols that appear in chart notes, with enough accuracy to obtain a satisfactory evaluation.

STUDY OUTLINE

Electronic Data Interchange
Electronic Claims
Advantages of Electronic Claim Submission
Clearinghouses
Transaction and Code Set Regulations: Streamlining Electronic Data Interchange
- Transaction and Code Set Standards

Transition from Paper CMS-1500 (08-05) to Electronic Standard HIPAA 837P
- Levels of Information for 837P Standard Transaction Format
- Accredited Standards Committee X12 (ASC X12) Version 5010

Claims Attachments Standards
- Standard Unique Identifiers

Practice Management System
Building the Claim
- Encounter or Multipurpose Billing Forms
- Scannable Encounter Form
- Keying Insurance Data for Claim Transmission
- Encoder
- Clean Electronic Claims Submission

Putting HIPAA Standard Transactions to Work
- Interactive Transactions

Electronic Remittance Advice
Driving the Data
Methods for Sending Claims
Computer Claims Systems
- Payer or Carrier-Direct
- Clearinghouses

Transmission Reports
- Electronic Processing Problems
- Billing and Account Management Schedule
- Administrative Simplification Enforcement Tool
- The Security Rule: Administrative, Physical, and Technical Safeguards

HIPAA: Application to the Practice Setting
Computer Confidentiality
- Confidentiality Statement
- Prevention Measures

Records Management
- Data Storage
- Data Disposal
- Electronic Power Protection

ASSIGNMENT 8-1 ▸ REVIEW QUESTIONS

Part I Fill in the Blank

Review the objectives, key terms, glossary definitions of key terms, chapter information, and figures before completing the following review questions.

1. Exchange of data in a standardized format through computer systems is a technology known as ______________________.

2. The act of converting computerized data into a code so that unauthorized users are unable to read it is a security system known as ______________________.

3. Payment to the provider of service of an electronically submitted insurance claim may be received in approximately ______________________.

4. List benefits of using HIPAA standard transactions and code sets.

   a. ______________________

   b. ______________________

   c. ______________________

   d. ______________________

   e. ______________________

   f. ______________________

5. Dr. Morgan has 10 or more full-time employees and submits insurance claims for his Medicare patients. Is his medical practice subject to the HIPAA transaction rules? ______________________

6. Dr. Maria Montez does not submit insurance claims electronically and has five full-time employees. Is she required to abide by HIPAA transaction rules? ______________________

7. Name the standard code sets used for the following:

   a. physician services

   ____

   b. diseases and injuries

   ____

   c. pharmaceuticals and biologics

   ____

8. Refer to Table 8-3 in the *Handbook* to complete these statements.

   a. The staff at College Clinic submits professional health care claims for each of their providers and must use the industry standard electronic format called ____________________ to transmit them electronically.

   b. The billing department at College Hospital must use the industry standard electronic format called ____________________ to transmit health care claims electronically.

   c. The Medicare fiscal intermediary (insurance carrier) uses the industry standard electronic format called ____________________ to transmit payment information to the College Clinic and College Hospital.

   d. It has been 3 weeks since Gordon Marshall's health care claim was transmitted to the XYZ insurance company and you wish to inquire about the status of the claim. The industry standard electronic format that must be used to transmit this inquiry is called ____________________.

   e. Dr. Practon's insurance billing specialist must use the industry standard electronic format called ____________________ to obtain information about Beatrice Garcia's health policy benefits and coverage from the insurance plan.

9. The family practice taxonomy code is ____________________.

10. A Medicare patient, Charles Gorman, signed a signature authorization form, which is on file. The patient's signature source code for data element #1351 is ____________________.

11. Name the levels for data collected to construct and submit an electronic claim.

    a. ____________________

    b. ____________________

    c. ____________________

    d. ____________________

    e. ____________________

    f. ____________________

12. The most important function of a practice management system is

    ____________________.

13. To look for and correct all errors before the health claim is transmitted to the insurance carrier, you may

    ____

    or ____________________.

14. Add-on software to a practice management system that can reduce the time it takes to build or review a claim before batching is known as a/an ______________________________.

15. Software that is used in a network that serves a group of users working on a related project allowing access to the same data is called a/an ______________________________.

Part II Multiple Choice

Choose the best answer.

16. An alert feature that may be incorporated into the software in a physician's office that finds errors so they may be corrected before transmitting an insurance claim is called a/an

    a. online error-edit process

    b. encoder

    c. clearing transaction

    d. edit code set

17. Under HIPAA, data elements that are used uniformly to document why patients are seen (diagnosis) and what is done to them during their encounter (procedure) are known as

    a. medical code sets

    b. information elements

    c. TCS standards

    d. National Standard Format (NSF).

18. The standard transaction that replaces the paper CMS-1500 (08-05) claim form and more than 400 versions of the electronic National Standard Format is called the

    a. 270

    b. 837I

    c. 837P

    d. 837D

19. A paperless computerized system that enables payments to be transferred automatically to a physician's bank account by a third-party payer may be done via

    a. electronic savings account

    b. electronic remittance advice (ERA)

    c. electronic funds transfer (EFT)

    d. electronic data interchange (EDI)

20. An electronic Medicare remittance advice that takes the place of a paper Medicare explanation of benefits (EOB) is referred to as

   a. ANSI 277

   b. ANSI 820

   c. ANSI 830

   d. ANSI 835

Part III True/False

Write "T" or "F" in the blank to indicate whether you think the statement is true or false.

_______ 21. When transmitting electronic claims, inaccuracies that violate the HIPAA standard transaction format are known as syntax errors.

_______ 22. An organization may file a complaint online against someone whose actions impact the ability of a transaction to be accepted or efficiently processed by using the Administration Simplification Enforcement Tool (ASET).

_______ 23. Incidental uses and disclosures of protected health information (PHI) are permissible under HIPAA when reasonable safeguards have been used to prevent inappropriate revelation of PHI.

_______ 24. Deleting files or formatting the hard drive is sufficient to keep electronic protected health information from being accessed.

_______ 25. Employees who handle sensitive computer documents should sign an annual confidentiality statement.

_______ 26. When an insurance billing specialist e-mails a colleague to ask a coding question, it is permissible to refer to the case using the patient's name.

ASSIGNMENT 8-2 ▶ CRITICAL THINKING FOR MEDICAL AND NONMEDICAL CODE SETS FOR 837P ELECTRONIC CLAIMS SUBMISSION

Performance Objective

Task: Decide whether keyed medical and nonmedical data elements are required, situational, or not used when electronically submitting the 837P health care claim.

Conditions: List of keyed data elements (Table 8-5 in *Handbook*) and pen or pencil.

Standards: Time: ____________________ minutes

Accuracy: ____________________

(Note: The time element and accuracy criteria may be given by your instructor.)

Directions: When submitting the 837P health care claim, supporting code sets of medical and nonmedical data are composed of "Required" and "Situational" data elements. Read each keyed data element and answer whether you think it is **R** for required, **S** for situational, or **N** for not used.

a. Patient's last menstrual period ____________________

b. Patient's telephone number ____________________

c. Insured's name ____________________

d. Diagnosis code ____________________

e. Provider's NPI ____________________

f. Procedure code ____________________

g. Provider's signature ____________________

h. Employer's name ____________________

i. Place of service ____________________

j. Procedure modifier ____________________

ASSIGNMENT 8-3 ▶ INPUT DATA INTO ELEMENT FOR PLACE OF SERVICE CODES FOR 837P ELECTRONIC CLAIMS SUBMISSIONS

Performance Objective

Task: Insert the correct place of service code for each location description where medical professional service was rendered.

Conditions: Place of service codes reference (Figure 8-1), list of places where medical care was rendered, and pen or pencil.

Standards: Time: ______________________ minutes

Accuracy: ______________________

(Note: The time element and accuracy criteria may be given by your instructor.)

Directions: When submitting the 837P electronic claim, place of service codes must be entered in data element 1331. Refer to the place of service codes reference list and insert the correct code for each place of service for the following locations.

a. Inpatient psychiatric facility ______________________________

b. Doctor's office ______________________________

c. Outpatient hospital ______________________________

d. Intermediate nursing facility ______________________________

e. Independent clinic ______________________________

f. Independent laboratory ______________________________

g. Birthing center ______________________________

h. End-stage renal disease treatment facility ______________________________

i. Inpatient hospital ______________________________

j. Hospice ______________________________

PLACE OF SERVICE CODES	
Codes	**Place of Service**
01	Pharmacy
00-02	Unassigned
03	School
04	Homeless shelter
05	Indian health service free -standing facility
06	Indian health service provider -based facility
07	Tribal 638 free -standing facility
08	Tribal 638 provide r-based facility
09	Prison/correctional facility
10	Unassigned
11	Doctor's office
12	Patient's home
13	Assisted living facility
14	Group home
15	Mobile unit
16	Temporary lodging
17-19	Unassigned
20	Urgent care facility
21	Inpatient hospital
22	Outpatient hospital or urgent care center
23	Emergency department —hospi tal
24	Ambulatory surgical center
25	Birthing center
26	Military treatment facility/uniformed service treatment facility
27-30	Unassigned
31	Skilled nursing facility (s wing bed visits)
32	Nursing facility (intermediate/long -term care facilities)
33	Custodial care facility (domiciliary or rest home services)
34	Hospice (domiciliary or rest home services)
35-40	Unassigned
41	Ambulance —land
42	Ambulance —air or water
43-48	Unassigned
49	Independent clinic
50	Federally qualified health center
51	Inpatient psychiatric facility
52	Psychiatric facility —partial hospitalization
53	Community mental health care (outpatient, twenty-four-hours-a-day services, admission screening, consultation, and educational services)
54	Intermediate care facility/ mentally retarded
55	Residential substance abuse treatment facility
56	Psychiatric residential treatment center
57	Non-residential substance abuse treatment facility
58-59	Unassigned
60	Mass immunization center
61	Comprehensive inpatient rehabilitation facility
62	Comprehensive outpatient rehabilitation facility
63-64	Unassigned
65	End-stage renal disease treatment facility
66-70	Unassigned
71	State or local public health clinic
72	Rural health clinic
73-80	Unassigned
81	Independent laboratory
82-98	Unassigned
99	Other unlisted facility

Figure 8-1

ASSIGNMENT 8-4 ▶ SELECT THE CORRECT INDIVIDUAL RELATIONSHIP CODE NUMBER FOR 837P ELECTRONIC CLAIMS SUBMISSION

Performance Objective

Task: Insert the correct individual relationship code for the patient's relationship to the insured.

Conditions: Individual relationship code number reference (Figure 8-2), list of individuals or entities, and pen or pencil.

Standards: Time: ____________________ minutes

Accuracy: ____________________

(Note: The time element and accuracy criteria may be given by your instructor.)

Directions: Refer to the individual relationship code number list, choose the correct code for the patient's relationship to the insured for the following persons, and insert it on the lines.

a. Mother ____________________

b. Spouse ____________________

c. Child ____________________

d. Father ____________________

e. Stepdaughter ____________________

f. Emancipated minor ____________________

g. Adopted child ____________________

h. Handicapped dependent ____________________

i. Stepson ____________________

j. Sponsored dependent ____________________

Individual Relationship Code	
Code	**Relationship**
01	Spouse
04	Grandfather or grandmother
05	Grandson or granddaughter
07	Nephew or niece
09	Adopted child
10	Foster child
15	Ward
17	Stepson or stepdaughter
19	Child
20	Employee
21	Unknown
22	Handicapped dependent
23	Sponsored dependent
24	Dependent of a minor dependent
29	Significant other
32	Mother
33	Father
34	Other adult
36	Emancipated minor
39	Organ donor
40	Cadaver donor
41	Injured plaintiff
43	Child where insured has no financial responsibility
53	Life partner
G8	Other relationship

Figure 8-2

ASSIGNMENT 8-5 ▶ SELECT THE CORRECT TAXONOMY CODES FOR MEDICAL SPECIALISTS FOR 837P ELECTRONIC CLAIMS SUBMISSION

Performance Objective

Task: Choose the correct taxonomy code for each specialist for submission of 837P electronic claims by referring to the Health Care Provider Taxonomy code list.

Conditions: Health Care Provider Taxonomy code list (Figure 8-3), list of providers of service, and pen or pencil.

Standards: Time: ____________________ minutes

Accuracy: ____________________

(Note: The time element and accuracy criteria may be given by your instructor.)

Directions: Refer to the Health Care Provider Taxonomy code list, choose the correct code for each of the following specialists, and insert the code numbers on the lines.

a. Raymond Skeleton, MD, orthopedist ____________________

b. Gaston Input, MD, gastroenterologist ____________________

c. Vera Cutis, MD, dermatologist ____________________

d. Gene Ulibarri, MD, urologist ____________________

e. Bertha Caesar, MD, obstetrician/gynecologist ____________________

f. Gerald Practon, MD, general practitioner ____________________

g. Pedro Atrics, MD, pediatrician ____________________

h. Astro Parkinson, MD, neurosurgeon ____________________

i. Brady Coccidioides, MD, pulmonary disease ____________________

j. Max Gluteus, RPT, physical therapist ____________________

College Clinic Staff		
Health Care Provider Taxonomy Codes		
Name	**Speciality**	**Taxonomy Code**
Concha Antrum, MD	Otolaryngologist	207Y00000X
Pedro Atrics, MD	Pediatrician	208000000X
Bertha Caesar, MD	Obstetrician/Gynecologist	207V00000X
Perry Cardi, MD	Cardiologist	207RC0000X
Brady Coccidioides, MD	Pulmonary disease	207RP1001X
Vera Cutis, MD	Dermatologist	207N00000X
Clarence Cutler, MD	General surgeon	208600000X
Dennis Drill, DDS	Dentist	122300000X
Max Gluteus, RPT	Physical therapist	208100000X
Cosmo Graff, MD	Plastic surgeon	208200000X
Malvern Grumose, MD	Pathologist	207ZP0105X
Gaston Input, MD	Gastroenterologist	207RG0100X
Adam Langerhans, MD	Endocrinologist	207RE0101X
Cornell Lenser, MD	Ophthalmologist	207W00000X
Michael Menter, MD	Psychiatrist	2084P0800X
Arthur O. Dont, DDS	Orthodontist	1223X0400X
Astro Parkinson, MD	Neurosurgeon	207T00000X
Nick Pedro, MD	Podiatrist	213E00000X
Gerald Practon, MD	General practitioner	208D00000X
Walter Radon, MD	Radiologst	2085R0202X
Rex Rumsey, MD	Proctologist	208C00000X
Sensitive E. Scott, MD	Anesthesiologist	207L00000X
Raymond Skeleton, MD	Orthopedist	207X00000X
Gene Ulibarri, MD	Urologist	208800000X

Figure 8-3

ASSIGNMENT 8-6 ▶ COMPOSE ELECTRONIC MAIL MESSAGES

Performance Objective

Task: Compose brief messages for electronic mail transmission after reading each scenario.

Conditions: List of scenarios, one sheet of 8½- × 11-inch plain typing paper, and a computer or a pen.

Standards: Time: ______________________ minutes

Accuracy: ______________________

(Note: The time element and accuracy criteria may be given by your instructor.)

Directions: Read each scenario. Compose polite, effective, and brief messages that, on the job, would be transmitted via electronic mail (e-mail). Use the guidelines for electronic mail presented on the Evolve website. Be sure to list a descriptive subject line as the first item in each composition. Single-space the message. Insert a short signature at the end of the message to include your name and affiliation, and create an e-mail address for yourself if you do not have one. Print hard copies of e-mail messages for Scenarios 1 through 5 to give to your instructor. After the instructor has returned your work, either make the necessary corrections and place your work in a three-ring notebook for future reference or, if you received a high score, place it in your portfolio for use when applying for a job.

Scenario 1:

Ask an insurance biller, Mary Davis, in a satellite office to locate and fax you a copy of the billing done on account number 43500 for services rendered to Margarita Sylva on March 2, 20xx. Explain that you must telephone the patient about her account. Mary Davis' e-mail address is mdavis@aal.com.

Scenario 2:

Patient Ellen Worth was recently hospitalized; her hospital number is 20-9870-11. Compose an e-mail message to the medical record department at College Hospital (collegehospmedrecords@rrv.net) for her final diagnosis and the assigned diagnostic code needed to complete the insurance claim form.

Scenario 3:

You are working for a billing service and receive an encounter form that is missing the information about the patient's professional service received on August 2, 20xx. The patient's account number is 45098. You have the diagnosis data. Compose an e-mail message to Dr. Mason (pmason@email.mc.com) explaining what you must obtain to complete the billing portion of the insurance claim form.

Scenario 4:

A new patient, John Phillips, has e-mailed your office to ask what the outstanding balance is on his account. The account number is 42990. You look up the financial record and note the service was for an office visit on June 14, 20xx. The charge was $106.11. Compose an e-mail response to Mr. Phillips, whose e-mail address is bphillips@hotmail.com.

Scenario 5:

You are having difficulty deciding whether the codes 13101, 13102, and 13132 with modifier -51 selected for a case are appropriate. Compose an e-mail message that will be posted on the Part B News Internet listserv (PartB-L@usa.net) asking for comments. The case involves a 12-year-old boy who fell against a bicycle, lacerating the left side of his chest to the pectoralis muscle through a 12-cm gaping wound. He also sustained a 5-cm laceration to his left cheek. Complex repairs were required for these two wounds and totaled 17 cm. Find out whether modifier -15 should be appended to the second code or to the third code.

ASSIGNMENT 8-7 ▶ PROOFREAD A COMPUTER-GENERATED HEALTH INSURANCE CLAIM FORM AND LOCATE INCORRECT AND MISSING DATA

Performance Objective

Task: Locate and designate blocks on the computer-generated insurance claim form that have incorrect information or need completion; correct or add data before submission to the insurance company.

Conditions: Use Brad E. Diehl's patient record (Figure 8-4), completed insurance claim (Figure 8-5), and a highlighter and a red ink pen.

Standards: Time: ____________________ minutes

Accuracy: ____________________

(Note: The time element and accuracy criteria may be given by your instructor.)

Directions: Proofread the insurance claim form (see Figure 8-5) and locate blocks that need correction or completion before submission to the insurance company. Highlight all errors you discover. Refer to the patient's record (see Figure 8-4) to verify pertinent demographic and insurance information. Refer to the progress notes to verify procedures and determine diagnoses. Verify all entries on the claim form, including dates, codes, rounded out fees, and physician identification numbers. Insert all corrections and missing information in red. If you cannot locate the necessary information but know it is mandatory, write "NEED" in the corresponding block.

Optional: Retype a blank CMS-1500 (08-05) claim form with all corrections and changes. Or if you have access to a computer, log on to your Evolve account at http://evolve.elsevier.com and access the student resources for Fordney: *Insurance Handbook for the Medical Office*, 12th edition. There you can fill out a CMS-1500 PDF file and print it or save it.

Additional Coding

1. Assume that Mr. Diehl followed Dr. Input's treatment plan. Refer to his record, abstract information, and locate procedure codes that would be billed by providers outside of the office.

Site	*Description of Service*	*Code*
a. ABC Radiology	____________	____________
b. College Hospital	____________	____________
c. Surgeon	____________	____________

2. Code the symptoms Mr. Diehl was complaining about when he presented for the January 6, 20XX, office visit.

Symptom	*ICD-9-CM Code*	*ICD-10-CM Code*
a. ____________	____________	____________
b. ____________	____________	____________
c. ____________	____________	____________
d. ____________	____________	____________
e. ____________	____________	____________

PATIENT RECORD NO. 8-7

LAST NAME	FIRST NAME	MIDDLE NAME	BIRTH DATE	SEX	HOME PHONE
Diehl	Brad	E.	09-21-46	M	555-222-0123

ADDRESS	CITY	STATE	ZIP CODE
3975 Hills Road	Woodland Hills	XY	12345

CELL PHONE	PAGER NO.	FAX NO.	E-MAIL ADDRESS
555-703-6600	555-321-0988	555-222-0123	Diehl@WB.net

PATIENT'S SOC. SEC. NO.	DRIVER'S LICENSE
561-XX-1501	M0983457

PATIENT'S OCCUPATION	NAME OF COMPANY
radio advertising salesman	KACY Radio

ADDRESS OF EMPLOYER	PHONE
4071 Mills Road, Woodland Hills, XY 12335	555-201-6666

SPOUSE OR PARENT	OCCUPATION
Tak E. Diehl (birthdate 4-7-45)	legal secretary

EMPLOYER	ADDRESS	PHONE
Attys. Dilman, Forewise & Gilson,	12 West Dix Street, Woodland Hills, XY 12345	555-222-6432

NAME OF INSURANCE	INSURED OR SUBSCRIBER
Aetna Insurance Co., 2412 Main Street, Woodland Hills, XY 12345	Brad E. Diehl

POLICY/CERTIFICATE NO.	GROUP NO.
403119	

REFERRED BY: Raymond Skeleton, MD

DATE	PROGRESS NOTES No. 8-7
1-6-20xx	NP pt comes in complaining of coughing and sneezing; some difficulty breathing.
	Occasional dizziness and epigastric abdominal pain with cramping. Symptoms started in
	July of last year. Performed a detailed history and physical examination with low
	complexity medical decision making. AP & lat chest x-rays taken; neg findings. BP 178/98.
	Pt to have cholecystography with oral contrast at ABC Radiology. Diagnostic colonoscopy
	(flexible) to be scheduled at College Hospital. Dx: hypertension and respiratory distress;
	R/O irritable colon. No disability at this time.
	GI/llf Gaston Input, MD
1-20-xx	Pt retns for a EPF hx/exam LC MDM. Oral cholecystography reveals a single 1.5 cm
	radiolucent calculus within the cholecyst. Colonoscopy confirmed irritable bowel
	syndrome. Blood drawn and CBC (auto with diff) performed in office indicates
	WBC 10,000. DX: cholecystitis with cholelithiasis. Adv. cholecystectomy
	(abdominal approach) as soon as possible; to be scheduled at College Hospital.
	GI/llf Gaston Input, MD

Figure 8-4

1500

HEALTH INSURANCE CLAIM FORM

APPROVED BY NATIONAL UNIFORM CLAIM COMMITTEE 08/05

PICA PICA

CARRIER

1. MEDICARE (Medicare #) MEDICAID (Medicaid #) TRICARE CHAMPUS (Sponsor's SSN) CHAMPVA (Member ID#) GROUP HEALTH PLAN (SSN or ID) [X] FECA BLK LUNG (SSN) OTHER (ID)

1a. INSURED'S I.D. NUMBER (For Program in Item 1): 403119

2. PATIENT'S NAME (Last Name, First Name, Middle Initial): DIEHL BRAD E

3. PATIENT'S BIRTH DATE MM DD YY: 09 21 1946 SEX M F

4. INSURED'S NAME (Last Name, First Name, Middle Initial): SAME

5. PATIENT'S ADDRESS (No., Street): 3975 HILLS ROAD

6. PATIENT RELATIONSHIP TO INSURED: Self Spouse Child Other

7. INSURED'S ADDRESS (No., Street)

CITY: WOODLAND HILLS STATE: XY

8. PATIENT STATUS: Single Married [X] Other; Employed [X] Full-Time Student Part-Time Student

CITY STATE

ZIP CODE: 12345 TELEPHONE (Include Area Code): (555) 2220123

ZIP CODE TELEPHONE (INCLUDE AREA CODE) ( )

9. OTHER INSURED'S NAME (Last Name, First Name, Middle Initial)

10. IS PATIENT'S CONDITION RELATED TO:

11. INSURED'S POLICY GROUP OR FECA NUMBER

a. OTHER INSURED'S POLICY OR GROUP NUMBER

a. EMPLOYMENT? (CURRENT OR PREVIOUS) YES [X] NO

a. INSURED'S DATE OF BIRTH MM DD YY SEX M F

b. OTHER INSURED'S DATE OF BIRTH MM DD YY SEX M F

b. AUTO ACCIDENT? YES [X] NO PLACE (State)

b. EMPLOYER'S NAME OR SCHOOL NAME

c. EMPLOYER'S NAME OR SCHOOL NAME

c. OTHER ACCIDENT? YES [X] NO

c. INSURANCE PLAN NAME OR PROGRAM NAME

d. INSURANCE PLAN NAME OR PROGRAM NAME

10d. RESERVED FOR LOCAL USE

d. IS THERE ANOTHER HEALTH BENEFIT PLAN? YES [X] NO *If yes, return to and complete item 9 a-d.*

READ BACK OF FORM BEFORE COMPLETING & SIGNING THIS FORM.

12. PATIENT'S OR AUTHORIZED PERSON'S SIGNATURE I authorize the release of any medical or other information necessary to process this claim. I also request payment of government benefits either to myself or to the party who accepts assignment below.

SIGNED ______ DATE ______

13. INSURED'S OR AUTHORIZED PERSON'S SIGNATURE I authorize payment of medical benefits to the undersigned physician or supplier for services described below.

SIGNED ______

PATIENT AND INSURED INFORMATION

14. DATE OF CURRENT: MM DD YY ILLNESS (First symptom) OR INJURY (Accident) OR PREGNANCY(LMP)

15. IF PATIENT HAS HAD SAME OR SIMILAR ILLNESS. GIVE FIRST DATE MM DD YY

16. DATES PATIENT UNABLE TO WORK IN CURRENT OCCUPATION FROM MM DD YY TO MM DD YY

17. NAME OF REFERRING PHYSICIAN OR OTHER SOURCE: RAYMOND SKELETON MD

17a. 17b. NPI 12678547XX

18. HOSPITALIZATION DATES RELATED TO CURRENT SERVICES FROM MM DD YY TO MM DD YY

19. RESERVED FOR LOCAL USE

20. OUTSIDE LAB? YES NO $ CHARGES

21. DIAGNOSIS OR NATURE OF ILLNESS OR INJURY. (RELATE ITEMS 1,2,3 OR 4 TO ITEM 24E BY LINE)

1. 574.10 3. 786.09

2. ___ . ___ 4. ___ . ___

22. MEDICAID RESUBMISSION CODE ORIGINAL REF. NO.

23. PRIOR AUTHORIZATION NUMBER

	24. A. DATE(S) OF SERVICE From MM DD YY	To MM DD YY	B. PLACE OF SERVICE	C. EMG	D. PROCEDURES, SERVICES, OR SUPPLIES (Explain Unusual Circumstances) CPT/HCPCS	MODIFIER	E. DIAGNOSIS POINTER	F. $ CHARGES	G. DAYS OR UNITS	H. EPSDT Family Plan	I. ID. QUAL.	J. RENDERING PROVIDER ID. #
1	01 06 20XX		11		99203		3 4	70 92	1		NPI	32783127XX
2	01 06 20XX		11		71020		3	40 97	1		NPI	32783127XX
3	1 20 20XX		11		99213		1 2	40 20	1		NPI	32783127XX
4	01 20 20XX		11		85025		1	25 00	1		NPI	32783127XX
5	01 20 20XX		11				1		1		NPI	32783127XX
6											NPI	

25. FEDERAL TAX I.D. NUMBER SSN EIN

26. PATIENT'S ACCOUNT NO.: 8

27. ACCEPT ASSIGNMENT? (For govt. claims, see back) [X] YES NO

28. TOTAL CHARGE $ 29. AMOUNT PAID $ 30. BALANCE DUE $

31. SIGNATURE OF PHYSICIAN OR SUPPLIER INCLUDING DEGREES OR CREDENTIALS (I certify that the statements on the reverse apply to this bill and are made a part thereof.)

SIGNED DATE 01/25/20XX

32. SERVICE FACILITY LOCATION INFORMATION: SAME

a. NPI b.

33. BILLING PROVIDER INFO & PH # (555) 4869002
COLLEGE CLINIC
4567 BROAD AVENUE
WOODLAND HILLS XY 12345 0001

a. 3664021CC NPI b.

PHYSICIAN OR SUPPLIER INFORMATION

NUCC Instruction Manual available at: www.nucc.org **PLEASE PRINT OR TYPE** APPROVED OMB-0938-0999 FORM CMS-1500 (08-05)

Figure 8-5

ASSIGNMENT 8-8 ▶ PROOFREAD A COMPUTER-GENERATED HEALTH INSURANCE CLAIM FORM AND LOCATE INCORRECT AND MISSING DATA

Performance Objective

Task: Locate and designate blocks on the computer-generated insurance claim form that have incorrect information or need completion; correct or add data before submission to the insurance company.

Conditions: Use Evert I. Strain's patient record (Figure 8-6), completed insurance claim (Figure 8-7), and a highlighter and a red ink pen.

Standards: Time: ____________________ minutes

Accuracy: ____________________

(Note: The time element and accuracy criteria may be given by your instructor.)

Directions: Proofread the insurance claim form (see Figure 8-7) and locate blocks that need correction or completion before submission to the insurance company. Highlight all errors you discover. Refer to the patient's record (see Figure 8-6) to verify pertinent demographic and insurance information. Refer to the progress notes to verify procedures and determine diagnoses. Verify all entries on the claim form, including dates, codes, rounded out fees, and physician identification numbers. Insert all corrections and missing information in red. If you cannot locate the necessary information but know it is mandatory, write "NEED" in the corresponding block.

Optional: Retype a blank CMS-1500 (08-05) claim form with all corrections and changes. Or if you have access to a computer, log on to your Evolve account at http://evolve.elsevier.com and access the student resources for Fordney: *Insurance Handbook for the Medical Office*, 12th edition. There you can fill out a CMS-1500 claim form and print it or save it. If your instructor tells you to also find the ICD-10-CM codes, a draft version may be downloaded from the following website: http://www.cdc.gov/nchs/icd/icd10cm.htm#10update.

Additional Coding

1. Refer to Mr. Strain's medical record, abstract information, and code procedures that would be billed by outside providers.

Site	*Description of Service*	*Code*
a. ABC Laboratory	____________________	____________________
b. ABC Radiology	____________________	____________________

PATIENT RECORD NO. 8-8

LAST NAME	FIRST NAME	MIDDLE NAME	BIRTH DATE	SEX	HOME PHONE
Strain,	Evert	I	09-11-46	M	555-678-0211

ADDRESS	CITY	STATE	ZIP CODE
7650 None Such Road	Woodland Hills	XY	12345

CELL PHONE	PAGER NO.	FAX NO.	E-MAIL ADDRESS
555-430-2101	555-320-9980	555-678-0211	Strain@WB.net

PATIENT'S SOC. SEC. NO.	DRIVER'S LICENSE
453-XX-4739	Y0923658

PATIENT'S OCCUPATION	NAME OF COMPANY
mechanical engineer	R & R Company

ADDRESS OF EMPLOYER	PHONE
2400 Davon Road, Woodland Hills, XY 12345	555-520-8977

SPOUSE OR PARENT	OCCUPATION
Ester I. Strain (wife)	administrative assistant

EMPLOYER	ADDRESS	PHONE
University College, 4021 Book Road, Woodland Hills, XY 12345		555-450-9908

NAME OF INSURANCE	INSURED OR SUBSCRIBER
ABC Insurance Co., P.O. Box 130, Woodland Hills, XY 12345	Evert I. Strain

POLICY/CERTIFICATE NO.	GROUP NO.
453-XX-4739	96476A

REFERRED BY: Gerald C. Jones, MD, 1403 Haven Street, Woodland Hills, XY 12345 NPI # 54754966XX

DATE	PROGRESS NOTES No. 8-8
1-8-20xx	Est pt comes in complaining of frequent urination, headaches, polyphagia; unable to
	remember current events. These problems have been present for almost a year.
	A comprehensive history is taken and compared to his last H & P 2 years ago.
	A com PX is performed. BP 160/110; pt was prescribed antihypertensive medication but
	discontinued it when the prescription ran out. Lab report, hand carried by pt from an
	urgent care center indicates SGOT in normal range and cholesterol elevated. Fasting blood
	sugar extremely high. Dx: diabetes mellitus, malignant hypertensive, and ASCVD.
	Pt to have 3 hour GTT tomorrow a.m. at ABC laboratory. STAT CT scan of head s̄ contrast
	ordered at ABC radiology to follow lab work. Arrangement will be made for pt to be
	admitted to College Hospital. Disability 1/9 through 1/31.
	GI/llf Gerald Practon, MD
1-9-xx	Admit to College Hospital (C hx/exam MC MDM).
	GI/llf Gerald Practon, MD
1-10-xx	Hosp visit (PF hx/exam SF MDM). CT scan of head reviewed, neg. findings. Pt alert and
	comfortable. If blood sugar and BP remain stable, discharge planned for tomorrow.
	BP 130/85.
	GI/llf Gerald Practon, MD
1-11-xx	DC from hosp. Pt to be seen in one week in ofc.
	GI/llf Gerald Practon, MD

Figure 8-6

(1500)

HEALTH INSURANCE CLAIM FORM

APPROVED BY NATIONAL UNIFORM CLAIM COMMITTEE 08/05

PICA | PICA

CARRIER

1. MEDICARE (Medicare #) ☐ MEDICAID (Medicaid #) ☐ TRICARE CHAMPUS (Sponsor's SSN) ☐ CHAMPVA (Member ID#) ☐ GROUP HEALTH PLAN (SSN or ID) ☒ FECA BLK LUNG (SSN) ☐ OTHER (ID) ☐

1a. INSURED'S I.D. NUMBER (For Program in Item 1): 453 XX 4739 96476A

2. PATIENT'S NAME (Last Name, First Name, Middle Initial): STRAIN EVERT I

3. PATIENT'S BIRTH DATE MM DD YY — SEX M ☒ F ☐

4. INSURED'S NAME (Last Name, First Name, Middle Initial): SAME

5. PATIENT'S ADDRESS (No., Street): 7650 NONE SUCH ROAD

6. PATIENT RELATIONSHIP TO INSURED: Self ☐ Spouse ☐ Child ☐ Other ☐

7. INSURED'S ADDRESS (No., Street)

CITY: WOODLAND HILLS STATE: XY

8. PATIENT STATUS: Single ☐ Married ☒ Other ☐; Employed ☒ Full-Time Student ☐ Part-Time Student ☐

CITY | STATE

ZIP CODE | TELEPHONE (Include Area Code) ( )

ZIP CODE | TELEPHONE (INCLUDE AREA CODE) ( )

9. OTHER INSURED'S NAME (Last Name, First Name, Middle Initial)

10. IS PATIENT'S CONDITION RELATED TO:

11. INSURED'S POLICY GROUP OR FECA NUMBER

a. OTHER INSURED'S POLICY OR GROUP NUMBER

a. EMPLOYMENT? (CURRENT OR PREVIOUS) ☐ YES ☒ NO

a. INSURED'S DATE OF BIRTH MM DD YY — SEX M ☐ F ☐

b. OTHER INSURED'S DATE OF BIRTH MM DD YY — SEX M ☐ F ☐

b. AUTO ACCIDENT? ☐ YES ☒ NO PLACE (State)

b. EMPLOYER'S NAME OR SCHOOL NAME

c. EMPLOYER'S NAME OR SCHOOL NAME

c. OTHER ACCIDENT? ☐ YES ☒ NO

c. INSURANCE PLAN NAME OR PROGRAM NAME

d. INSURANCE PLAN NAME OR PROGRAM NAME

10d. RESERVED FOR LOCAL USE

d. IS THERE ANOTHER HEALTH BENEFIT PLAN? ☐ YES ☐ NO *If yes*, return to and complete item 9 a-d.

READ BACK OF FORM BEFORE COMPLETING & SIGNING THIS FORM.

12. PATIENT'S OR AUTHORIZED PERSON'S SIGNATURE I authorize the release of any medical or other information necessary to process this claim. I also request payment of government benefits either to myself or to the party who accepts assignment below.

SIGNED ______ DATE ______

13. INSURED'S OR AUTHORIZED PERSON'S SIGNATURE I authorize payment of medical benefits to the undersigned physician or supplier for services described below.

SIGNED ______

PATIENT AND INSURED INFORMATION

14. DATE OF CURRENT: MM DD YY ILLNESS (First symptom) OR INJURY (Accident) OR PREGNANCY(LMP)

15. IF PATIENT HAS HAD SAME OR SIMILAR ILLNESS. GIVE FIRST DATE MM DD YY

16. DATES PATIENT UNABLE TO WORK IN CURRENT OCCUPATION FROM MM DD YY TO MM DD YY

17. NAME OF REFERRING PHYSICIAN OR OTHER SOURCE: GERALD C JONES

17a. | 17b. NPI 54754966XX

18. HOSPITALIZATION DATES RELATED TO CURRENT SERVICES FROM 01 09 20XX TO 01 11 20XX

19. RESERVED FOR LOCAL USE

20. OUTSIDE LAB? ☐ YES ☒ NO $ CHARGES

21. DIAGNOSIS OR NATURE OF ILLNESS OR INJURY. (RELATE ITEMS 1,2,3 OR 4 TO ITEM 24E BY LINE)

1. 250.00 3. ___.__
2. 401.0 4. ___.__

22. MEDICAID RESUBMISSION CODE | ORIGINAL REF. NO.

23. PRIOR AUTHORIZATION NUMBER

	24. A. DATE(S) OF SERVICE From MM DD YY	To MM DD YY	B. PLACE OF SERVICE	C. EMG	D. PROCEDURES, SERVICES, OR SUPPLIES (Explain Unusual Circumstances) CPT/HCPCS	MODIFIER	E. DIAGNOSIS POINTER	F. $ CHARGES	G. DAYS OR UNITS	H. EPSDT Family Plan	I. ID. QUAL.	J. RENDERING PROVIDER ID. #
1	01 08 20XX		11		99215			96 97	1		NPI	46278897XX
2	01 09 20XX		21		99222			120 80	1		NPI	46278897XX
3	1 10 20XX		21		99231			37 74	1		NPI	46278897XX
4	01 11 20XX		21		99231			65 26	1		NPI	46278897XX
5											NPI	
6											NPI	

25. FEDERAL TAX I.D. NUMBER: 7034597 SSN ☐ EIN ☒

26. PATIENT'S ACCOUNT NO.: 8

27. ACCEPT ASSIGNMENT? (For govt. claims, see back) ☒ YES ☐ NO

28. TOTAL CHARGE $ 320 77

29. AMOUNT PAID $

30. BALANCE DUE $ 320 77

31. SIGNATURE OF PHYSICIAN OR SUPPLIER INCLUDING DEGREES OR CREDENTIALS (I certify that the statements on the reverse apply to this bill and are made a part thereof.)

GERALD PRACTON MD 01/25/20XX

SIGNED DATE

32. SERVICE FACILITY LOCATION INFORMATION

a. NPI b.

33. BILLING PROVIDER INFO & PH # (555) 4869002

COLLEGE CLINIC
4567 BROAD AVENUE
WOODLAND HILLS XY 12345 0001

a. 3664021CC NPI b.

PHYSICIAN OR SUPPLIER INFORMATION

NUCC Instruction Manual available at: www.nucc.org **PLEASE PRINT OR TYPE** APPROVED OMB-0938-0999 FORM CMS-1500 (08-05)

Figure 8-7

ASSIGNMENT 8-9 ▶ DEFINE PATIENT RECORD ABBREVIATIONS

Performance Objective

Task: Insert definitions of abbreviations.

Conditions: Use pencil or pen.

Standards: Time: ____________________ minutes

Accuracy: ____________________

(Note: The time element and accuracy criteria may be given by your instructor.)

Directions: After completing the assignments in this chapter, you will be able to define the abbreviations shown here.

Abbreviations pertinent to the record of Brad E. Diehl:

NP	____________________	R/O	____________________
LC	____________________	auto	____________________
pt	____________________	retn	____________________
MDM	____________________	diff	____________________
AP	____________________	EPF	____________________
cm	____________________	WBC	____________________
lat	____________________	hx	____________________
neg	____________________	DX	____________________
BP	____________________	exam	____________________
CBC	____________________	adv	____________________

Abbreviations pertinent to the record of Evert I. Strain:

est	____________________	comp	____________________
CT	____________________	exam	____________________
pt	____________________	PX	____________________
C	____________________	MC	____________________
H & P	____________________	BP	____________________
hx	____________________	MDM	____________________

lab	______	ASCVD	______
hosp	______	neg	______
SGOT	______	GTT	______
PF	______	DC	______
Dx	______	STAT	______
SF	______	ofc	______

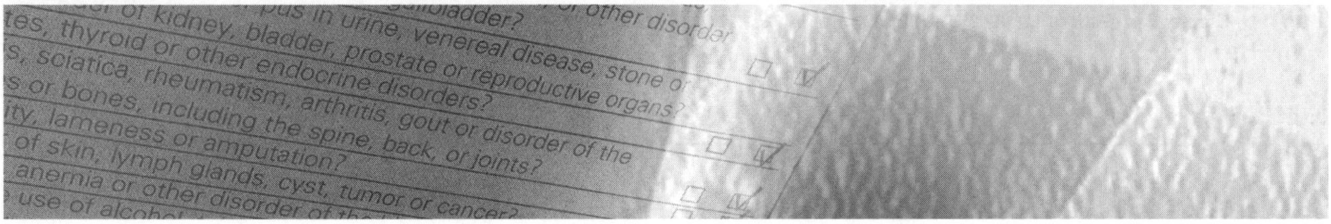

CHAPTER

9

Receiving Payments and Insurance Problem Solving

KEY TERMS

Your instructor may wish to select some words pertinent to this chapter for a test. For definitions of the terms, further study, and/or reference, the words, phrases, and abbreviations may be found in the glossary at the end of the Handbook. *Key terms for this chapter follow.*

appeal
delinquent claim
denied paper or electronic claim
explanation of benefits
inquiry
lost claim
overpayment
peer review
rebill (resubmit)
rejected claim
remittance advice
review
suspended claim
suspense
tracer

KEY ABBREVIATIONS

See how many abbreviations and acronyms you can translate and then use this as a handy reference list. Definitions for the key abbreviations are located near the back of the Handbook *in the glossary.*

ALJ ____________________
CMS ____________________
DAB ____________________
EOB ____________________
ERISA ____________________
FTC ____________________
HIPAA ____________________
HMO ____________________
HO ____________________
NPI ____________________
RA ____________________

PERFORMANCE OBJECTIVES

The student will be able to:

- Define and spell the key terms and key abbreviations for this chapter, given the information from the *Handbook* glossary, within a reasonable time period and with enough accuracy to obtain a satisfactory evaluation.
- After reading the chapter, answer the fill-in-the-blank, multiple choice, and true/false review questions with enough accuracy to obtain a satisfactory evaluation.
- Complete the insurance claim tracer form, given a request for an insurance claim trace and the patient's insurance claim, within a reasonable time period, and with enough accuracy to obtain a satisfactory evaluation.
- Locate the errors on each claim, given three returned insurance claims, within a reasonable time period and with enough accuracy to obtain a satisfactory evaluation.
- Complete form CMS-1965, Request for Hearing, Part B, Medicare Claim, within a reasonable time period and with enough accuracy to obtain a satisfactory evaluation.
- File an appeal by composing and typing a letter with envelope, within a reasonable time period, and with enough accuracy to obtain a satisfactory evaluation.

STUDY OUTLINE

Follow-Up after Claim Submission

Claim Policy Provisions

- Insured
- Payment Time Limits

Explanation of Benefits

- Components of an EOB
- Interpretation of an EOB
- Posting an EOB

Claim Management Techniques

- Insurance Claims Register
- Tickler File
- Aging Reports
- Insurance Company Payment History

Claim Inquiries

Problem Paper and Electronic Claims

- Types of Problems

Rebilling

Review and Appeal Process

Filing an Appeal

- Medicare Review and Redetermination Process
- TRICARE Review and Appeal Process

State Insurance Commissioner

- Commission Objectives
- Types of Problems

Commission Inquiries

Procedure: Trace an Unpaid Insurance Claim

Procedure: File an Appeal

ASSIGNMENT 9-1 ▶ REVIEW QUESTIONS

Part I Fill in the Blank

Review the objectives, key terms, and chapter information before completing the following review questions.

1. Name provisions seen in health insurance policies.

   a. ____________________

   b. ____________________

   c. ____________________

   d. ____________________

2. After an insurance claim is processed by the insurance carrier (paid, suspended, rejected, or denied),

   a document known as a/an ____________________
   is sent to the patient and to the provider of professional medical services.

3. Name other items that indicate the patient's responsibility to pay that may appear on the document explaining the payment and check issued by the insurance carrier.

   a. ____________________

   b. ____________________

   c. ____________________

   d. ____________________

   e. ____________________

   f. ____________________

4. After receiving an explanation of benefits (EOB) document and posting insurance payment, the copy of the

   insurance claim form is put into a file marked ____________________.

5. To locate delinquent insurance claims on an insurance claims register quickly, which column should be looked at first?

   ____

   Would it appear blank or completed? ____________________

6. Name some of the principal procedures that should be followed in good bookkeeping and record-keeping practice when a payment has been received from an insurance company.

   ____

   ____

   ____

7. In good office management, a manual method used to track submitted pending or resubmitted insurance claims, a/an ______________________________ is used.

8. Two procedures to include in a manual reminder system to track pending claims are:

   a. ______________________________

   b. ______________________________

9. In making an inquiry about a claim by telephone, efficient secretarial procedure would be to ______________________________

   ____

   ______________________________.

10. Denied paper or electronic claims are those denied because of ______________________________

    or ______________________________.

11. State the solution if a claim has been denied because the professional service rendered was for an injury that is being considered as compensable under workers' compensation.

    ____

    ____

    ____

12. At the time of his first office visit, Mr. Doi signed an Assignment of Benefits, and Dr. James' office submitted a claim to ABC Insurance Company. Mr. Doi received, in error, a check from the insurance company and cashed it. What steps should be taken by Dr. James' office after this error is discovered?

    a. ______________________________

    b. ______________________________

    c. ______________________________

13. If an appeal of an insurance claim is not successful, the next step to proceed with is a/an ______________________________.

14. Name the five levels for appealing a Medicare claim.

a. ______

b. ______

c. ______

d. ______

e. ______

15. Medicare reconsideration by the insurance carrier is usually completed

within ______ to ______ days.

16. A Medicare patient has insurance with United American (a Medigap policy), and payment has not been received from the Medigap insurer within a reasonable length of time. State the action to take in this case.

______

______

______

17. A TRICARE EOB is received stating that the allowable charge for Mrs. Dayton's office visit is $30. Is it possible to appeal this for additional payment? Answer "yes" or "no," and explain.

______

______

18. A state department or agency that helps resolve complaints about insurance policies, medical claims, or insurance agents or brokers and that verifies that insurance contracts are carried out in good faith is known as a/an

______.

19. When an insurance company consistently pays slowly on insurance claims, it may help speed up payments if a formal written complaint is made to the

______.

Part II Multiple Choice

Choose the best answer.

20. If the insurance carrier is a self-insured plan, a Medicaid or Medicare health maintenance organization, or an Employee Retirement Income Security Act (ERISA)–based plan, the insurance commissioner

    a. is able to assist with carrier issues

    b. is not able to assist with carrier issues

    c. is able to assist on specific problem issues related to payment

    d. is able to give help on denied insurance claims

21. A written request made to an insurance company to locate the status of an insurance claim is often referred to as

    a. inquiry

    b. follow-up

    c. tracer

    d. all of the above

22. An insurance claim transmitted to the third-party payer that is rejected because it contains a technical error, such as missing the insured's birth date, is also known as a/an

    a. soft denial

    b. suspended claim

    c. delinquent claim

    d. downcoded claim

23. When an electronic claim is transmitted for several services and one service is rejected for incomplete information, the solution is to

    a. resubmit a paper claim with the needed data for the rejected services only

    b. add the required information in Field 19 that it is a retransmission

    c. add the required information and retransmit the rejected claim

    d. not retransmit a rejected claim

24. A request for payment to a third-party payer asking for a review of an insurance claim that has been denied is referred to as a/an

    a. review

    b. appeal

    c. request

    d. demand

Part III True/False

Write "T" or "F" in the blank to indicate whether you think the statement is true or false.

_______ 25. If the provider has no contract with the insurance carrier, the provider is not obligated to the carrier's deadline.

_______ 26. A patient should be asked to sign an Advance Beneficiary Notice if he or she has decided to undergo plastic surgery that is not related to a medical condition.

_______ 27. An *overpayment* is receipt of less than the contract rate from a managed care plan for a patient who has received medical services.

_______ 28. In the Medicare reconsideration Level 2 process, the request must be within 9 months from the date of the original determination shown on the remittance advice.

_______ 29. A decision to appeal a claim should be based on whether there is sufficient data to back up the claim and if there is a large amount of money in question.

ASSIGNMENT 9-2 ▶ CRITICAL THINKING: LOCATE AND EXPLAIN CHOICE OF DIAGNOSTIC CODES

Performance Objective

Task: Locate the correct diagnostic code for the case scenario presented.

Conditions: Use a pen or pencil and the *International Classification of Diagnoses, Ninth Revision, Clinical Modification* (ICD-9-CM) diagnostic code book.

Standards: Time: ______________ minutes

Accuracy: ______________

(Note: The time element and accuracy criteria may be given by your instructor.)

Directions: Using your critical thinking skills, answer the following questions after reading the scenario. Record your answer on the blank lines. These questions are presented to enhance your skill in critical thinking.

Scenario: Using your diagnostic code book, look up the ICD-9-CM diagnostic code for a patient being treated for bacillary dysentery. How would you code this case and why?

1. Locate the main term or condition in the Alphabetic Index, Volume 2. What is the main term or condition? ______________
2. Refer to any notes under the main term. What is the subterm? ______________
3. Read any notes or terms enclosed in parentheses after the main term. What is the code number listed after the main term and subterm? ______________
4. What is the appropriate subterm after that? ______________
5. Look for the appropriate sub-subterm and follow any cross-reference instructions. What does it say?

   ____

   ____
6. What is the generic code? ______________
7. Verify the code number in the Tabular List, Volume 1, and list it here. ______________
8. Read and be guided by any instructional terms in the Tabular List. It reads: ______________
9. Read the complete description and then code to the highest specificity. (Assign the code and write it here.) ______________
10. Write justification of chosen code(s). ____

    ____

ASSIGNMENT 9-3 ▶ POST TO A FINANCIAL ACCOUNTING RECORD (LEDGER) FROM AN EXPLANATION OF BENEFITS DOCUMENT

Performance Objective

Task: Post data from an EOB document to a patient's financial accounting record (ledger).

Conditions: Use a blank financial accounting record (ledger) (Figure 9-1), an EOB document (Figure 9-2), and a pen or computer.

Standards: Time: ____________________ minutes

Accuracy: ____________________

(Note: The time element and accuracy criteria may be given by your instructor.)

Directions: Post in ink the payment received and preferred provider organization (PPO) adjustment to a patient's financial accounting record (ledger) (see Figure 9-1) by referring to an EOB document (see Figure 9-2). An example of financial accounting record (ledger) entries is shown in Figure 3-14 in the *Handbook*. An EOB document is defined in Figure 9-1 in the *Handbook*.

After the instructor has returned your work to you, either make the necessary corrections and place your work in a three-ring notebook for future reference or, if you received a high score, place it in your portfolio for reference when applying for a job.

1. Locate patient's financial accounting record (ledger) and EOB.

   Note: Refer to the step-by-step procedures at the end of Chapter 3 in the Handbook and graphic examples in Figures 3-14 and 10-3.

2. Ledger lines 6 and 7: Insert date of service (DOS), reference (CPT code number, check number, or dates of service for posting adjustments or when insurance was billed), description of the transaction, charge amounts, payments, adjustments, and running current balance. The posting date is the actual date the transaction is recorded. If the DOS differs from the posting date, list the DOS in the reference or description column.

   Note: A good bookkeeping practice is to take a red pen and draw a line across the financial accounting record (ledger) from left to right to indicate the last entry billed to the insurance company.

Acct No. 9-3

STATEMENT
Financial Account
COLLEGE CLINIC
4567 Broad Avenue
Woodland Hills, XY 12345-0001
Tel. 555-486-9002
Fax No. 555-487-8976

Mr. Jabe Bortolussi
989 Moorpark Road
Woodland Hills, XY 12345

Phone No. (H) (555) 230-8870 (W) (555) 349-6689 Birthdate 04-07-71

Primary Insurance Co. ABC Insurance Company Policy/Group No. 4206/010

DATE	REFERENCE	DESCRIPTION	CHARGES		CREDITS PYMNTS.		CREDITS ADJ.		BALANCE	
	BALANCE FORWARD →									
6-3-xx	99204	E/M NP Level 4	250	00					250	00
6-3-xx	94375	Respiratory flow vol loop	40	00					290	00
6-3-xx	94060	Spirometry	75	00					365	00
6-3-xx	94664	Aerosol inhalation	50	00					415	00
6-3-xx	94760	Pulse oximetry	50	00					465	00

PLEASE PAY LAST AMOUNT IN BALANCE COLUMN

THIS IS A COPY OF YOUR FINANCIAL ACCOUNT AS IT APPEARS ON OUR RECORDS

Figure 9-1

ABC Insurance Company
P.O. Box 4300
Woodland Hills, XY 12345-0001

Claim No.:	1-00-16987087-00-zmm
Group Name:	COLLEGE CLINIC
Group No.:	010
Employee:	JABE V. BORTOLUSSI
Patient:	JABE V. BORTOLUSSI
SSN:	554-XX-8876
Plan No.:	4206
Prepared by:	M. SMITH
Prepared on:	07/04/20XX

GERALD PRACTON MD
4567 BROAD AVENUE
WOODLAND HILLS XY 12345

Patient Responsibility	
Amount not covered:	00
Co-pay amount:	00
Deductible:	00
Co-insurance:	64.61
Patient's total responsibility:	64.61
Other insurance payment:	00

EXPLANATION OF BENEFITS

Treatment Dates	Service Code	CPT Code	Charge Amount	Not Covered	Reason Code	PPO Discount	Covered Amount	Deductible Amount	Co-pay Amount	Paid At	Payment Amount
06/03/xx	200	99204	250.00	00	48	136.00	114.00	00	00	80%	91.20
06/03/xx	540	94375	40.00	00	48	00	40.00	00	00	80%	32.00
06/03/xx	540	94060	75.00	00	48	00	75.00	00	00	80%	60.00
06/03/xx	200	94664	50.00	00	48	1.55	48.45	00	00	80%	38.76
06/03/xx	540	94760	50.00	00	48	4.40	45.60	00	00	80%	36.48
		TOTAL	465.00	00		141.95	323.05	00	00		258.44

Other Insurance Credits or Adjustments 00

Total Payment Amount 258.44

CPT Code
99204 OFFICE/OUTPT VISIT E&M NEW MOD-HI SEVERIT
94375 RESPIRATORY FLOW VOLUM LOOP
94060 BRONCHOSPSM EVAL SPIROM PRE & POST BRON
94664 AEROSOL/VAPOR INHALA; INIT DEMO & EVAL
94760 NONINVASIVE EAR/PULSE OXIMETRY-02 SAT

Reason Code
48 CON DISCOUNT/PT NOT RESPONSIBLE

Participant		Date
GERALD PRACTON MD		07-04-xx
Patient		ID Number
JABE V. BORTOLUSSI		554-XX-8876
Plan Number	Patient Number	Office No.
4206		010

GC 1234567890

258.44

PAY TO THE ORDER OF

COLLEGE CLINIC
4567 BROAD AVENUE
WOODLAND HILLS XY 12345

J M Smith
ABC Insurance Company

Figure 9-2

ASSIGNMENT 9-4 ▶ TRACE AN UNPAID INSURANCE CLAIM

Performance Objective

Task: Complete an insurance claim tracer form and attach to this document a photocopy of the claim.

Conditions: Use an Insurance Claim Tracer form (Figure 9-3), an insurance claim form from the *Handbook* (Figure 7-3), and a computer.

Standards: Time: ________________________ minutes

Accuracy: ________________________

(Note: The time element and accuracy criteria may be given by your instructor.)

Directions: You discover that the insurance claim you submitted to Blue Shield, 146 Main Street, Woodland Hills, XY 12345, on Harry N. Forehand 3 months ago was never paid. Complete an insurance claim tracer form (see Figure 9-3). Make a photocopy of Harry Forehand's insurance claim form from the *Handbook* in Chapter 7 to attach to the tracer form. Mr. Forehand's employer is Acme Electrical Company at 450 South Orange Street, Woodland Hills, XY 12345. Place your name on the tracer form as the person to contact at Dr. Antrum's office.

After the instructor has returned your work to you, either make the necessary corrections and place your work in a three-ring notebook for future reference or, if you received a high score, place it in your portfolio for reference when applying for a job.

COLLEGE CLINIC
4567 Broad Avenue
Woodland Hills, XY 12345-0001
Telephone (555) 486-9002
Fax (555) 487-8976

INSURANCE CLAIM TRACER

INSURANCE COMPANY NAME ______________________ DATE: ______________.

ADDRESS ____.

Patient name: ______________________

Date of birth: ______________________

Employer: ______________________

Insured: ______________________

Policy/certificate No. ______________________

Group name/No. ______________________

Date of initial claim submission: ______________________

Date(s) of service: ______________________

Total charges submitted: ______________________

An inordinate amount of time has passed since submission of our original claim. We have not received a request for additional information and still await payment of this assigned claim. Please review the attached duplicate and process for payment within 7 days.

DETAILS OF INQUIRY

Please check the claim status and return this letter to our office. Thank you.

- ☐ No record of claim.
- ☐ Claim received and payment is in process.
- ☐ Claim is in suspense (comment please).
- ☐ Claim is in review (comment please).
- ☐ Additional information needed (comment please).
- ☐ Applied to deductible. Amount: $ ________
- ☐ Patient not eligible for benefits.
- ☐ Determination issued to beneficiary.
- ☐ Claim paid. Date: ______ Amount: $ _______ To whom: ______________________
- ☐ Claim denied (comment please).

Comments: ____

____

Thank you for your assistance in this important matter. Please contact the insurance specialist named below if you have any questions regarding this claim.

Insurance Specialist: ______________________ (555) 486-9002 Ext. ____________.

Treating Physician: ______________________ State license number ____________.

Provider Number: ______________________ Provider's IRS number ____________.

Figure 9-3

ASSIGNMENT 9-5 ▶ LOCATE ERRORS ON A RETURNED INSURANCE CLAIM

Performance Objective

Task: Highlight the blocks on the insurance claim form where errors are discovered.

Conditions: Use an insurance claim form (Figure 9-4) and a highlighter or red pen.

Standards: Time: ______________________ minutes

Accuracy: ______________________

(Note: The time element and accuracy criteria may be given by your instructor.)

Directions: An insurance claim (see Figure 9-4) was returned by the Prudential Insurance Company. Highlight or circle in red all blocks on the claim form where errors are discovered.

Option 1: Retype the claim and either insert the correction if data are available to fix the error or insert the word "NEED" in the block of the claim form.

Option 2: On a separate sheet of paper, list the blocks from 1 to 33 and state where errors occur.

A Performance Evaluation Checklist may be reproduced from the "Instruction Guide to the Workbook" chapter if your instructor wishes you to submit it to assist with scoring and comments.

After the instructor has returned your work to you, either make the necessary corrections and place your work in a three-ring notebook for future reference or, if you received a high score, place it in your portfolio for reference when applying for a job.

PRUDENTIAL INSURANCE COMPANY
500 SOUTH BEND STREET
WOODLAND HILLS XY 12345

CARRIER

1500

HEALTH INSURANCE CLAIM FORM

APPROVED BY NATIONAL UNIFORM CLAIM COMMITTEE 08/05

PICA | PICA

1. MEDICARE (Medicare #) | MEDICAID (Medicaid #) | TRICARE CHAMPUS (Sponsor's SSN) | CHAMPVA (Member ID#) | GROUP HEALTH PLAN (SSN or ID) | FECA BLK LUNG (SSN) | OTHER [X] (ID)

1a. INSURED'S I.D. NUMBER (For Program in Item 1)

2. PATIENT'S NAME (Last Name, First Name, Middle Initial): JOHNSON EMILY B.

3. PATIENT'S BIRTH DATE MM DD YY: 02 12 1963 SEX M [ ] F [ ]

4. INSURED'S NAME (Last Name, First Name, Middle Initial): JOHNSON ERRON T.

5. PATIENT'S ADDRESS (No., Street): 4391 EVERETT STREET

CITY: WOODLAND HILLS STATE: XY

ZIP CODE: 12345 TELEPHONE (Include Area Code): ( )

6. PATIENT RELATIONSHIP TO INSURED: Self [ ] Spouse [X] Child [ ] Other [ ]

7. INSURED'S ADDRESS (No., Street): SAME

CITY STATE

ZIP CODE TELEPHONE (INCLUDE AREA CODE) ( )

8. PATIENT STATUS: Single [ ] Married [X] Other [ ]
Employed [ ] Full-Time Student [ ] Part-Time Student [ ]

9. OTHER INSURED'S NAME (Last Name, First Name, Middle Initial)

a. OTHER INSURED'S POLICY OR GROUP NUMBER

b. OTHER INSURED'S DATE OF BIRTH MM DD YY SEX M [ ] F [ ]

c. EMPLOYER'S NAME OR SCHOOL NAME

d. INSURANCE PLAN NAME OR PROGRAM NAME

10. IS PATIENT'S CONDITION RELATED TO:
a. EMPLOYMENT? (CURRENT OR PREVIOUS) [ ] YES [ ] NO
b. AUTO ACCIDENT? [ ] YES [ ] NO PLACE (State)
c. OTHER ACCIDENT? [ ] YES [ ] NO
10d. RESERVED FOR LOCAL USE

11. INSURED'S POLICY GROUP OR FECA NUMBER
a. INSURED'S DATE OF BIRTH MM DD YY SEX M [ ] F [ ]
b. EMPLOYER'S NAME OR SCHOOL NAME
c. INSURANCE PLAN NAME OR PROGRAM NAME
d. IS THERE ANOTHER HEALTH BENEFIT PLAN? [ ] YES [X] NO *If yes*, return to and complete item 9 a-d.

PATIENT AND INSURED INFORMATION

READ BACK OF FORM BEFORE COMPLETING & SIGNING THIS FORM.

12. PATIENT'S OR AUTHORIZED PERSON'S SIGNATURE I authorize the release of any medical or other information necessary to process this claim. I also request payment of government benefits either to myself or to the party who accepts assignment below.

SIGNED *Emily B. Johnson* DATE 1/4/2020

13. INSURED'S OR AUTHORIZED PERSON'S SIGNATURE I authorize payment of medical benefits to the undersigned physician or supplier for services described below.

SIGNED *Emily B. Johnson*

14. DATE OF CURRENT: MM DD YY ILLNESS (First symptom) OR INJURY (Accident) OR PREGNANCY(LMP)

15. IF PATIENT HAS HAD SAME OR SIMILAR ILLNESS. GIVE FIRST DATE MM DD YY

16. DATES PATIENT UNABLE TO WORK IN CURRENT OCCUPATION FROM MM DD YY TO MM DD YY

17. NAME OF REFERRING PHYSICIAN OR OTHER SOURCE 17a. 17b. NPI 67805027XX

18. HOSPITALIZATION DATES RELATED TO CURRENT SERVICES FROM MM DD YY TO MM DD YY

19. RESERVED FOR LOCAL USE

20. OUTSIDE LAB? [ ] YES [X] NO $ CHARGES

21. DIAGNOSIS OR NATURE OF ILLNESS OR INJURY. (RELATE ITEMS 1,2,3 OR 4 TO ITEM 24E BY LINE)
1. ___ . __ 3. ___ . __
2. ___ . __ 4. ___ . __

22. MEDICAID RESUBMISSION CODE ORIGINAL REF. NO.

23. PRIOR AUTHORIZATION NUMBER

	24. A. DATE(S) OF SERVICE From MM DD YY	To MM DD YY	B. PLACE OF SERVICE	C. EMG	D. PROCEDURES, SERVICES, OR SUPPLIES (Explain Unusual Circumstances) CPT/HCPCS	MODIFIER	E. DIAGNOSIS POINTER	F. $ CHARGES	G. DAYS OR UNITS	H. EPSDT Family Plan	I. ID. QUAL.	J. RENDERING PROVIDER ID. #
1	01 04 20XX		11		99213		1	25 00	1		NPI	705687717XX
2	01 04 20XX		11		99213		1	25 00			NPI	
3											NPI	
4											NPI	
5											NPI	
6											NPI	

PHYSICIAN OR SUPPLIER INFORMATION

25. FEDERAL TAX I.D. NUMBER SSN EIN: 7180561XX

26. PATIENT'S ACCOUNT NO.: 9

27. ACCEPT ASSIGNMENT? (For govt. claims, see back) [X] YES [ ] NO

28. TOTAL CHARGE $ 60 00

29. AMOUNT PAID $

30. BALANCE DUE $ 60 00

31. SIGNATURE OF PHYSICIAN OR SUPPLIER INCLUDING DEGREES OR CREDENTIALS (I certify that the statements on the reverse apply to this bill and are made a part thereof.)

Vera Cutis, MD 01/06/20XX
SIGNED DATE

32. SERVICE FACILITY LOCATION INFORMATION
a. NPI b.

33. BILLING PROVIDER INFO & PH # (555) 4869002
COLLEGE CLINIC
4567 BROAD AVENUE
WOODLAND HILLS XY 12345
a. 3664021XX NPI b.

NUCC Instruction Manual available at: www.nucc.org **PLEASE PRINT OR TYPE** APPROVED OMB-0938-0999 FORM CMS-1500 (08-05)

Figure 9-4

ASSIGNMENT 9-6 ▶ LOCATE ERRORS ON A RETURNED INSURANCE CLAIM

Performance Objective

Task: Highlight the blocks on the insurance claim form where errors are discovered.

Conditions: Use an insurance claim form (Figure 9-5) and a highlighter or red pen.

Standards: Time: ______________________ minutes

Accuracy: ______________________

(Note: The time element and accuracy criteria may be given by your instructor.)

Directions: An insurance claim was returned by the Healthtech Insurance Company. Highlight or circle in red all blocks on the claim form where errors are discovered.

Option 1: Retype the claim and either insert the correction if data are available to fix the error or insert the word "NEED" in the block of the claim form.

Option 2: On a separate sheet of paper, list the blocks from 1 to 33 and state where errors occur.

A Performance Evaluation Checklist may be reproduced from the "Instruction Guide to the Workbook" chapter if your instructor wishes you to submit it to assist with scoring and comments.

After the instructor has returned your work to you, either make the necessary corrections and place your work in a three-ring notebook for future reference or, if you received a high score, place it in your portfolio for reference when applying for a job.

1500

HEALTH INSURANCE CLAIM FORM

APPROVED BY NATIONAL UNIFORM CLAIM COMMITTEE 08/05

HEALTHTECH INSURANCE COMPANY
4821 WEST LAKE AVENUE
WOODLAND HILLS XY 12345

CARRIER

PICA PICA

1. MEDICARE (Medicare #) MEDICAID [X] (Medicaid #) TRICARE CHAMPUS [X] (Sponsor's SSN) CHAMPVA (Member ID#) GROUP HEALTH PLAN (SSN or ID) FECA BLK LUNG (SSN) OTHER [X] (ID)

1a. INSURED'S I.D. NUMBER (For Program in Item 1): 433 12 9870ANC

2. PATIENT'S NAME (Last Name, First Name, Middle Initial): DUGAN CHARLES C

3. PATIENT'S BIRTH DATE MM DD YY: 12 24 1968 SEX M [X] F

4. INSURED'S NAME (Last Name, First Name, Middle Initial): SAME

5. PATIENT'S ADDRESS (No., Street): 5900 ELM STREET

6. PATIENT RELATIONSHIP TO INSURED: Self [X] Spouse Child Other

7. INSURED'S ADDRESS (No., Street): SAME

CITY: WOODLAND HILLS STATE: XY

8. PATIENT STATUS: Single Married [X] Other

CITY STATE

ZIP CODE: 12345 TELEPHONE (Include Area Code): (555) 559 3300

Employed Full-Time Student Part-Time Student

ZIP CODE TELEPHONE (INCLUDE AREA CODE) ( )

9. OTHER INSURED'S NAME (Last Name, First Name, Middle Initial)

10. IS PATIENT'S CONDITION RELATED TO:

11. INSURED'S POLICY GROUP OR FECA NUMBER

a. OTHER INSURED'S POLICY OR GROUP NUMBER

a. EMPLOYMENT? (CURRENT OR PREVIOUS) YES [X] NO

a. INSURED'S DATE OF BIRTH MM DD YY SEX M F

b. OTHER INSURED'S DATE OF BIRTH MM DD YY SEX M F

b. AUTO ACCIDENT? YES [X] NO PLACE (State)

b. EMPLOYER'S NAME OR SCHOOL NAME

c. EMPLOYER'S NAME OR SCHOOL NAME

c. OTHER ACCIDENT? YES [X] NO

c. INSURANCE PLAN NAME OR PROGRAM NAME

d. INSURANCE PLAN NAME OR PROGRAM NAME

10d. RESERVED FOR LOCAL USE

d. IS THERE ANOTHER HEALTH BENEFIT PLAN? YES NO *If yes*, return to and complete item 9 a-d.

PATIENT AND INSURED INFORMATION

READ BACK OF FORM BEFORE COMPLETING & SIGNING THIS FORM.

12. PATIENT'S OR AUTHORIZED PERSON'S SIGNATURE I authorize the release of any medical or other information necessary to process this claim. I also request payment of government benefits either to myself or to the party who accepts assignment below.

SIGNED ______ DATE ______

13. INSURED'S OR AUTHORIZED PERSON'S SIGNATURE I authorize payment of medical benefits to the undersigned physician or supplier for services described below.

SIGNED ______

14. DATE OF CURRENT: MM DD YY ILLNESS (First symptom) OR INJURY (Accident) OR PREGNANCY(LMP)

15. IF PATIENT HAS HAD SAME OR SIMILAR ILLNESS. GIVE FIRST DATE MM DD YY

16. DATES PATIENT UNABLE TO WORK IN CURRENT OCCUPATION FROM MM DD YY TO MM DD YY

17. NAME OF REFERRING PHYSICIAN OR OTHER SOURCE

17a.

17b. NPI 67805027XX

18. HOSPITALIZATION DATES RELATED TO CURRENT SERVICES FROM MM DD YY TO MM DD YY

19. RESERVED FOR LOCAL USE

20. OUTSIDE LAB? YES [X] NO $ CHARGES

21. DIAGNOSIS OR NATURE OF ILLNESS OR INJURY. (RELATE ITEMS 1,2,3 OR 4 TO ITEM 24E BY LINE)

1. 881 00
2. ___ . __
3. ___ . __
4. ___ . __

22. MEDICAID RESUBMISSION CODE ORIGINAL REF. NO.

23. PRIOR AUTHORIZATION NUMBER

	24. A. DATE(S) OF SERVICE From MM DD YY	To MM DD YY	B. PLACE OF SERVICE	C. EMG	D. PROCEDURES, SERVICES, OR SUPPLIES (Explain Unusual Circumstances) CPT/HCPCS	MODIFIER	E. DIAGNOSIS POINTER	F. $ CHARGES	G. DAYS OR UNITS	H. EPSDT Family Plan	I. ID. QUAL.	J. RENDERING PROVIDER ID. #
1	09 55 20XX		11		99203		1	70 92	1		NPI	46278897XX
2	09 55 20XX		11		12001		1				NPI	46278897XX
3											NPI	
4											NPI	
5											NPI	
6											NPI	

PHYSICIAN OR SUPPLIER INFORMATION

25. FEDERAL TAX I.D. NUMBER SSN EIN [X]: 7034597XX

26. PATIENT'S ACCOUNT NO.: 9

27. ACCEPT ASSIGNMENT? (For govt. claims, see back) [X] YES NO

28. TOTAL CHARGE $

29. AMOUNT PAID $

30. BALANCE DUE $

31. SIGNATURE OF PHYSICIAN OR SUPPLIER INCLUDING DEGREES OR CREDENTIALS (I certify that the statements on the reverse apply to this bill and are made a part thereof.)

Gerald Practon, MD 09/30/20XX

SIGNED DATE

32. SERVICE FACILITY LOCATION INFORMATION
COLLEGE HOSPITAL
4500 BROAD AVENUE
WOODLAND HILLS XY 12345
a. 937310XX NPI b.

33. BILLING PROVIDER INFO & PH # (555) 4869002
COLLEGE CLINIC
4567 BROAD AVENUE
WOODLAND HILLS XY 12345 0001
a. 3664021XX NPI b.

NUCC Instruction Manual available at: www.nucc.org **PLEASE PRINT OR TYPE** APPROVED OMB-0938-0999 FORM CMS-1500 (08-05)

Figure 9-5

ASSIGNMENT 9-7 ▶ LOCATE ERRORS ON A RETURNED INSURANCE CLAIM

Performance Objective

Task: Highlight the blocks on the insurance claim form where errors are discovered.

Conditions: Use an insurance claim form (Figure 9-6) and a highlighter or red pen.

Standards: Time: ______________________ minutes

Accuracy: ______________________

(Note: The time element and accuracy criteria may be given by your instructor.)

Directions: An insurance claim (see Figure 9-6) was returned by an insurance plan. Highlight or circle in red all blocks on the claim form where errors are discovered.

Option 1: Retype the claim and either insert the correction if data are available to fix the error or insert the word "NEED" in the block of the claim form.

Option 2: On a separate sheet of paper, list the blocks from 1 to 33 and state where errors occur.

A Performance Evaluation Checklist may be reproduced from the "Instruction Guide to the Workbook" chapter if your instructor wishes you to submit it to assist with scoring and comments.

After the instructor has returned your work to you, either make the necessary corrections and place your work in a three-ring notebook for future reference or, if you received a high score, place it in your portfolio for reference when applying for a job.

AMERICAN INSURANCE COMPANY
509 MAIN STREET
WOODLAND HILLS XY 12345

CARRIER

1500

HEALTH INSURANCE CLAIM FORM

APPROVED BY NATIONAL UNIFORM CLAIM COMMITTEE 08/05

PICA PICA

1. MEDICARE (Medicare #) MEDICAID (Medicaid #) TRICARE CHAMPUS (Sponsor's SSN) CHAMPVA (Member ID#) GROUP HEALTH PLAN (SSN or ID) FECA BLK LUNG (SSN) OTHER [X] (ID)

1a. INSURED'S I.D. NUMBER (For Program in Item 1)

2. PATIENT'S NAME (Last Name, First Name, Middle Initial): MARY T AVERY

3. PATIENT'S BIRTH DATE MM DD YY: 05 07 1980 SEX M [ ] F [ ]

4. INSURED'S NAME (Last Name, First Name, Middle Initial): SAME

5. PATIENT'S ADDRESS (No., Street): 4309 MAIN STREET

6. PATIENT RELATIONSHIP TO INSURED: Self [X] Spouse [ ] Child [ ] Other [ ]

7. INSURED'S ADDRESS (No., Street)

CITY: WOODLAND HILLS STATE: XY

8. PATIENT STATUS: Single [ ] Married [ ] Other [ ]; Employed [ ] Full-Time Student [ ] Part-Time Student [ ]

CITY STATE

ZIP CODE: 12345 TELEPHONE (Include Area Code): (555) 450-9899

ZIP CODE TELEPHONE (INCLUDE AREA CODE) ( )

9. OTHER INSURED'S NAME (Last Name, First Name, Middle Initial)

10. IS PATIENT'S CONDITION RELATED TO:

11. INSURED'S POLICY GROUP OR FECA NUMBER

a. OTHER INSURED'S POLICY OR GROUP NUMBER

a. EMPLOYMENT? (CURRENT OR PREVIOUS) [ ] YES [X] NO

a. INSURED'S DATE OF BIRTH MM DD YY SEX M [ ] F [ ]

b. OTHER INSURED'S DATE OF BIRTH MM DD YY SEX M [ ] F [ ]

b. AUTO ACCIDENT? [ ] YES [X] NO PLACE (State)

b. EMPLOYER'S NAME OR SCHOOL NAME

c. EMPLOYER'S NAME OR SCHOOL NAME

c. OTHER ACCIDENT? [ ] YES [X] NO

c. INSURANCE PLAN NAME OR PROGRAM NAME

d. INSURANCE PLAN NAME OR PROGRAM NAME

10d. RESERVED FOR LOCAL USE

d. IS THERE ANOTHER HEALTH BENEFIT PLAN? [ ] YES [ ] NO *If yes*, return to and complete item 9 a-d.

READ BACK OF FORM BEFORE COMPLETING & SIGNING THIS FORM.

12. PATIENT'S OR AUTHORIZED PERSON'S SIGNATURE I authorize the release of any medical or other information necessary to process this claim. I also request payment of government benefits either to myself or to the party who accepts assignment below.

SIGNED Mary T. Avery DATE 11/20/2007

13. INSURED'S OR AUTHORIZED PERSON'S SIGNATURE I authorize payment of medical benefits to the undersigned physician or supplier for services described below.

SIGNED Mary T. Avery

PATIENT AND INSURED INFORMATION

14. DATE OF CURRENT: MM DD YY ILLNESS (First symptom) OR INJURY (Accident) OR PREGNANCY(LMP)

15. IF PATIENT HAS HAD SAME OR SIMILAR ILLNESS. GIVE FIRST DATE MM DD YY

16. DATES PATIENT UNABLE TO WORK IN CURRENT OCCUPATION FROM 11 09 20XX TO 11 30 20XX

17. NAME OF REFERRING PHYSICIAN OR OTHER SOURCE: GERALD PRACTON MD 17a. 17b. NPI

18. HOSPITALIZATION DATES RELATED TO CURRENT SERVICES FROM 11 11 20XX TO 11 12 20XX

19. RESERVED FOR LOCAL USE

20. OUTSIDE LAB? [ ] YES [X] NO $ CHARGES

21. DIAGNOSIS OR NATURE OF ILLNESS OR INJURY. (RELATE ITEMS 1,2,3 OR 4 TO ITEM 24E BY LINE)

1. 463 . 3. . 2. . 4. .

22. MEDICAID RESUBMISSION CODE ORIGINAL REF. NO.

23. PRIOR AUTHORIZATION NUMBER

	24. A. DATE(S) OF SERVICE From MM DD YY	To MM DD YY	B. PLACE OF SERVICE	C. EMG	D. PROCEDURES, SERVICES, OR SUPPLIES CPT/HCPCS	MODIFIER	E. DIAGNOSIS POINTER	F. $ CHARGES	G. DAYS OR UNITS	H. EPSDT Family Plan	I. ID. QUAL.	J. RENDERING PROVIDER ID. #
1	11 10 20XX		11		99203		1	50 00			NPI	43050047XX
2	11 11 20XX		21		99222		1	120 80			NPI	43050047XX
3	11 11 20XX		21		42821		1	410 73			NPI	43050047XX
4	11 22 20XX		21		99231		1	20 00			NPI	
5											NPI	
6											NPI	

PHYSICIAN OR SUPPLIER INFORMATION

25. FEDERAL TAX I.D. NUMBER: 715737291XX SSN [ ] EIN [X]

26. PATIENT'S ACCOUNT NO.

27. ACCEPT ASSIGNMENT? (For govt. claims, see back) [ ] YES [ ] NO

28. TOTAL CHARGE $ 29. AMOUNT PAID $ 30. BALANCE DUE $

31. SIGNATURE OF PHYSICIAN OR SUPPLIER INCLUDING DEGREES OR CREDENTIALS (I certify that the statements on the reverse apply to this bill and are made a part thereof.)

SIGNED DATE 11/15/20XX

32. SERVICE FACILITY LOCATION INFORMATION
COLLEGE HOSPITAL
4500 BROAD AVENUE
WOODLAND HILLS XY 12345
a. 9507310XX NPI b.

33. BILLING PROVIDER INFO & PH # (555) 4869002
COLLEGE CLINIC
4567 BROAD AVENUE
WOODLAND HILLS XY 12345
a. 3664021XX NPI b.

NUCC Instruction Manual available at: www.nucc.org **_PLEASE PRINT OR TYPE_** APPROVED OMB-0938-0999 FORM CMS-1500 (08-05)

Figure 9-6

ASSIGNMENT 9-8 ▶ REQUEST FOR MEDICARE HEARING BY AN ADMINISTRATIVE LAW JUDGE

Performance Objective

Task: Insert information on a Request for Medicare Hearing by an Administrative Law Judge CMS-5011 A/B form.

Conditions: Request for Medicare Hearing by an Administrative Law Judge CMS-5011 A/B form (Figure 9-7), and a computer with a printer.

Standards: Time: ________________________ minutes

Accuracy: ________________________

(Note: The time element and accuracy criteria may be given by your instructor.)

Directions: After Medicare processes the tracer on the insurance claim for Bill Hutch, you receive a Medicare EOB and payment check, but the amount is incorrect because of an excessive reduction in the allowed payment. An appeal was made in September and denied; the document control number assigned by Medicare Blue Shield is 240-577-9008. Dr. Brady Coccidioides believes that a mistake has been made and wishes to request a hearing.

Complete the Request for Medicare Hearing by an Administrative Law Judge CMS-5011 A/B form for this case (see Figure 9-7) by referring to the tracer form (Figure 9-8) and Figure 7-6 in the *Handbook*. Mr. Hutch's e-mail address is bhutch@gmail.net. Complete the form as the appellant and do not fill in the representative's portion. As you will learn in the chapter on Medicare, the Health Insurance Claim Number is the patient's Medicare identification number as shown in Figure 7-6, Block 1a. No additional evidence is to be presented, and the doctor does not wish to appear for the hearing. Date the form December 5, 20xx. The beneficiary has assigned his appeal rights to the provider.

After the instructor has returned your work to you, either make the necessary corrections and place your work in a three-ring notebook for future reference or, if you received a high score, place it in your portfolio for reference when applying for a job.

DEPARTMENT OF HEALTH AND HUMAN SERVICES
OFFICE OF MEDICARE HEARINGS AND APPEALS

REQUEST FOR MEDICARE HEARING BY AN ADMINISTRATIVE LAW JUDGE

Effective July 1, 2005. For use by party to a reconsideration/fair hearing determination issued by a Fiscal Intermediary (FI), Carrier, or Quality Improvement Organization (QIO)
(Amount in controversy must be $100 or more.)

❑ **Part A**
❑ **Part B**

Send copies of this completed form to:
Original *— The FI, Carrier, or QIO that issued the Reconsideration/Fair Hearing Notice*
Copy *— Appellant*

Appellant *(The party appealing the reconsideration determination)*

Beneficiary *(Leave blank if same as the appellant.)*	Provider or Supplier *(Leave blank if same as the appellant.)*
Address	Address
City / State / Zip Code	City / State / Zip Code
Area Code/Telephone Number / E-mail Address	Area Code/Telephone Number / E-mail Address
Health Insurance (Medicare) Claim Number	Document control number assigned by the FI, Carrier, or QIO

FI, Carrier, or QIO that made the reconsideration/fair hearing determination | Dates of Service From | To

I DISAGREE WITH THE DETERMINATION MADE ON MY APPEAL BECAUSE:

____

____

You have a right to be represented at the hearing. If you are not represented but would like to be, your Office of Medicare Hearings and Appeals Field Office will give you a list of legal referral and service organizations. *(If you are represented and have not already done so, complete form CMS-1696.)*

Check **Only One** Statement:
- ❑ I **wish** to have a hearing.
- ❑ I **do not wish** to have a hearing and I request that a decision be made on the basis of the evidence in my case. *(Complete form HHS-723, "Waiver of Right to an ALJ Hearing.")*

Check **Only One** Statement:
- ❑ I **have** additional evidence to submit.
- ❑ I **have no** additional evidence to submit.

The appellant should complete No. 1 and the representative, if any, should complete No. 2. If a representative is not present to sign, print his or her name in No. 2. Where applicable, check to indicate if appellant will accompany the representative at the hearing. ❑ Yes ❑ No

1. (Appellant's Signature) / Date	**2.** (Representative's Signature/Name) / Date
Address	Address ❑ Attorney ❑ Non-Attorney
City / State / Zip Code	City / State / Zip Code
Area Code/Telephone Number / E-mail Address	Area Code/Telephone Number / E-mail Address

Answer the following questions that apply:

A) Does request involve multiple claims? ❑ Yes ❑ No
(If yes, a list of all the claims must be attached.)

B) Does request involve multiple beneficiaries? ❑ Yes ❑ No
(If yes, a list of beneficiaries, their HICNs and the dates of the applicable reconsideration determinations must be attached.)

C) Did the beneficiary assign his or her appeal rights to you as the provider/supplier? ❑ Yes ❑ No
(If yes, you must complete and attach form CMS-20031. Failure to do so will prevent approval of the assignment.)

D) If there was no assignment, are you a physician being held liable pursuant to 1842(l)(1)(A) of the Social Security Act? ❑ Yes ❑ No

CMS-5011A/B U2 (08/05) EF 08/2005 ATTACH A COPY OF THE RECONSIDERATION/FAIR HEARING DETERMINATION (IF AVAILABLE) TO THIS COPY.

Figure 9-7 CMS 5011 A/B form Request for Medicare Hearing by an Administration Law Judge

College Clinic
4567 Broad Avenue
Telephone (555) 486-9002 Woodland Hills, XY 12345-0001 Fax (555) 487-8976

INSURANCE CLAIM TRACER

INSURANCE COMPANY NAME Medicare Blue Shield DATE 06-10-20xx

ADDRESS 146 Main Street, Woodland Hills, XY 12345

Patient name: Bill Hutch
Date of birth: 02-17-1944
Employer: Retired
Insured: Bill Hutch
Policy/certificate no. 123XX6789A
Group name/no. None
Date of initial claim submission: 03-10-20XX
Date(s) of service: 03-10-20XX
Total charges submitted: $132.00

An inordinate amount of time has passed since submission of our original claim. We have not received a request for additional information and still await payment of this assigned claim. Please review the attached duplicate and process for payment within 7 days.

DETAILS OF INQUIRY

Please check the claim status and return this letter to our office. Thank you.

- ☐ No record of claim.
- ☐ Claim received and payment is in process.
- ☐ Claim is in suspense (comment please).
- ☐ Claim is in review (comment please).
- ☐ Additional information needed (comment please)
- ☐ Applied to deductible. Amount: $ ________
- ☐ Patient not eligible for benefits.
- ☐ Determination issued to beneficiary.
- ☐ Claim paid. Date: _______ Amount: $ _______ To whom: ____________________
- ☐ Claim denied (comment please).

Comments: ____

____

Thank you for your assistance in this important matter. Please contact the insurance specialist named below if you have any questions regarding this claim.

Insurance Specialist: Student's name (555) 486-9002 Ext. ________
Treating Physician: Brady Coccidioides, MD State license number ________
Provider Number: 64211067XX Provider's IRS number ________

Figure 9-8

ASSIGNMENT 9-9 ▶ FILE AN APPEAL

Performance Objective

Task: Compose, format, key, proofread, and print a letter of appeal, and attach to this document photocopies of information to substantiate reimbursement requested.

Conditions: Computer, printer, letterhead paper, envelope, attachments, thesaurus, English dictionary, medical dictionary, and pen or pencil.

Standards: Time: ________________________ minutes

Accuracy: ________________________

(Note: The time element and accuracy criteria may be given by your instructor.)

Scenario: After retyping and resubmitting Mary T. Avery's insurance claim in Assignment 9-7, the insurance company sends an EOB/RA (health insurance claim number 123098) with a check in the amount of $300 to the College Clinic for payment of the claim. Dr. Cutler wishes an appeal to be made for an increase of the payment to an additional $100. Note: This patient's marital status is single and the insured's identification number is T45098.

Directions: Use the retyped claim to Assignment 9-7 for Mary T. Avery. Follow these basic step-by-step procedures.

1. Refer to the end of Chapter 4 in the *Handbook* and follow the procedure to compose, format, key, proofread, and print a letter.

2. Include the beneficiary's name, health insurance claim number, dates of service in question, and items or services in question with name, address, and signature of the provider.

3. Compose a letter with an introduction that stresses the medical practice's qualifications, the physician's commitment to complying with regulations and providing appropriate services, and the importance of the practice to the payer's panel of physicians or specialists.

4. Provide a detailed account of the necessity of the treatment given and its relationship to the patient's problems and chief complaint. You might cross-reference the medical record and emphasize parts of it that the reviewer may have missed.

5. Explain the reason why the provider does not agree with the payment. Use a blank sheet labeling it "Explanation of Benefits" because you do not have this printed document to attach.

6. Abstract excerpts from the coding resource book if necessary.

7. Direct the correspondence to Mr. Donald Pearson, a claims adjuster at the American Insurance Company, 509 Main Street, Woodland Hills, XY 12345.

8. Type an envelope for the letter.

9. Retain copies of all data sent for the physician's files.

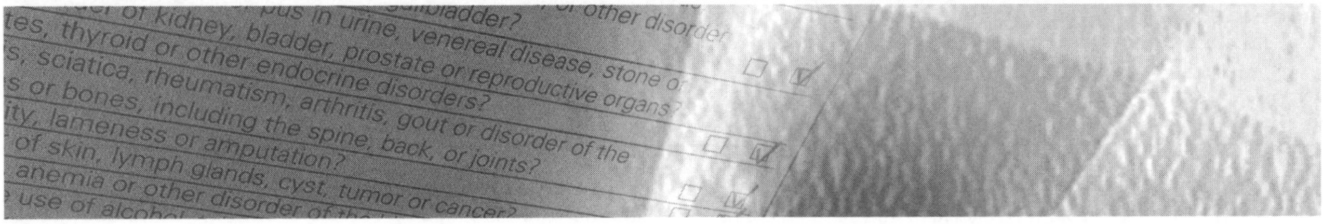

CHAPTER

10

Office and Insurance Collection Strategies

KEY TERMS

Your instructor may wish to select some words pertinent to this chapter for a test. For definitions of the terms, further study, and/or reference, the words, phrases, and abbreviations may be found in the glossary at the end of the Handbook. *Key terms for this chapter follow.*

accounts receivable
age analysis
AMA Code of Medical Ethics
automatic stay
balance
bankruptcy
bonding
cash flow
Code of Medical Ethics
collateral
collection ratio
credit
credit card
creditor
cycle billing
debit card
debt
debtor
discount
dun messages
embezzlement
estate administrator
estate executor
fee schedule
financial accounting record
garnishment
insurance balance billing
itemized statement
lien
manual billing
netback
no charge
nonexempt assets
professional courtesy
reimbursement
secured debt
skip
statute of limitations
unsecured debt
write-off

KEY ABBREVIATIONS

See how many abbreviations and acronyms you can translate and then use this as a handy reference list. Definitions for the key abbreviations are located near the back of the Handbook *in the glossary.*

A/R ______________________

ATM ______________________

CMS ______________________

e-check ______________________

ERISA ______________________

FACT ______________________

FCBA ______________________

FCRA ______________________

FDCPA ______________________

FEHBA ______________________

FTC ______________________

HMO ______________________

N/A ______________________

NC ______________________

NSF ______________________

TILA ______________________

W2 ______________________

PERFORMANCE OBJECTIVES

The student will be able to:

- Define and spell the key terms and key abbreviations for this chapter, given the information from the *Handbook* glossary, within a reasonable time period and with enough accuracy to obtain a satisfactory evaluation.
- After reading the chapter, answer the fill-in-the-blank, mix and match, multiple choice, and true/false review questions with enough accuracy to obtain a satisfactory evaluation.
- Select an appropriate dun message for a patient's bill, given a patient's ledger/statement, within a reasonable time period and with enough accuracy to obtain a satisfactory evaluation.
- Post a courtesy adjustment, given a patient's ledger/statement, within a reasonable time period and with enough accuracy to obtain a satisfactory evaluation.
- Post a patient's charges and payment to the patient's financial accounting record, using the Mock Fee Schedule in Appendix A in this *Workbook*, within a reasonable time period and with enough accuracy to obtain a satisfactory evaluation.
- Compose a collection letter for a delinquent account, given letterhead stationery, within a reasonable time period and with enough accuracy to obtain a satisfactory evaluation.
- Complete a credit card voucher, given a patient's ledger/statement, within a reasonable time period and with enough accuracy to obtain a satisfactory evaluation.
- Complete a financial agreement, given a patient's ledger/statement, within a reasonable time period and with enough accuracy to obtain a satisfactory evaluation.

ASSIGNMENT **10-3 ▶ MANUALLY POST A COURTESY ADJUSTMENT**

Performance Objective

Task: Post a courtesy adjustment to a patient's financial accounting record (ledger card).

Conditions: Use the patient's financial accounting record (Figure 10-2) and a pen.

Standards: Time: ______________________ minutes

Accuracy: ______________________

(Note: The time element and accuracy criteria may be given by your instructor.)

Directions: Read the case scenario and refer to the patient's financial accounting record (see Figure 10-2). You may wish to refer to Figure 10-3 in the *Handbook*. Post a courtesy adjustment to her financial accounting record.

Scenario: Maria Smith recently lost her job and is raising two children as a single parent. It is September 1 (current year). A discussion with Dr. Gerald Practon leads to a decision to write off the balance of the current charges on the account but not the balance forward.

After the instructor has returned your work to you, either make the necessary corrections and place your work in a three-ring notebook for future reference or, if you received a high score, place it in your portfolio for reference when applying for a job.

Acct No. 10-3

STATEMENT
Financial Account
COLLEGE CLINIC
4567 Broad Avenue
Woodland Hills, XY 12345-0001
Tel. 555-486-9002
Fax No. 555-487-8976

Ms. Maria Smith
3737 Unser Road
Woodland Hills, XY 12345

Phone No. (H) (555) 430-8877 (W) (555) 908-1233 Birthdate 06-11-80

Primary Insurance Co. Metropolitan Insurance Company Policy/Group No. 4320870

	REFERENCE	DESCRIPTION	CHARGES		CREDITS PYMNTS.		CREDITS ADJ.		BALANCE	
		BALANCE FORWARD →							20	00
5-19-xx	99214	OV DX 582	61	51					81	51
5-20-xx		Metropolitan billed (5-19-xx)							81	51
6-20-xx		Rec'd ins ck #6778			25	00			56	51
7-1-xx		Pt billed							56	51
8-1-xx		Pt billed							56	51

PLEASE PAY LAST AMOUNT IN BALANCE COLUMN

THIS IS A COPY OF YOUR FINANCIAL ACCOUNT AS IT APPEARS ON OUR RECORDS

Figure 10-2

ASSIGNMENT 10-4 ▶ MANUALLY POST A PATIENT'S CHARGES AND PAYMENT

Performance Objective

Task: Post a payment to a patient's financial accounting record (ledger card).

Conditions: Use the patient's financial accounting record (Figure 10-3), the Mock Fee Schedule in Appendix A in this *Workbook*, and a pen.

Standards: Time: ______________________ minutes

Accuracy: ______________________

(Note: The time element and accuracy criteria may be given by your instructor.)

Directions: Read the case scenario, refer to the patient's financial accounting record (see Figure 10-3), and refer to the Mock Fee Schedule in Appendix A in this *Workbook*. You may wish to refer to Figure 10-3 in the *Handbook*. Post the charges for the services rendered and payment to the patient's financial accounting record.

Scenario: On October 12 (current year), new patient Kenneth Brown came in for a Level III office visit and electrocardiogram (ECG). He has no insurance and paid $50 on his account with check number 3421.

After the instructor has returned your work to you, either make the necessary corrections and place your work in a three-ring notebook for future reference or, if you received a high score, place it in your portfolio for reference when applying for a job.

Acct No. 10-4

STATEMENT
Financial Account
COLLEGE CLINIC
4567 Broad Avenue
Woodland Hills, XY 12345-0001
Tel. 555-486-9002
Fax No. 555-487-8976

Mr. Kenneth Brown
8896 Aster Drive
Woodland Hills, XY 12345

Phone No. (H) (555) 760-5211 (W) (555) 987-3355 Birthdate 01-15-82

Primary Insurance Co. none Policy/Group No. ____

	REFERENCE	DESCRIPTION	CHARGES	CREDITS		BALANCE
				PYMNTS.	ADJ.	
			BALANCE FORWARD →			

PLEASE PAY LAST AMOUNT IN BALANCE COLUMN

THIS IS A COPY OF YOUR FINANCIAL ACCOUNT AS IT APPEARS ON OUR RECORDS

Figure 10-3

ASSIGNMENT 10-5 ▶ COMPOSE A COLLECTION LETTER

Performance Objective

Task: Key a letter for the physician's signature and post the entry on the patient's financial accounting record (ledger card).

Conditions: Use the patient's financial accounting record (Figure 10-4), one sheet of letterhead (Figure 10-5), a number 10 envelope, English dictionary, thesaurus, medical dictionary, computer, printer, and a pen.

Standards: Time: ______________________ minutes

Accuracy: ______________________

(Note: The time element and accuracy criteria may be given by your instructor.)

Directions: Read the case scenario, refer to the patient's financial accounting record (see Figure 10-4), and compose a collection letter, using your signature and requesting payment. Type this letter on letterhead stationery in full block format (paragraphs to left margin). Include a paragraph stating that a copy of the delinquent statement is enclosed. You may wish to refer to Figure 10-15 in the *Handbook*. Post an entry on the patient's financial accounting record.

Scenario: It is December 1 (current year), and you have sent Mr. Ron Kelsey two statements with no response. You tried to reach him by telephone without success and have decided to send him a collection letter (see Figure 10-5).

After the instructor has returned your work to you, either make the necessary corrections and place your work in a three-ring notebook for future reference or, if you received a high score, place it in your portfolio for reference when applying for a job.

Acct No. 10-5

STATEMENT
Financial Account
COLLEGE CLINIC
4567 Broad Avenue
Woodland Hills, XY 12345-0001
Tel. 555-486-9002
Fax No. 555-487-8976

Mr. Ron Kelsey
6321 Ocean Street
Woodland Hills, XY 12345

Phone No. (H) (555) 540-9800 (W) (555) 890-7766 Birthdate 03-25-75

Primary Insurance Co. XYZ Insurance Company Policy/Group No. 8503Y

	REFERENCE	DESCRIPTION	CHARGES		CREDITS PYMNTS.		CREDITS ADJ.		BALANCE	
		BALANCE FORWARD →								
07-09-xx	99283	ER new pt EPF hx/exam MC DM	66	23					66	23
07-10-xx		XYZ Insurance billed (3-9-xx)							66	23
09-20-xx		EOB rec'd pt has not met deductible							66	23
10-01-xx		Billed pt							66	23
11-01-xx		Billed pt							66	23

PLEASE PAY LAST AMOUNT IN BALANCE COLUMN

THIS IS A COPY OF YOUR FINANCIAL ACCOUNT AS IT APPEARS ON OUR RECORDS

Figure 10-4

COLLEGE CLINIC
4567 Broad Avenue
Woodland Hills, XY 12345-0001
Tel. (555) 486-9002
FAX (555) 487-8976

Figure 10-5

ASSIGNMENT 10-6 ▸ COMPLETE A CREDIT CARD VOUCHER

Performance Objective

Task: Complete a credit card voucher and post an entry on the patient's ledger.

Conditions: Use the patient's ledger card (Figure 10-6), a credit card voucher (Figure 10-7), and a pen.

Standards: Time: ______________________ minutes

Accuracy: ______________________

(Note: The time element and accuracy criteria may be given by your instructor.)

Directions: Read the case scenario and refer to the patient's ledger/statement (see Figure 10-6). Fill in the credit card voucher (see Figure 10-7) and post an appropriate entry on the ledger/statement. You may wish to refer to Figure 10-12 in the *Handbook*.

Scenario: It is November 6 (current year), and you receive a telephone call at the College Clinic. It is Kevin Long, who has an unpaid balance, and it is up to you to discuss this delinquency with Mr. Long and come to an agreement on how the account can be paid. After discussion, Mr. Long decides to pay the total balance due by MasterCard credit card, giving you his authorization and account number: 5676 1342 5437 XXX0 (expiration date, December 31, 20xx). His name is listed on the card as Kevin O. Long. You call the bank, and the authorization number given is 534889.

After the instructor has returned your work to you, either make the necessary corrections and place your work in a three-ring notebook for future reference or, if you received a high score, place it in your portfolio for reference when applying for a job.

Acct No. 10-6

STATEMENT
Financial Account
COLLEGE CLINIC
4567 Broad Avenue
Woodland Hills, XY 12345-0001
Tel. 555-486-9002
Fax No. 555-487-8976

Mr. Kevin O. Long
2443 Davis Street
Woodland Hills, XY 12345

Phone No. (H) (555) 244-5600 (W) (555) 970-4466 Birthdate 08-15-76

Primary Insurance Co. Blue Cross Policy/Group No. 130-XX-0987

	REFERENCE	DESCRIPTION	CHARGES		CREDITS PYMNTS.		CREDITS ADJ.		BALANCE	
		BALANCE FORWARD →								
09-08-xx	99205	OV Level V DX 582	132	28					132	28
09-09-xx		Blue Cross billed (9-8-xx)							132	28
10-12-xx		BC EOB rec'd pt has not met deductible							132	28
10-23-xx		Not covered by insurance. Balance due							132	28

PLEASE PAY LAST AMOUNT IN BALANCE COLUMN

THIS IS A COPY OF YOUR FINANCIAL ACCOUNT AS IT APPEARS ON OUR RECORDS

Figure 10-6

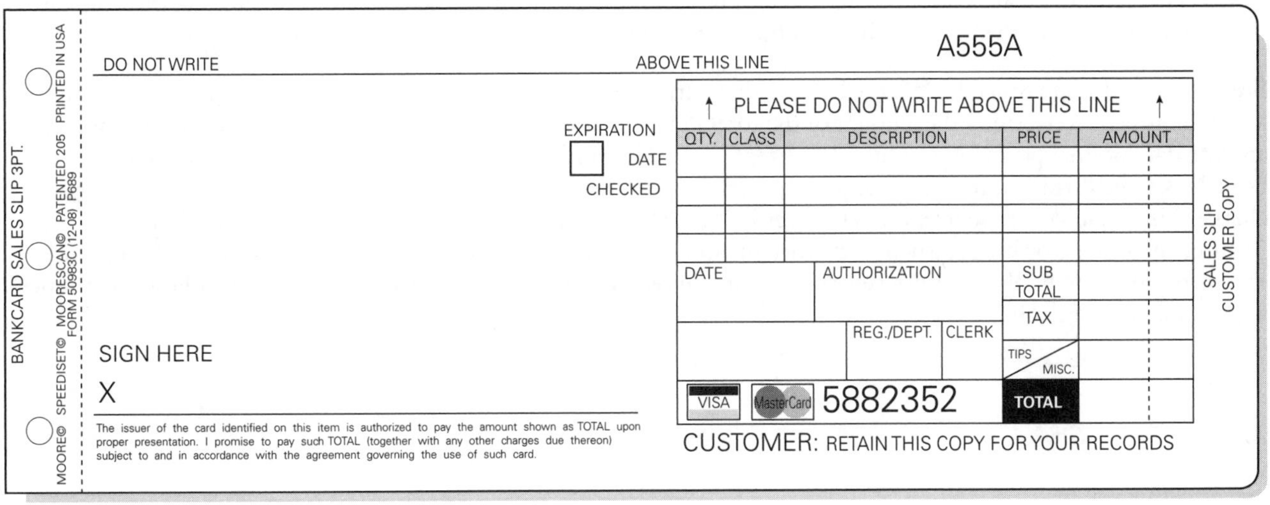
BANKCARD SALES SLIP 3PT.

MOORE© SPEEDISET© MOORESCAN© PATENTED 205 PRINTED IN USA

FORM 50983C (12-08) P689

DO NOT WRITE ABOVE THIS LINE

A555A

EXPIRATION DATE CHECKED

↑ PLEASE DO NOT WRITE ABOVE THIS LINE ↑

QTY.	CLASS	DESCRIPTION	PRICE	AMOUNT
DATE	AUTHORIZATION		SUB TOTAL	
	REG./DEPT.	CLERK	TAX	
			TIPS / MISC.	
VISA	MasterCard	5882352	TOTAL	

SIGN HERE

X

The issuer of the card identified on this item is authorized to pay the amount shown as TOTAL upon proper presentation. I promise to pay such TOTAL (together with any other charges due thereon) subject to and in accordance with the agreement governing the use of such card.

CUSTOMER: RETAIN THIS COPY FOR YOUR RECORDS

SALES SLIP CUSTOMER COPY

Figure 10-7

ASSIGNMENT 10-7 ▶ COMPLETE A FINANCIAL AGREEMENT

Performance Objective

Task: Complete a financial agreement and post an entry on the patient's ledger.

Conditions: Use the patient's ledger card (Figure 10-8), a financial statement form (Figure 10-9), and a pen.

Standards: Time: ______________________ minutes

Accuracy: ______________________

(Note: The time element and accuracy criteria may be given by your instructor.)

Directions: Read the case scenario. Complete a financial agreement (see Figure 10-9) by subtracting the down payment from the total debt. Refer to the patient's ledger/statement (see Figure 10-8) and post an appropriate entry to the ledger/statement using a pen. You may wish to refer to Figure 10-7 in the *Handbook*. Review the completed financial agreement with the patient (role played by another student). Ask the patient (role played by another student) to sign the financial agreement. Make a photocopy of the form for the patient to retain. File the original financial agreement in the patient's financial files in the office.

Scenario: Mr. Joseph Small has a large balance due. Create a payment plan for this case. You have discussed the installment plan concerning the amount of the total debt, the down payment, amount and date of each installment, and the date of final payment. On June 1 (current year), Mr. Small is paying $500 cash as a down payment, and the balance is to be divided into five equal payments, due on the first of each month. There will be no monthly finance charge. Mr. Small's daytime telephone number is 555-760-5502. He is a patient of Dr. Brady Coccidioides.

After the instructor has returned your work to you, either make the necessary corrections and place your work in a three-ring notebook for future reference or, if you received a high score, place it in your portfolio for reference when applying for a job.

Acct No. 10-7

STATEMENT
Financial Account
COLLEGE CLINIC
4567 Broad Avenue
Woodland Hills, XY 12345-0001
Tel. 555-486-9002
Fax No. 555-487-8976

Mr. Joseph Small
655 Sherry Street
Woodland Hills, XY 12345

Phone No. (H) (555) 320-8801 (W) (555) 760-5502 Birthdate 11-04-77

Primary Insurance Co. Blue Shield Policy/Group No. 870-XX-4398

	REFERENCE	DESCRIPTION	CHARGES		CREDITS PYMNTS.		CREDITS ADJ.		BALANCE	
		BALANCE FORWARD →							20	00
04-19-xx	99215	OV Level	96	97					116	97
04-30-xx	99218	Adm hosp	74	22					191	19
04-30-xx	32440	Pneumonectomy, total	1972	10					2163	29
05-20-xx		Blue Shield billed (1-19 to 30-xx)							2163	29
05-15-xx		BS EOB Pt deductible $2000 rec'd ck #544			163	29			2000	00

PLEASE PAY LAST AMOUNT IN BALANCE COLUMN

THIS IS A COPY OF YOUR FINANCIAL ACCOUNT AS IT APPEARS ON OUR RECORDS

Figure 10-8

College Clinic
4567 Broad Avenue
Woodland Hills, XY 12345-0001
Phone: 555/486-9002
Fax: 555/487-8976

FINANCIAL PAYMENT PLAN AGREEMENT

For medical professional services rendered to:

Patient Name ______________________ Account No. __________

Responsible Party ______________________________

Address ______________________________

____

Telephones: Home ______________________________
Mobile ______________________________
Business ______________________________

1. Cash price of total medical treatment $________
2. Down payment (partial payment) $________
3. Amount covered by insurance plan $________
4. Unpaid balance due $________
5. **ANNUAL PERCENTAGE RATE** (interest rate) ________%
6. **FINANCE CHARGE** ($ amt of cost to patient) $________
7. Total amount of unpaid balance due ________
8. Monthly payment amount $________

TERMS:

1. ALL PAYMENTS ARE DUE ON OR BEFORE YOUR DUE DATE EACH MONTH.
2. The patient agrees to be fully responsible for the total payment of medical services performed in this office including any amounts not covered by any health insurance plan.
3. The patient has the right at any time to pay the unpaid balance due without penalty.
4. First payment due ___/___/___ and subsequent payments on the same day of each consecutive month until paid in full.

____
Signature of Patient/Responsible Party Date

____
Physician's signature or Authorized representative Date

Figure 10-9

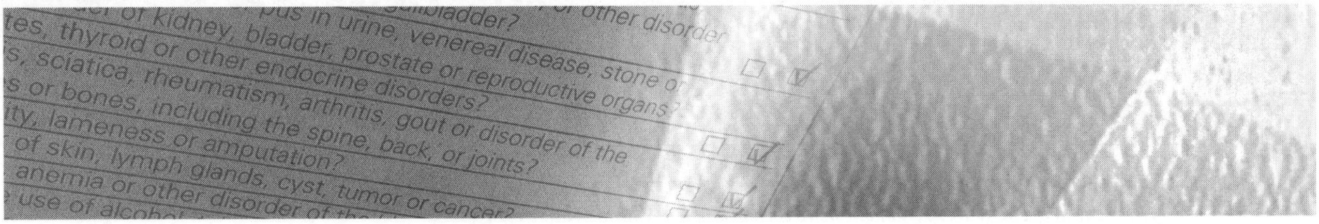

CHAPTER

11

The Blue Plans, Private Insurance, and Managed Care Plans

KEY TERMS

Your instructor may wish to select some words pertinent to this chapter for a test. For definitions of the terms, further study, and/or reference, the words, phrases, and abbreviations may be found in the glossary at the end of the Handbook. *Key terms for this chapter follow.*

ancillary services
buffing
capitation
carve outs
churning
claims-review type of foundation
closed panel program
comprehensive type of foundation
copayment
deductible
direct referral
disenrollment
exclusive provider organization
fee-for-service
formal referral
foundation for medical care
gatekeeper
health maintenance organization
in-area
independent (or individual) practice association
managed care organizations
participating physician
per capita
physician provider group
point-of-service plan
preferred provider organization
prepaid group practice model
primary care physician
self-referral
service area
staff model
stop loss
tertiary care
turfing
utilization review
verbal referral
withhold

KEY ABBREVIATIONS

See how many abbreviations and acronyms you can translate and then use this as a handy reference list. Definitions for the key abbreviations are located near the back of the Handbook *in the glossary.*

copay ____________
EBP ____________
EPO ____________
ERISA ____________
FMC ____________
HEDIS ____________
HMO ____________
IPA ____________
MCO ____________
NCQA ____________
PCP ____________
POS ____________
PPG ____________
PPO ____________
QIO ____________
QISMC ____________
UR ____________

PERFORMANCE OBJECTIVES

The student will be able to:

- Define and spell the key terms and key abbreviations for this chapter, given the information from the *Handbook* glossary, within a reasonable time period and with enough accuracy to obtain a satisfactory evaluation.
- After reading the chapter, answer the fill-in-the-blank, multiple choice, and true/false review questions with enough accuracy to obtain a satisfactory evaluation.
- Complete treatment authorization forms of managed care plans, given completed new patient information forms, within a reasonable time period and with enough accuracy to obtain a satisfactory evaluation.

STUDY OUTLINE

Private Insurance
- Blue Cross and Blue Shield Plans

Managed Care
- Prepaid Group Practice Health Plans
- Benefits
- Health Care Reform

Managed Care Systems
- Health Maintenance Organizations
- Exclusive Provider Organizations
- Foundations for Medical Care
- Independent Practice Associations
- Preferred Provider Organizations
- Physician Provider Groups
- Point-of-Service Plans
- Triple-Option Health Plans
- Provider-Sponsored Organization
- Religious Fraternal Benefit Society
- Employee Retirement Income Security Act

Medical Review
- Quality Improvement Organization
- Utilization Review of Management

Management of Plans
- Contracts
- Carve Outs

Plan Administration
- Patient Information Letter
- Preauthorization of Prior Approval
- Diagnostic Tests
- Managed Care Guide

Financial Management
- Payment
- Statement of Remittance
- Accounting
- Fee-for-Service
- Year-End Evaluation
- Bankruptcy

College Clinic
4567 Board Avenue
Woodland Hills, XY 12345-0001
Telephone No. (555) 487-8976
Fax No. (555) 487-8976

MANAGED CARE PLAN AUTHORIZATION REQUEST

❑ Health Net ❑ Met Life
❑ Pacificare ❑ Travelers
❑ Secure Horizons ❑ Pru Care
❑ Other

Member/Group No.

TO BE COMPLETED BY PRIMARY CARE PHYSICIAN OR OUTSIDE PROVIDER

Patient Name__________ Date__________
❑ Male ❑ Female Birthdate__________ Home Telephone Number __________
Address __________
Primary Care Physician__________ NPI__________
Referring Physician __________ NPI__________
Referred to __________ NPI__________
Address __________ Telephone No. __________
Diagnosis Code__________ Diagnosis__________
Diagnosis Code__________ Diagnosis__________
Treatment Plan __________
Authorization requested for: ❑ Consult only ❑ Treatment only ❑ Consult/Treatment
❑ Consult/Procedure/Surgery ❑ Diagnostic Tests
Procedure Code: __________ Description: __________
Procedure Code: __________ Description: __________
Place of service ❑ Office ❑ Outpatient ❑ Inpatient ❑ Other Number of visits: __________
Facility: __________ Length of stay: __________
Physician's signature: __________

TO BE COMPLETED BY PRIMARY CARE PHYSICIAN

PCP Recommendations: __________ PCP Initials: __________
Date eligibility checked: __________

TO BE COMPLETED BY UTILIZATION MANAGEMENT
Authorized: __________ Auth. No: __________ Not Authorized __________
Deferred: __________ Modified: __________
Effective Date: __________ Expiration Date: __________ No. of visits: __________

Figure 11-3

ASSIGNMENT 11-4 ▶ OBTAIN AUTHORIZATION FOR DIAGNOSTIC ARTHROSCOPY FROM A MANAGED CARE PLAN

Performance Objective

Task:	Complete a treatment authorization form to obtain permission for diagnostic arthroscopy with débridement for a patient covered by a managed care plan.
Conditions:	Use a treatment authorization form (Figure 11-4), computer, and printer.
Standards:	Time: ______________________ minutes
	Accuracy: ______________________
	(Note: The time element and accuracy criteria may be given by your instructor.)

Directions: Complete the treatment authorization form for this patient (see Figure 11-4), date it August 12 of the current year, and submit it to the managed care plan. Refer to Figure 11-2 in the *Handbook* for visual guidance.

Scenario: Daniel Chan has been referred by his primary care physician, Dr. Gerald Practon, to an orthopedic surgeon, Dr. Raymond Skeleton. Both physicians are members of his managed care plan, Metropolitan Life. The patient comes into Dr. Skeleton's office complaining of pain, swelling, and crepitus of the right knee. The patient is having difficulty walking but indicates no recent injury to the knee.

Mr. Chan lives at 226 West Olive Avenue, Woodland Hills, XY, 12340-0329, and his telephone number is 555-540-6700. His plan identification number is FTW90876, effective February 1, 20xx, and he was born February 23, 1971.

After taking a history, completing a physical examination, and taking and reviewing radiographs, Dr. Skeleton suspects the patient has a tear of the medial meniscus and may require débridement of articular cartilage. This procedure will be performed on an outpatient basis at College Hospital. Authorization must be obtained for the surgical arthroscopy with débridement of articular cartilage. Dr. Practon's Metropolitan Life provider number is ML C01402X and Dr. Skeleton's Metropolitan Life provider number is ML C4561X.

After the instructor has returned your work to you, either make the necessary corrections and place your work in a three-ring notebook for future reference or, if you received a high score, place it in your portfolio for reference when applying for a job.

College Clinic
4567 Board Avenue
Woodland Hills, XY 12345-0001
Telephone No. (555) 487-8976
Fax No. (555) 487-8976

MANAGED CARE PLAN AUTHORIZATION REQUEST

❑ Health Net ❑ Met Life
❑ Pacificare ❑ Travelers
❑ Secure Horizons ❑ Pru Care
❑ Other

Member/Group No.

TO BE COMPLETED BY PRIMARY CARE PHYSICIAN OR OUTSIDE PROVIDER

Patient Name__________ Date__________
❑ Male ❑ Female Birthdate__________ Home Telephone Number __________
Address __________
Primary Care Physician __________ NPI __________
Referring Physician __________ NPI __________
Referred to __________ NPI __________
Address __________ Telephone No. __________
Diagnosis Code__________ Diagnosis __________
Diagnosis Code__________ Diagnosis __________
Treatment Plan __________
Authorization requested for: ❑ Consult only ❑ Treatment only ❑ Consult/Treatment ❑ Consult/Procedure/Surgery ❑ Diagnostic Tests
Procedure Code: __________ Description: __________
Procedure Code: __________ Description: __________
Place of service ❑ Office ❑ Outpatient ❑ Inpatient ❑ Other Number of visits: __________
Facility: __________ Length of stay: __________
Physician's signature: __________

TO BE COMPLETED BY PRIMARY CARE PHYSICIAN

PCP Recommendations: __________ PCP Initials: __________
Date eligibility checked: __________

TO BE COMPLETED BY UTILIZATION MANAGEMENT
Authorized: __________ Auth. No: __________ Not Authorized __________
Deferred: __________ Modified: __________
Effective Date: __________ Expiration Date: __________ No. of visits: __________

Figure 11-4

ASSIGNMENT 11-5 ▶ OBTAIN AUTHORIZATION FOR CONSULTATION FROM A MANAGED CARE PLAN

Performance Objective

Task: Complete a treatment authorization form to obtain permission for consultation for a patient from a managed care plan.

Conditions: Use a treatment authorization form (Figure 11-5), computer, and printer.

Standards: Time: ____________________ minutes

Accuracy: ____________________

(Note: The time element and accuracy criteria may be given by your instructor.)

Directions: Complete the treatment authorization form for this patient (see Figure11-5), date it September 3 of the current year, and submit it to the managed care plan. Refer to Figure 11-2 in the *Handbook* for visual guidance.

Scenario: Frederico Fellini, with a history of getting up four times during the night with a slow urinary stream, was seen by his primary care physician, Dr. Gerald Practon. An intravenous pyelogram yielded negative results except for distention of the urinary bladder. Physical examination of the prostate showed an enlargement. The preliminary diagnosis is benign prostatic hypertrophy (BPH).

The patient will be referred to Dr. Douglas Lee, a urologist, for consultation (Level 4) and cystoscopy. Transurethral resection of the prostate is possible at a future date. Dr. Lee's address is 4300 Cyber Street, Woodland Hills, XY, 12345, and his office telephone number is 555-675-3322. His NPI is 55026717XX.

Dr. Practon's managed care contract is with PruCare, identification number PC C01402X, of which this patient is a member.

Mr. Fellini lives at 476 Miner Street, Woodland Hills, XY, 12345, and his telephone number is 555-679-0098. His PruCare plan identification number is VRG87655, effective January 1, 20xx. His birth date is May 24, 1944.

After the instructor has returned your work to you, either make the necessary corrections and place your work in a three-ring notebook for future reference or, if you received a high score, place it in your portfolio for reference when applying for a job.

College Clinic
4567 Board Avenue
Woodland Hills, XY 12345-0001
Telephone No. (555) 487-8976
Fax No. (555) 487-8976

MANAGED CARE PLAN AUTHORIZATION REQUEST

❑ Health Net ❑ Met Life
❑ Pacificare ❑ Travelers
❑ Secure Horizons ❑ Pru Care
❑ Other

Member/Group No.

TO BE COMPLETED BY PRIMARY CARE PHYSICIAN OR OUTSIDE PROVIDER

Patient Name ______ Date ______
❑ Male ❑ Female Birthdate ______ Home Telephone Number ______
Address ______
Primary Care Physician ______ NPI ______
Referring Physician ______ NPI ______
Referred to ______ NPI ______
Address ______ Telephone No. ______
Diagnosis Code ______ Diagnosis ______
Diagnosis Code ______ Diagnosis ______
Treatment Plan ______
Authorization requested for: ❑ Consult only ❑ Treatment only ❑ Consult/Treatment
❑ Consult/Procedure/Surgery ❑ Diagnostic Tests
Procedure Code: ______ Description: ______
Procedure Code: ______ Description: ______
Place of service ❑ Office ❑ Outpatient ❑ Inpatient ❑ Other Number of visits: ______
Facility: ______ Length of stay: ______
Physician's signature: ______

TO BE COMPLETED BY PRIMARY CARE PHYSICIAN

PCP Recommendations: ______ PCP Initials: ______
Date eligibility checked: ______

TO BE COMPLETED BY UTILIZATION MANAGEMENT
Authorized: ______ Auth. No: ______ Not Authorized ______
Deferred: ______ Modified: ______
Effective Date: ______ Expiration Date: ______ No. of visits: ______

Figure 11-5

ASSIGNMENT 11-6 ▶ OBTAIN AUTHORIZATION FOR DIAGNOSTIC BODY SCAN FROM A MANAGED CARE PLAN

Performance Objective

Task: Complete a treatment authorization form to obtain permission for diagnostic complete body bone scan and mammogram for a patient covered by a managed care plan.

Conditions: Use a treatment authorization form (Figure 11-6), computer, and printer.

Standards: Time: ____________________ minutes

Accuracy: ____________________

(Note: The time element and accuracy criteria may be given by your instructor.)

Directions: Complete the treatment authorization form for this patient (see Figure 11-6), date it October 23 of the current year, and submit it to the managed care plan. Refer to Figure 11-2 in the *Handbook* for visual guidance.

Scenario: A patient, Debbie Dye, sees her primary care physician, Dr. Gerald Practon, for complaint of midback pain. She underwent a lumpectomy 2 years ago for a malignant neoplasm of the lower left breast; thus she has a history of breast cancer. She has been referred by Dr. Practon (PacifiCare identification number PC C01402X) to Dr. Donald Patos, an oncologist, for a complete workup. He finds that her complaint of midback pain warrants the need to refer her to XYZ Radiology for bilateral diagnostic mammography and a complete body bone scan.

Dr. Patos' address is 4466 East Canter Drive, Woodland Hills, XY, 12345, and his office telephone number is 555-980-5566. Dr. Patos' PacifiCare identification number is PC 5673X. His NPI is 6520101678XX.

Ms. Dye lives at 6700 Flora Road, Woodland Hills, XY, 12345, and her telephone number is 555-433-6755. Her PacifiCare plan identification number is SR45380, effective January 1, 20xx. Her birth date is August 6, 1952.

XYZ Radiology's address is 4767 Broad Avenue, Woodland Hills, XY, 12345-0001, and the office telephone number is 555-486-9162.

After the instructor has returned your work to you, either make the necessary corrections and place your work in a three-ring notebook for future reference or, if you received a high score, place it in your portfolio for reference when applying for a job.

College Clinic
4567 Board Avenue
Woodland Hills, XY 12345-0001
Telephone No. (555) 487-8976
Fax No. (555) 487-8976

MANAGED CARE PLAN AUTHORIZATION REQUEST

❑ Health Net ❑ Met Life
❑ Pacificare ❑ Travelers
❑ Secure Horizons ❑ Pru Care
❑ Other

Member/Group No.

TO BE COMPLETED BY PRIMARY CARE PHYSICIAN OR OUTSIDE PROVIDER

Patient Name__________ Date__________
❑ Male ❑ Female Birthdate__________ Home Telephone Number __________
Address __________
Primary Care Physician __________ NPI __________
Referring Physician __________ NPI __________
Referred to __________ NPI __________
Address __________ Telephone No. __________
Diagnosis Code__________ Diagnosis __________
Diagnosis Code__________ Diagnosis __________
Treatment Plan __________
Authorization requested for: ❑ Consult only ❑ Treatment only ❑ Consult/Treatment
❑ Consult/Procedure/Surgery ❑ Diagnostic Tests
Procedure Code: __________ Description: __________
Procedure Code: __________ Description: __________
Place of service ❑ Office ❑ Outpatient ❑ Inpatient ❑ Other Number of visits: __________
Facility: __________ Length of stay: __________
Physician's signature: __________

TO BE COMPLETED BY PRIMARY CARE PHYSICIAN

PCP Recommendations: __________ PCP Initials: __________
Date eligibility checked: __________

TO BE COMPLETED BY UTILIZATION MANAGEMENT

Authorized: __________ Auth. No: __________ Not Authorized: __________
Deferred: __________ Modified: __________
Effective Date: __________ Expiration Date: __________ No. of visits: __________

Figure 11-6

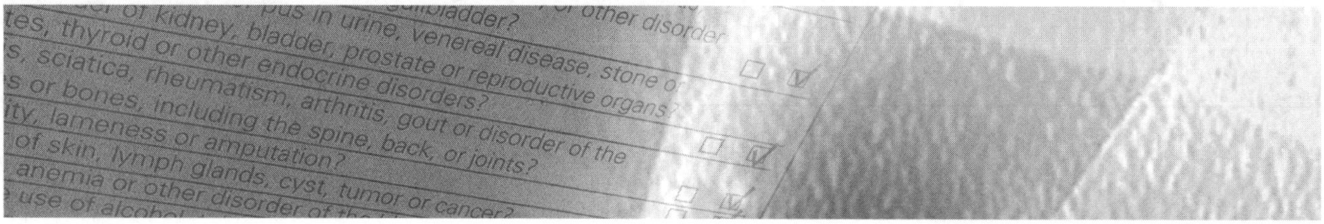

CHAPTER

12 Medicare

KEY TERMS

Your instructor may wish to select some words pertinent to this chapter for a test. For definitions of the terms, further study, and/or reference, the words, phrases, and abbreviations may be found in the glossary at the end of the Handbook. *Key terms for this chapter follow.*

Advance Beneficiary Notice of Noncoverage
approved charges
assignment
benefit period
Centers for Medicare and Medicaid Services
Correct Coding Initiative
crossover claim
diagnostic cost groups
disabled
end-stage renal disease
formulary
hospice
hospital insurance
intermediate care facilities
limiting charge
medical necessity
Medicare
Medicare administrative contractor
Medicare Part A
Medicare Part B
Medicare Part C
Medicare Part D
Medicare/Medicaid
Medicare Secondary Payer
Medicare Summary Notice
Medigap
national alphanumeric codes
nonparticipating physician
nursing facility
participating physician
Physician Quality Reporting Initiative
premium
prospective payment system
Quality Improvement Organization
qui tam action
reasonable fee
Recovery Audit Contractor Initiative
relative value unit
remittance advice
resource-based relative value scale
respite care
Supplemental Security Income
supplementary medical insurance
volume performance standard
whistleblowers

KEY ABBREVIATIONS

See how many abbreviations and acronyms you can translate and then use this as a handy reference list. Definitions for the key abbreviations are located near the back of the Handbook *in the glossary.*

ABN ______
CAP ______
CCI ______
CLIA ______
CMS ______
COBRA ______
DC ______
DCGs ______
DEFRA ______
DME ______
EGHP ______
ERA ______
ESRD ______
GPCI ______
ICFs ______
ICU ______
LCD ______
LGHP ______
LMRP ______
MAAC ______
MACs ______
Medi-Medi ______
MG ______
MMA ______
MSA ______
MSN ______
MSP ______
NCDs ______
NEMB ______
NF ______
nonpar physician ______
OASDI ______
OBRA ______
OCNA ______
OIG ______
OR ______
par physician ______
PAYRID ______
PFFS plan ______
PIN ______
PPS ______
PQRI ______
PSO ______
QIO ______
RA ______
RAC ______
RBRVS ______
RFBS ______
RVU ______
SMI ______
SOF ______
SSI ______
TEFRA ______
VPS ______

PERFORMANCE OBJECTIVES

The student will be able to:

- Define and spell the key terms and key abbreviations for this chapter, given the information from the *Handbook* glossary, within a reasonable time period and with enough accuracy to obtain a satisfactory evaluation.
- After reading the chapter, answer the fill-in-the-blank, multiple choice, and true/false review questions, with enough accuracy to obtain a satisfactory evaluation.
- Fill in the correct meaning of each abbreviation, given a list of common medical abbreviations and symbols that appear in chart notes, within a reasonable time period and with enough accuracy to obtain a satisfactory evaluation.
- Complete each CMS-1500 (08-05) Health Insurance Claim Form for billing, given the patients' medical chart notes, ledger cards, and blank insurance claim forms, within a reasonable time period and with enough accuracy to obtain a satisfactory evaluation.
- Post payments, adjustments, and balances on the patients' ledger cards, using the Medicare Mock Fee Schedule in Appendix A in this, within a reasonable time period and with enough accuracy to obtain a satisfactory evaluation.
- Compute mathematical calculations, given Medicare problem situations, within a reasonable time period and with enough accuracy to obtain a satisfactory evaluation.
- Using the *Current Procedural Terminology* (CPT) code book or the Mock Fee Schedule in Appendix A in this *Workbook* and the Healthcare Common Procedure Coding System (HCPCS) list of codes in Appendix B in this *Workbook*, select the HCPCS and/or procedural code numbers, given a series of medical services, procedures, or supplies, within a reasonable time period and with enough accuracy to obtain a satisfactory evaluation.

STUDY OUTLINE

Background

Policies and Regulations

- Eligibility Requirements
- Health Insurance Card
- Enrollment Status
- Benefits and Nonbenefits

Additional Insurance Programs

- Medicare/Medicaid
- Medicare/Medigap
- Medicare Secondary Payer
- Automobile or Liability Insurance Coverage

Medicare Managed Care Plans

- Health Maintenance Organizations
- Carrier Dealing Prepayment Organization

Utilization and Quality Control

- Quality Improvement Organizations
- Federal False Claims Amendment Act

Medicare Billing Compliance Issues

- Clinical Laboratory Improvement Amendments

Payment Fundamentals

- Provider
- Prior Authorization
- Waiver of Liability Provision
- Elective Surgery Estimate
- Prepayment Screens
- Correct Coding Initiative

Medicare Reimbursement

- Chronology of Prospective Payment System
- Reasonable Fee
- Resource-Based Relative Value Scale
- Healthcare Common Procedure Coding System (HCPCS)
- Physician Quality Reporting Initiative

Claim Submission

- Local Coverage Determination
- Medicare Administrative Contractors and Fiscal Intermediaries
- Provider Identification Numbers
- Patient's Signature Authorization
- Time Limit
- Paper Claims
- Electronic Claims
- Medicare/Medicaid Claims
- Medicare/Medigap Claims
- Medicare/Employer Supplemental Insurance Claims
- Medicare/Supplemental and MSP Claims
- Claims for Deceased Patients
- Physician Substitute Coverage

After Claim Submission

- Remittance Advice
- Medicare Summary Notice

Beneficiary Representative/Representative Payee

- Posting Payments
- Review and Redetermination Process

Procedure: Determine Whether Medicare is Primary or Secondary and Determine Additional Benefits

Procedure: Complete an Advance Beneficiary Notice of Noncoverage (ABN) Form CMS-R-131

ASSIGNMENT 12-1 ▶ REVIEW QUESTIONS

Part I Fill in the Blank

Review the objectives, key terms, glossary definitions of key terms, chapter information, and figures before completing the following review questions.

1. An individual becomes eligible for Medicare Parts A and B at age ____________________.

2. Medicare Part A is ____________ coverage, and Medicare Part B is ____________ coverage.

3. Name an eligibility requirement that would allow aliens to receive Medicare benefits.

____

4. Funding for the Medicare Part A program is obtained from

____

and funding for the Medicare Part B program is obtained equally from

____.

5. Define a Medicare Part A hospital benefit period. ____________________

____

____

6. A program designed to provide pain relief, symptom management, and supportive services to terminally ill individuals and their families is known as

____.

7. Short-term inpatient medical care for terminally ill individuals to give temporary relief to the caregiver is known as ____.

8. The frequency of Pap tests for Medicare patients is ____________________, and that for mammograms is ____________________.

9. Some third-party payers offer policies that fall under guidelines issued by the federal government and may cover prescription costs, Medicare deductibles, and copayments;

these secondary or supplemental policies are known as ____________________ insurance policies.

10. Name two types of health maintenance organization (HMO) plans that may have Medicare Part B contracts.

    a. ______________________________

    b. ______________________________

11. The federal laws establishing standards of quality control and safety measures in clinical laboratories are known as ______________________________.

12. Acceptance of assignment by a participating physician means that he or she agrees to ______________________________ after the $ __________ annual deductible has been met.

13. Philip Lenz is seen by Dr. Doe, who schedules an operative procedure in 1 month. This type of surgery is known as ______________________________, because it does not have to be performed immediately.

14. A Medicare insurance claim form showed an alphanumeric code, J0540, for an injection of 600,000 U of penicillin G. This number is referred to as a/an ______________________________.

15. Organizations or claims processors under contract to the federal government that handle insurance claims and payments for hospitals under Medicare Part A are known as ______________________________, and those that process claims for physicians and other suppliers of services under Medicare Part B are called ______________________________.

16. A Centers for Medicare and Medicaid Services (CMS)–assigned provider identification number is known as a/an ______________________________.

    Physicians who supply durable medical equipment must have a/an ______________________________ number.

17. If circumstances make it impossible to obtain a signature each time a paper claim is submitted or an electronic claim is transmitted, the Medicare patient's signature may be obtained either ______________________________ or ______________________________, thus indicating the signature is on file.

18. The time limit for sending in a Medicare insurance claim is ______________________________.

19. Mrs. Davis, a Medicare/Medicaid (Medi-Medi) patient, has a cholecystectomy. In completing the insurance claim form, the assignment portion is left blank in error. What will happen in this case?

____

____

20. If an individual is 65 years of age and is a Medicare beneficiary but is working and has a group insurance policy, where is the insurance claim form sent initially?

____

21. If a Medicare beneficiary is injured in an automobile accident, the physician submits the claim form to

____.

Part II Multiple Choice

Choose the best answer.

22. Medicare prescription drug benefits for individuals who purchase the insurance are available under

   a. Medicare part A

   b. Medicare part B

   c. Medicare part C

   d. Medicare part D

23. Medicare secondary payer (MSP) cases may involve

   a. Medicare-aged workers under group health plans of more than 20 covered employees

   b. Medicare-aged or disabled individuals who also receive benefits under the Department of Veterans Affairs and Medicare

   c. A Medicare patient who is involved in an automobile accident

   d. All of the above

24. If a Medicare patient is to receive a medical service that may be denied payment either entirely or partially, the provider should

   a. Transmit a claim for adjudication to receive an official notice of denial

   b. Have the patient sign an Advance Beneficiary Notice of Noncoverage form

   c. Have the patient make a partial payment

   d. Ask the patient for payment

25. A decision by a Medicare administrative contractor (MAC) whether to cover (pay) a particular medical service on a contractor-wide basis in accordance with whether it is reasonable and necessary is known as a/an

a. Local Coverage Determination

b. Correct Coding Initiative edit

c. Prepayment screen

d. Redetermination process

26. According to regulations, a Medicare patient must be billed for a copayment

a. At least once before a balance is adjusted off as uncollectible

b. At least two times before a balance is adjusted off as uncollectible

c. At least three times before a balance is adjusted off as uncollectible

d. No more than four times before a balance is adjusted off as uncollectible

Part III True/False

Write "T" or "F" in the blank to indicate whether you think the statement is true or false.

_______ 27. All patients who have a Medicare health insurance card have Part A hospital and Part B medical coverage.

_______ 28. Prescription drug plans refer to the drugs in their formularies by tier numbers.

_______ 29. Nonparticipating physicians may decide on a case-by-case basis whether to accept assignment when providing medical services to Medicare patients.

_______ 30. Medicare's Correct Coding Initiative was implemented by the Centers for Medicare and Medicaid Services to eliminate unbundling of CPT codes.

_______ 31. A Medicare/Medigap claim is not called a crossover claim.

ASSIGNMENT 12-2 ▶ CALCULATE MATHEMATICAL PROBLEMS

Performance Objective

Task: Calculate and insert the correct amounts for seven Medicare scenarios.

Conditions: Use a pen or pencil, the description of problem, and, for Problem 7, Figures 12-1 and 12-2.

Standards: Time: ____________________ minutes

Accuracy: ____________________

(Note: The time element and accuracy criteria may be given by your instructor.)

Directions: Submitting insurance claims, particularly Medicare claims, involves a bit of arithmetic. Several problems are given here so that you will gain experience with situations encountered daily in your work. The Medicare deductible is always subtracted from the allowed amount first before mathematic computations continue.

Problem 1: Mr. Doolittle has Medicare Parts A and B coverage. He was well during the entire past year. On January 1, Mr. Doolittle is rushed to the hospital, where Dr. Input performs an emergency gastric resection. The hospital bills Medicare under the Part A coverage and under the Part B coverage, the physician bills $450 for surgical services. The doctor agrees to accept assignment. The patient has not paid any deductible. Complete the following statements by putting in the correct amounts.

Original Bill

a. Medicare allows $400. Medicare payment: ____________________

b. Patient owes Dr. Input: ____________________

c. Dr. Input's courtesy adjustment: ____________________

Mathematical computations:

Problem 2: Mrs. James has Medicare Parts A and B coverage. She met her deductible when she was ill in March of this year. On November 1, Dr. Caesar performs a bilateral salpingo-oophorectomy. The hospital bills Medicare under the Part A coverage, and under Part B coverage, the physician bills $300 for surgical services. The doctor agrees to accept a Medicare assignment.

Original Bill

a. Medicare allows $275. Medicare payment: ____________________

b. Patient owes Dr. Caesar: ____________________

c. Dr. Caesar's courtesy adjustment: ____________________

Mathematical computations for surgeon:

The assistant surgeon charged Mrs. James $60 (the Medicare limiting charge) and does not accept assignment. After receiving her check from Medicare, Mrs. James sends the surgeon his $60. Medicare has allowed $55 for the fee.

a. How much of the money was from Mrs. James' private funds? $____________________.

b. How much did Medicare pay? $ ____________________.

Mathematical computations:

Problem 3: You work for Dr. Coccidioides. He does not accept assignment. He is treating Mr. Robinson for allergies. Mr. Robinson has Medicare Part A. You send in a bill to Medicare for the $135 that Mr. Robinson owes you. What portion of the bill will Medicare pay? ______________________________

Problem 4: In June, Mr. Fay has an illness that incurs $89 in medical bills. He asks you to bill Medicare, and the physician does not accept assignment. He has paid the deductible at another physician's office.

a. If Medicare allows the entire amount of your fees, the Medicare check to the patient is

$____________________ (which comes to you).

b. The patient's part of the bill to you is $ ____________________.

Mathematical computations:

Problem 5: Mr. Iba, a Medicare patient with a Medigap insurance policy, is seen for an office visit and the fee is $80. The Medicare-approved amount is $54.44. The patient has met his deductible for the year.

a. The Medicare payment check is $ ____________________.

b. After the claim is submitted to the Medigap insurance, the Medigap payment check is

$ ____________________.

c. To zero out the balance, the Medicare courtesy adjustment is $ ______________________.

Mathematical computations:

Problem 6: Mrs. Smith, a Medicare patient, had surgery, and the participating physician's fee is $1250. This patient is working part-time, and her employer group health plan (primary insurance) allowed $1100, applied $500 to the deductible, and paid 80% of $600.

a. Amount paid by this plan: $______________________.

b. The spouse's employer group health plan (secondary insurance) is billed for the balance, which is

$______________________. This program also has a $500 deductible. This plan pays 100% of the fee billed, minus the deductible.

c. The spouse's employer group plan makes a payment of $______________________.

You send copies of remittance advice from the two group health plans and submit a claim to Medicare

(the third insurance) for $1250. The balance at this point is $______________________

Mathematical computations:

Problem 7: Beverly James has Medicare Part B coverage. She has $242 in medical bills and has met $100 of the $162 (2011 deductible). Dr. Practon agrees to accept assignment.

Original Bill

a. Medicare allows $200. Medicare payment: ______________________

b. Beverly James owes Dr. Practon: ______________________

c. Dr. Practon's courtesy adjustment: ______________________

Mathematical computations:

Problem 8: Oliver Mills has Medicare Part B coverage. He fell at home and suffered a sprain and Dr. Skeleton treated him. His medical bill totaled $370 and he has met $60 of the $162 (2011 deductible). Dr. Skeleton agrees to accept assignment.

Original Bill

a. Medicare allows $280. Medicare payment: ____________________

b. Oliver Mills owes Dr. Skeleton: ____________________

c. Dr. Skeleton's courtesy adjustment: ____________________

Mathematical computations:

Problem 9: Maria Sanchez has Medicare Part B coverage. She has $565 in medical bills at Dr. Cardi's office and met $45 of the $162 (2011 deductible) at another physician's office. Dr. Cardi agrees to accept assignment.

Original Bill

a. Medicare allows $480. Medicare payment: ____________________

b. Maria Sanchez owes Dr. Cardi: ____________________

c. Dr. Cardi's courtesy adjustment: ____________________

Mathematical computations:

Problem 10: In the late 1980s, Medicare's Resource-Based Relative Value System (RBRVS) became the way payment was determined each year. However, since the early 1990s, annual fee schedules have been supplied by local fiscal intermediaries, and so the RBRVS has become more useful in determining practice cost to convert patients to capitation in negotiations of managed care contracts. Because physicians may request determination of fees for certain procedures to discover actual cost and what compensation ratios should be, it is important to know how Medicare fees are determined. Each year the *Federal Register* publishes geographic practice cost indices by Medicare carrier and locality as well as relative value units and related information. This assignment will give you some mathematical practice in using figures for annual conversion factors to determine fees for given procedures in various regions of the United States. Refer to Figures 12-1 and 12-2, which are pages of the *Federal Register*.

a. HCPCS Code 47600: Removal of gallbladder. The medical practice is located in Phoenix, Arizona.

	Work	*Overhead*	*Malpractice*
RVUs	________	________	________
GPCI	× ________	× ________	× ________

+ ________ + ________ + ________ = Total adjusted RVUs

2011 Conversion factor \$33.9764 × Total adjusted RVUs ________ = allowed amount \$________.

b. HCPCS Code 47715: Excision of bile duct cyst. The medical practice is located in Arkansas.

	Work	*Overhead*	*Malpractice*
RVUs	________	________	________
GPCI	× ________	× ________	× ________

+ ________ + ________ + ________ = Total adjusted RVUs ________

2011 Conversion factor \$33.9764 × Total adjusted RVUs ________ = allowed amount \$________.

c. HCPCS Code 48146: Pancreatectomy. The medical practice is located in Fresno, California.

	Work	*Overhead*	*Malpractice*
RVUs	________	________	________
GPCI	× ________	× ________	× ________

+ ________ + ________ + ________ = Total adjusted RVUs ________

2011 Conversion factor \$33.9764 × Total adjusted RVUs × ________ = allowed amount \$________.

ADDENDUM D.---GEOGRAPHIC PRACTICE COST INDICES BY MEDICARE CARRIER AND LOCALITY						
Carrier number	Locality number	Locality name	Work	Practice expense	Mal-practice	
510	5	Birmingham, AL	0.981	0.913	0.824	
510	4	Mobile, AL	0.964	0.911	0.824	
510	2	North Central AL	0.970	0.867	0.824	
510	1	Northwest AL	0.985	0.869	0.824	
510	6	Rest of AL	0.975	0.851	0.824	
510	3	Southeast AL	0.972	0.869	0.824	
1020	1	Alaska	1.106	1.255	1.042	
1030	5	Flagstaff (city), AZ	0.983	0.911	1.255	
1030	1	Phoenix, AZ	1.003	1.016	1.255	
1030	7	Prescott (city), AZ	0.983	0.911	1.255	
1030	99	Rest of Arizona	0.987	0.943	1.255	
1030	2	Tucson (city), AZ	0.987	0.989	1.255	
1030	8	Yuma (city), AZ	0.983	0.911	1.255	
520	13	Arkansas	0.960	0.856	0.302	
2050	26	Anaheim-Santa Ana, CA	1.046	1.220	1.370	
542	14	Bakersfield, CA	1.028	1.050	1.370	
542	11	Fresno/Madera, CA	1.006	1.009	1.370	
542	13	Kings/Tulare, CA	0.999	1.001	1.370	
2050	18	Los Angeles, CA (1st of 8)	1.060	1.196	1.370	
2050	19	Los Angeles, CA (2nd of 8)	1.060	1.196	1.370	

Figure 12-1

ADDENDUM B.—RELATIVE VALUE UNITS (RVUs) AND RELATED INFORMATION

HCPCS[1]	MOD	Status	Description	Work RVUs	Practice expense RVUs[2]	Mal-practice RVUs	Total	Global period	Update
47399	....	C	Liver surgery procedure	0.00	0.00	0.00	0.00	YYY	S
47400	....	A	Incision of liver duct	19.11	8.62	1.38	29.11	090	S
47420	....	A	Incision of bile duct	15.48	9.59	2.01	27.08	090	S
47425	....	A	Incision of bile duct	14.95	11.84	2.48	29.27	090	S
47440	....	A	Incision of bile duct	18.51	10.61	2.23	31.35	090	S
47460	....	A	Incision of bile duct sphincter	14.57	15.71	1.84	32.12	090	N
47480	....	A	Incision of gallbladder	8.14	7.68	1.61	17.43	090	S
47490	....	A	Incision of gallbladder	6.11	3.61	0.38	10.10	090	N
47500	....	A	Injection for liver x-rays	1.98	1.53	0.14	3.65	000	N
47505	....	A	Injection for liver x-rays	0.77	1.34	0.14	2.25	000	N
47510	....	A	Insert catheter, bile duct	7.47	2.90	0.25	10.62	090	N
47511	....	A	Insert bile duct drain	10.02	2.90	0.25	13.17	090	N
47525	....	A	Change bile duct catheter	5.47	1.61	0.16	7.24	010	N
47530	....	A	Revise, reinsert bile tube	5.47	1.53	0.19	7.19	090	N
47550	....	A	Bile duct endoscopy	3.05	1.58	0.35	4.98	000	S
47552	....	A	Biliary endoscopy, thru skin	6.11	1.38	0.21	7.70	000	S
47553	....	A	Biliary endoscopy, thru skin	6.42	3.84	0.63	10.89	000	N
47554	....	A	Biliary endoscopy, thru skin	9.16	3.97	0.68	13.81	000	S
47555	....	A	Biliary endoscopy, thru skin	7.64	2.66	0.30	10.60	000	N
47556	....	A	Biliary endoscopy, thru skin	8.66	2.66	0.30	11.62	000	N
47600	....	A	Removal of gallbladder	10.80	7.61	1.60	20.01	090	S
47605	....	A	Removal of gallbladder	11.66	8.23	1.77	21.66	090	S
47610	....	A	Removal of gallbladder	14.01	9.47	2.02	25.50	090	S
47612	....	A	Removal of gallbladder	14.91	14.39	3.08	32.38	090	S
47620	....	A	Removal of gallbladder	15.97	11.35	2.39	29.71	090	S
47630	....	A	Removal of bile duct stone	8.40	3.79	0.40	12.59	090	N
47700	....	A	Exploration of bile ducts	13.90	7.71	1.60	23.21	090	S
47701	....	A	Bile duct revision	26.87	8.30	1.92	37.09	090	S
47710	....	A	Excision of bile duct tumor	18.64	12.19	2.49	33.32	090	S
47715	....	A	Excision of bile duct cyst	14.66	8.31	1.73	24.70	090	S
47716	....	A	Fusion of bile duct cyst	12.67	6.63	1.55	20.85	090	S
47720	....	A	Fuse gallbladder and bowel	12.03	9.26	1.95	23.34	090	S
47721	....	A	Fuse upper gi structures	14.57	11.55	2.50	28.62	090	S
47740	....	A	Fuse gallbladder and bowel	14.08	10.32	2.16	26.56	090	S
47760	....	A	Fuse bile ducts and bowel	20.15	11.74	2.56	34.45	090	S
47765	....	A	Fuse liver ducts and bowel	19.25	14.77	3.00	37.02	090	S
47780	....	A	Fuse bile ducts and bowel	20.63	13.22	2.76	36.61	090	S
47800	....	A	Reconstruction of bile ducts	17.91	13.37	2.46	33.74	090	S
47801	....	A	Placement, bile duct support	11.41	5.54	0.82	17.77	090	S
47802	....	A	Fuse liver duct and intestine	16.19	10.38	1.77	28.34	090	S
47999	....	C	Bile tract surgery procedure	0.00	0.00	0.00	0.00	YYY	S
48000	....	A	Drainage of abdomen	13.25	7.13	1.42	21.80	090	S
48001	....	A	Placement of drain, pancreas	15.71	8.22	1.91	25.84	090	S
48005	....	A	Resect/debride pancreas	17.77	9.29	2.16	29.22	090	S
48020	....	A	Removal of pancreatic stone	13.12	6.86	1.59	21.57	090	S
48100	....	A	Biopsy of pancreas	10.30	4.26	0.80	15.36	090	S
48102	....	A	Needle biopsy, pancreas	4.48	2.44	0.25	7.17	010	N
48120	....	A	Removal of pancreas lesion	12.93	9.83	2.09	24.85	090	S
48140	....	A	Partial removal of pancreas	18.47	13.44	2.86	34.77	090	S
48145	....	A	Partial removal of pancreas	19.30	15.88	3.20	38.38	090	S
48146	....	A	Pancreatectomy	21.97	16.67	1.94	40.58	090	S
48148	....	A	Removal of pancrearic duct	14.57	8.32	1.70	24.59	090	S
48150	....	A	Partial removal of pancreas	34.55	22.79	4.80	62.14	090	S
48151	....	D	Partial removal of pancreas	0.00	0.00	0.00	0.00	090	0
48152	....	A	Pancreatectomy	31.33	22.79	4.80	58.92	090	S
48153	....	A	Pancreatectomy	34.55	22.79	4.80	62.14	090	S
48154	....	A	Pancreatectomy	31.33	22.79	4.80	58.92	090	S
48155	....	A	Removal of pancreas	19.65	20.63	4.31	44.59	090	S
48160	....	N	Pancreas removal, transplant	0.00	0.00	0.00	0.00	XXX	0
48180	....	A	Fuse pancreas and bowel	21.11	12.74	2.66	36.51	090	S
48400	....	A	Injection, intraoperative	1.97	1.04	0.24	3.25	ZZZ	S
48500	....	A	Surgery of pancreas cyst	12.17	8.62	1.68	22.47	090	S
48510	....	A	Drain pancreatic pseudocyst	11.34	7.62	1.46	20.42	090	S
48520	....	A	Fuse pancreas cyst and bowel	13.11	11.43	2.46	27.00	090	S
48540	....	A	Fuse pancreas cyst and bowel	15.95	12.80	2.68	31.43	090	S
48545	....	A	Pancreatorrhaphy	14.81	7.75	1.81	24.37	090	S
48547	....	A	Duodenal exclusion	21.42	11.20	2.61	35.23	090	S

[1] All numeric CPT HCPCS Copyright 1993 American Medical Association.
[2] *Indicates reduction of Practice Expense RVUs as a result of OBRA 1993.

Figure 12-2

ASSIGNMENT 12-3 ▶ LOCATE HCPCS ALPHANUMERIC CODES

Performance Objective

Task: Insert the correct HCPCS codes for the problems presented.

Conditions: Use a pen or pencil, the HCPCS code book or Appendix B in this *Workbook*.

Standards: Time: ______________________ minutes

Accuracy: ______________________

(Note: The time element and accuracy criteria may be given by your instructor.)

Directions: As you have learned from the *Handbook*, it is necessary to use three levels of codes (CPT, HCPCS, and regional codes) when submitting Medicare claims. Refer to Appendix B in this *Workbook* to complete this HCPCS coding exercise for Medicare claims.

1. Cellular therapy ____________
2. Injection amygdalin, laetrile, vitamin B_{17} ____________
3. Lidocaine (Xylocaine) injection for local anesthetic ____________
4. Splint, wrist ____________
5. Crutches ____________
6. Cervical head harness ____________
7. 1 mL gamma globulin ____________
8. Injection, vitamin B_{12} ____________
9. Contraceptives (unclassified drugs) ____________
10. Surgical tray ____________
11. Penicillin, procaine, aqueous, injection ____________

ASSIGNMENT 12-4 ▶ LOCATE CPT CODES AND HCPCS ALPHANUMERIC MODIFIERS

Performance Objective

Task: Insert the correct CPT codes and HCPCS modifiers for problems presented.

Conditions: Use a pen or pencil, the CPT code book, and a HCPCS code book or Appendix B in this *Workbook*.

Standards: Time: ______________________ minutes

Accuracy: ______________________

(Note: The time element and accuracy criteria may be given by your instructor.)

Directions: Now get some practice in selecting CPT codes with HCPCS modifiers. For this assignment, in addition to referring to a CPT code book and Appendix A in this *Workbook*, you will need to refer to either a HCPCS code book or Appendix B in this *Workbook* to complete these Medicare problems.

1. Second surgical opinion ordered by a professional review organization, detailed history and examination, low-complexity decision-making ____________

2. Chiropractic manipulation of spine, one region, acute treatment ____________

3. Office visit by a locum tenens physician of established patient, problem-focused history and examination with straightforward decision-making ____________

4. Strapping of thumb of left hand ____________

Insurance Claim Assignments

Assignments presented in this section are to give you hands-on experience in completing a variety of Medicare insurance cases by using the CMS-1500 (08-05) claim form. Periodically, newsletters are issued by Medicare fiscal intermediaries relaying new federal policies and guidelines. This may change block requirements on the claim form, codes (procedural and diagnostic) that are covered in the Medicare program, or mean lower reimbursement or denial of reimbursement for a particular code number. Cases shown do not reflect payment policies for a particular procedure or service; this depends on federal guidelines and local medical review policies (LMRPs) at the time of claim submission.

The cases presented in this section are:

Assignment 12-5	Medicare
Assignment 12-6	Medicare/Medicaid (Medi-Medi)
Assignment 12-7	Medicare Secondary Payer (MSP) [advanced]
Assignment 12-8	Medicare/Medigap
Assignment 12-9	Medicare Railroad, Retiree with Advance Beneficiary Notice of Noncoverage [advanced]
Assignment 12-10	Medicare/Medicaid (Medi-Medi)

Additional cases presented on the Student Software Challenge (located on Evolve) are:

Computer Case 8	Medicare
Computer Case 9	Medicare/Medigap
Computer Case 10	Medicare/Medicaid

ASSIGNMENT 12-5 ▸ COMPLETE A CLAIM FORM FOR A MEDICARE CASE

Performance Objective

Task: Complete a CMS-1500 (08-05) claim form for a Medicare case, post transactions to the financial accounting record, and define patient record abbreviations.

Conditions: Use the patient's medical record (Figure 12-3) and financial statement (Figure 12-4), one health insurance claim form (print from Evolve website), a computer, procedural and diagnostic code books, and Appendixes A and B in this *Workbook*.

Standards: Claim Productivity Measurement

Time: ________________________ minutes

Accuracy: ________________________

(Note: The time element and accuracy criteria may be given by your instructor.)

Directions:

1. Complete the CMS-1500 (08-05) claim form, using Office for Civil Rights (OCR) guidelines for a Medicare case. If your instructor wants you to direct it to your local fiscal intermediary, obtain the name and address by going to the Evolve website listed in Internet Resources at the end of Chapter 12 in the *Handbook*. Refer to Elsa M. Mooney's patient record for information. Refer to Appendix A in this *Workbook* to locate the fees to be recorded on the claim and posted to the financial statement. Date the claim December 21. Dr. Cardi is a participating physician who is accepting assignment, and Mrs. Mooney has already met her deductible for the year owing to previous medical expenses with another physician. Use the participating provider Medicare fee.

2. Refer to Chapter 7 (Figure 7-6) of the *Handbook* for instructions on how to complete this claim form and a Medicare template.

3. Use your CPT code book or Appendix A in this *Workbook* to determine the correct five-digit code number and modifiers for each professional service rendered. Use your HCPCS Level II code book or refer to Appendix B in this *Workbook* for HCPCS procedure codes and modifiers. If your instructor tells you to also find the ICD-10-CM codes, a draft version may be downloaded from the following website: http://www.cdc.gov/nchs/icd/icd10cm.htm#10update.

4. Record all transactions on the financial accounting record and indicate when you have billed Medicare.

5. On January 12, Medicare sent check No. 115620 and paid 80% of the approved amount for services rendered on December 15, 20xx. Note: For this case, the approved amount will be the participating amount. Post this amount to the patient's financial account and indicate the balance due from the patient.

6. A Performance Evaluation Checklist may be reproduced from the "Instruction Guide to the Workbook" chapter if your instructor wishes you to submit it to assist with scoring and comments.

After the instructor has returned your work to you, either make the necessary corrections and place your work in a three-ring notebook for future reference or, if you received a high score, place it in your portfolio for reference when applying for a job.

Abbreviations pertinent to this record:

Pt	________________	LC	________________
N	________________	MDM	________________
EKG	________________	adv	________________
STAT	________________	rtn	________________
CPK	________________	ofc	________________
Dx	________________	echo	________________
ASCVD	________________	RTO	________________

Additional Coding and Fee Calculations

1. Refer to Mrs. Mooney's medical record, abstract information, and code procedures that would be billed by outside providers.

Site	*Description of Service*	*Code*
a. College Hospital Laboratory	________________	________________
b. College Hospital Physiology	________________	________________
c. College Hospital Radiology	________________	________________

2. Refer to the Mock Fee Schedule shown in Appendix A in this *Workbook* and complete the following questions:

A. If Dr. Cardi is not participating in the Medicare program, what is the maximum (limiting charge) he can bill for the professional services rendered?

Office visit $ ________________ ECG $________________

B. In the case of a nonparticipating physician, how much will Medicare pay for these services? Note: Use the nonparticipating fees as the allowed amount.

Office visit $________________ ECG $________________

C. How much is the patient's responsibility for these services?

Office visit $________________ ECG $________________

D. How much will the courtesy adjustment be on the patient's financial record?

Office visit $________________ ECG $________________

PATIENT RECORD NO. 12-5

LAST NAME	FIRST NAME	MIDDLE NAME	BIRTH DATE	SEX	HOME PHONE
Mooney	Elsa	M.	02-06-30	F	555-452-4968

ADDRESS	CITY	STATE	ZIP CODE
5750 Canyon Road	Woodland Hills	XY	12345

CELL PHONE	PAGER NO.	FAX NO.	E-MAIL ADDRESS
555-806-3244			Mooney@wb.net

PATIENT'S SOC. SEC. NO.	DRIVER'S LICENSE
321-XX-2653	R9865549

PATIENT'S OCCUPATION	NAME OF COMPANY
retired secretary	

ADDRESS OF EMPLOYER	PHONE

SPOUSE OR PARENT	OCCUPATION
husband deceased	

EMPLOYER	ADDRESS	PHONE

NAME OF INSURANCE	INSURED OR SUBSCRIBER
Medicare	self

POLICY/CERTIFICATE NO.	GROUP NO.
321-XX-2653A	

REFERRED BY: George Gentle, MD, 1000 N. Main Street, Woodland Hills, XY 12345 NPI# 40213102XX

DATE	PROGRESS NOTES
12-15-xx	New pt referred by Dr. Gentle comes in complaining of chest pain and shortness of
	breath; a detailed history was taken. A detailed examination was essentially N. EKG done
	to rule out myocardial infarction; normal sinus rhythm, no abnormalities noted. Pt sent to
	College Hospital for STAT cardiac enzymes (CPK), 2D echocardiogram
	(transthoracic/real-time with Doppler), and complete chest x-ray.
	Working Dx: angina—ASCVD (LC MDM). Pt adv to rtn to ofc this afternoon for test results.
	PC/llf Perry Cardi, MD

Figure 12-3

Acct No. 12-5

STATEMENT
Financial Account
COLLEGE CLINIC
4567 Broad Avenue
Woodland Hills, XY 12345-0001
Tel. 555-486-9002
Fax No. 555-487-8976

Mrs. Elsa M. Mooney
5750 Canyon Road
Woodland Hills, XY 12345-0001

Phone No. (H) (555) 452-4968 (W) ____________ Birthdate 02-06-30

Primary Insurance Co. Medicare Policy/Group No. 321-XX-2653A

	REFERENCE	DESCRIPTION	CHARGES	CREDITS PYMNTS.	CREDITS ADJ.	BALANCE
		BALANCE FORWARD →				
12-15-xx		Init OV, D hx/exam, LC decision making				
12-15-xx		EKG with interpret & report				

PLEASE PAY LAST AMOUNT IN BALANCE COLUMN

THIS IS A COPY OF YOUR FINANCIAL ACCOUNT AS IT APPEARS ON OUR RECORDS

Figure 12-4

ASSIGNMENT 12-6 ▶ COMPLETE A CLAIM FORM FOR A MEDICARE/MEDICAID CASE

Performance Objective

Task: Complete a CMS-1500 (08-05) claim form for a Medicare/Medicaid case, post transactions to the financial accounting record, and define patient record abbreviations.

Conditions: Use the patient's medical record (Figure 12-5) and financial statement (Figure 12-6), one health insurance claim form (print from Evolve website), a computer, procedural and diagnostic code books, and Appendixes A and B in this *Workbook*.

Standards: Claim Productivity Measurement

Time: ________________________ minutes

Accuracy: ________________________

(Note: The time element and accuracy criteria may be given by your instructor.)

Directions:

1. Complete the CMS-1500 (08-05) claim form, using OCR guidelines for a Medicare/Medicaid case. If your instructor wants you to direct it to your local Medicare fiscal intermediary, obtain the name and address by going to the Evolve website listed in Internet Resources at the end of Chapter 12 in the *Handbook*. Refer to Mrs. Helen P. Nolan's patient record for information. Refer to Appendix A in this *Workbook* to locate the fees to be recorded on the claim and posted to the financial statement. Date the claim May 31.

2. Refer to Chapter 7 and Figure 7-7 of the *Handbook* for instructions on how to complete the CMS-1500 (08-05) claim form.

3. Use your CPT code book or Appendix A in this *Workbook* to determine the correct five-digit code number and modifiers for each professional service rendered. Use your HCPCS Level II code book or refer to Appendix B in this *Workbook* for HCPCS procedure codes and modifiers. If your instructor tells you to also find the ICD-10-CM codes, a draft version may be downloaded from the following website: http://www.cdc.gov/nchs/icd/icd10cm.htm#10update.

4. Record all transactions on the financial record and indicate the proper information when you have billed Medicare/Medicaid. On July 1, you receive a check (number 107621) from Medicare for $600, and on July 15 you receive a voucher (number 3571) from Medicaid for $200. Record these payments on the account, and show a courtesy adjustment to zero the account.

5. A Performance Evaluation Checklist may be reproduced from the "Instruction Guide to the Workbook" chapter if your instructor wishes you to submit it to assist with scoring and comments.

After the instructor has returned your work to you, either make the necessary corrections and place your work in a three-ring notebook for future reference or, if you received a high score, place it in your portfolio for reference when applying for a job.

Abbreviations pertinent to this record:

Pt	______	phys	______
hx	______	prep	______
BP	______	hosp	______
ext	______	EPF	______
Dx	______	exam	______
int	______	MC	______
adv	______	MDM	______
Pre-op	______	slt	______
adm	______	PF	______
UA	______	SF	______
auto	______	RTO	______
FBS	______	wk	______
micro	______	OV	______
CXR	______	p.r.n.	______

Additional Coding and Fee Calculations

1. Refer to Mrs. Nolan's medical record, abstract information, and code procedures that would be billed by outside providers.

Site	*Description of Service*	*Code*
a. College Hospital Laboratory	______	______
b. College Hospital Laboratory	______	______
c. College Hospital Laboratory	______	______
d. College Hospital Radiology	______	______

2. Calculate Dr. Cutler's assistant surgeon fee, which is 18.5% of the primary surgeon's fee:

   Hemorrhoidectomy with fistulectomy: $______

PATIENT RECORD NO. 12-6

LAST NAME	FIRST NAME	MIDDLE NAME	BIRTH DATE	SEX	HOME PHONE
Nolan	Helen	P.	05-10-37	F	555-660-9878

ADDRESS	CITY	STATE	ZIP CODE
2588 Cedar Street	Woodland Hills	XY	12345

CELL PHONE	PAGER NO.	FAX NO.	E-MAIL ADDRESS
		555-660-9878	Nolan@wb.net

PATIENT'S SOC. SEC. NO.	DRIVER'S LICENSE
732-XX-1573	J4022876

PATIENT'S OCCUPATION	NAME OF COMPANY
homemaker	

ADDRESS OF EMPLOYER	PHONE

SPOUSE OR PARENT	OCCUPATION	BIRTH DATE
James J. Nolan (deceased)		

EMPLOYER	ADDRESS	PHONE

NAME OF INSURANCE	INSURED OR SUBSCRIBER
Medicare/Medicaid	

MEDICARE NO.	MEDICAID NO.
732-XX-1573B	19-60-2358490-1-XX

REFERRED BY: James B. Jeffers, MD, 100 S. Broadway, Woodland Hills, XY 12345 NPI# 12345069XX

DATE	PROGRESS NOTES
5-1-xx	New pt comes in complaining of constipation, rectal bleeding, and rectal pain. Detailed
	hx taken, BP 120/80. A detailed exam revealed ext hemorrhoids. Diagnostic proctoscopy
	done to further evaluate the hemorrhoids and control bleeding using bipolar cautery.
	Dx: int & ext bleeding hemorrhoids and anorectal fistula. Adv hospitalization for removal
	of hemorrhoids and fistula repair.
	RR/llf Rex Rumsey, MD
5-8-xx	Pre-op testing done prior to adm to College Hospital (UA auto/with micro., hemogram
	auto, FBS quantitative, CXR single frontal view). Admit, phys exam & prep of hospital
	records. Hemorrhoidectomy with fistulectomy performed (authorization no. 7699220012).
	Dr. Clarence Cutler assisted.
	RR/llf Rex Rumsey, MD
5-9-xx	Hosp visit (EPF hx/exam MC MDM). Pt comfortable, slt pain.
	RR/llf Rex Rumsey, MD
5-10-xx	Hosp visit (PF hx/exam SF MDM). No pain.
	RR/llf Rex Rumsey, MD
5-11-xx	Discharged pt to home. RTO in 1 wk.
	RR/llf Rex Rumsey, MD
5-17-xx	OV (PF hx/exam SF MDM). Pt doing well, surgical site healed. Return p.r.n.
	RR/llf Rex Rumsey, MD

Figure 12-5

Acct. No. 12-6

STATEMENT
Financial Account
COLLEGE CLINIC
4567 Broad Avenue
Woodland Hills, XY 12345-0001
Tel. 555-486-9002
Fax No. 555-487-8976

Helen P. Nolan
2588 Cedar Street
Woodland Hills, XY 12345

Phone No. (H) (555) 660-9878 (W) ______ Birthdate 05-10-37

Primary Insurance Co. Medicare/Medicaid Policy/Group No. 732-XX-1573B

	REFERENCE	DESCRIPTION	CHARGES	CREDITS PYMNTS.	CREDITS ADJ.	BALANCE
20XX		BALANCE FORWARD →				
05-01-xx		NP OV				
05-01-xx		Proctoscopy				
05-08-xx		Hemorrhoidectomy with fistulectomy				
05-09-xx		HV				
05-10-xx		HV				
05-11-xx		Discharge				
05-17-xx		OV				

PLEASE PAY LAST AMOUNT IN BALANCE COLUMN

THIS IS A COPY OF YOUR FINANCIAL ACCOUNT AS IT APPEARS ON OUR RECORDS

Figure 12-6

ASSIGNMENT 12-7 ▶ COMPLETE A CLAIM FORM FOR A MEDICARE/SECONDARY PAYER CASE

Performance Objective

Task: Complete a CMS-1500 (08-05) claim form for an MSP case, post transactions to the financial accounting record, and define patient record abbreviations.

Conditions: Use the patient's medical record (Figure 12-7) and financial statement (Figure 12-8), one health insurance claim form (print from Evolve website), a computer, procedural and diagnostic code books, and Appendixes A and B in this *Workbook*.

Standards: Claim Productivity Measurement

Time: ________________________ minutes

Accuracy: ________________________

(Note: The time element and accuracy criteria may be given by your instructor.)

Directions:

1. Complete the CMS-1500 (08-05) claim form, using OCR guidelines for an MSP case, and direct it to the primary insurance carrier. This assignment requires two claim forms, so make a photocopy of the CMS-1500 (08-05) claim form for the second claim. Refer to Peter F. Donlon's patient record for information. Refer to Appendix A in this *Workbook* to locate the fees to be recorded on the claim and posted to the financial statement. Date the claim May 14. Dr. Antrum is not accepting assignment in this case. For a nonparticipating physician, use the limiting charge column of the mock fee schedule. This should also be considered the allowed amount.

2. See Chapter 7 (Figure 7-9) of the *Handbook* for help in completing these forms.

3. Use your CPT code book or Appendix A in this *Workbook* to determine the correct five-digit code number and modifiers for each professional service rendered. Refer to your HCPCS Level II code book or Appendix B in this *Workbook* for HCPCS procedure codes and modifiers. If your instructor tells you to also find the ICD-10-CM codes, a draft version may be downloaded from the following website: http://www.cdc.gov/nchs/icd/icd10cm.htm#10update.

4. Record all transactions on the financial record and indicate when you have billed the primary insurance carrier.

5. On June 5, Coastal Health Insurance Company paid $800 (check number 45632) on this claim. Post this payment to the patient's financial account and indicate the balance that will be billed to Medicare the following day. Note: The explanation of benefits from Coastal Health would be sent to Medicare with a completed CMS-1500 (08-05) claim form.

6. A Performance Evaluation Checklist may be reproduced from the "Instruction Guide to the Workbook" chapter if your instructor wishes you to submit it to assist with scoring and comments.

After the instructor has returned your work to you, either make the necessary corrections and place your work in a three-ring notebook for future reference or, if you received a high score, place it in your portfolio for reference when applying for a job.

Abbreviations pertinent to this record:

ER	________	adm	________
p.m.	________	MC	________
EPF	________	imp	________
hx	________	PF	________
exam	________	SF	________
LC	________	hosp	________
MDM	________	RTO	________
est	________	OV	________
pts	________	surg	________
cm	________	sched	________
consult	________	ofc	________
c̄	________	post-op	________
MRI	________	wk	________
px	________		

Additional Coding and Fee Calculations

1. Refer to Mr. Donlon's medical record, abstract information, and code procedures that would be billed by outside providers.

Site	*Description of Service*	*Code*
a. Emergency room (ER) physician	________	________
b. ER consult	________	________
c. College Hospital Radiology	________	________
d. College Hospital Radiology	________	________

2. Use your diagnostic code book and code the symptoms that the patient presented with in the ER.

Symptom	*ICD-9-CM Code*	*ICD-10-CM Code*
a. ______	______	______
b. ______	______	______
c. ______	______	______

3. On the septoplasty surgery (May 10, 20xx), assume that Coastal Health Insurance Company paid $459.74.

   a. What would the Medicare payment be? ______

   b. What would the patient responsibility be? ______

   c. What would the courtesy adjustment be? ______

PATIENT RECORD NO. 12-7

Donlon	Peter	F	08-09-38	M	555-762-3580
LAST NAME	FIRST NAME	MIDDLE NAME	BIRTH DATE	SEX	HOME PHONE

1840 East Chevy Chase Drive	Woodland Hills	XY	12345
ADDRESS	CITY	STATE	ZIP CODE

CELL PHONE	PAGER NO.	FAX NO.	E-MAIL ADDRESS

987-XX-4321 — PATIENT'S SOC. SEC. NO.
Y2100968 — DRIVER'S LICENSE

chef — PATIENT'S OCCUPATION
Harbor Town Eatery — NAME OF COMPANY

1116 Harbor Way, Woodland Hills, XY 12345 — ADDRESS OF EMPLOYER
555-762-0050 — PHONE

wife deceased — SPOUSE OR PARENT
OCCUPATION

Coastal Health Insurance Co., 10 N. Main Street, Woodland Hills, XY 12345 — NAME OF PRIMARY INSURANCE / ADDRESS
555-369-4401 — PHONE

NAME OF INSURANCE
INSURED OR SUBSCRIBER

34276 — POLICY/CERTIFICATE NO.
45A — GROUP NO.

Medicare — NAME OF SECONDARY INSURANCE
987-XX-4321A — MEDICARE NO.

REFERRED BY:

DATE	PROGRESS NOTES
5-1-xx	Called to ER on Sunday, 11 p.m. ER physician, Dr. Rene Whitney (NPI # 77 536222XX) performed an EPF hx/exam with LC MDM on one of my est pts who was injured at home while walking across lawn pushing garbage can; tripped and hit his head on curb. Pt complains of acute headache, nausea, and nasal pain caused by impact and skin laceration. I sutured a 2.0 cm simple laceration of nose. Pt vomited twice in ER. Requested ER consult c̄ neurologist, Dr. Parkinson (C hx/exam M MDM), who ordered MRI of brain (without contrast) and complete skull series. I performed a C hx and px & adm pt to College Hospital; MDM MC. Imp: Concussion without skull fracture, no loss of consciousness; nasal laceration; deviated septum which may need reconstruction. Disability from work from 5-1 to 5-17.
	CA/IIf — Concha Antrum, MD
5-2-xx	Hospital visit (PF hx/exam LC MDM).
	CA/IIf — Concha Antrum, MD
5-3-xx	Hospital visit (PF hx/exam SF MDM).
	CA/IIf — Concha Antrum, MD
5-4-xx	Discharge from hospital. See hosp records for daily notes. RTO in 2 day for suture removal.
	CA/IIf — Concha Antrum, MD
5-6-xx	OV. Sutures removed; wound healed. Discussed deviated septum and recommended septoplasty. Surg sched for 5/10/xx at College Hospital.
	CA/IIf — Concha Antrum, MD
5-10-xx	Adm to College Hospital (D hx/exam LC MDM). Performed septoplasty. Pt doing well; moved to recovery room.
	CA/IIf — Concha Antrum, MD
5-11-xx	Pt doing well, no hemorrhage, discharged home.
	CA/IIf — Concha Antrum, MD
5-12-xx	Pt comes into ofc with postop anterior nasal hemorrhage. Cauterized rt side. RTO in 1 wk.
	CA/IIf — Concha Antrum, MD

Figure 12-7

Acct. No. 12-7

STATEMENT
Financial Account
COLLEGE CLINIC
4567 Broad Avenue
Woodland Hills, XY 12345-0001
Tel. 555-486-9002
Fax No. 555-487-8976

Peter F. Donlon
1840 East Chevy Chase Drive
Woodland Hills, XY 12345

Phone No. (H) (555) 762-3580 (W) (555)762-0050 Birthdate 08-09-38

Insurance Co. Coastal Health Insurance Co./Medicare Policy/Group No. 34276 Grp. 45A
Medicare No. 987-XX-4321A

	REFERENCE	DESCRIPTION	CHARGES	CREDITS PYMNTS.	CREDITS ADJ.	BALANCE
20XX		BALANCE FORWARD →				
05-01-xx		Initial hospital care				
05-01-xx		Skin repair				
05-02-xx		HV				
05-03-xx		HV				
05-04-xx		Discharge				
05-06-xx		Suture removal				
05-10-xx		Admit-Septoplasty				
05-11-xx		Discharge				
05-12-xx		Postop OV				

PLEASE PAY LAST AMOUNT IN BALANCE COLUMN

THIS IS A COPY OF YOUR FINANCIAL ACCOUNT AS IT APPEARS ON OUR RECORDS

Figure 12-8

ASSIGNMENT 12-8 ▶ COMPLETE A CLAIM FOR A MEDICARE/MEDIGAP CASE

Performance Objective

Task: Complete a CMS-1500 (08-05) claim form for a Medicare/Medigap case, post transactions to the financial accounting record, and define patient record abbreviations.

Conditions: Use the patient's medical record (Figure 12-9) and financial statement (Figure 12-10), one health insurance claim form (print from Evolve website), a computer, procedural and diagnostic code books, and Appendixes A and B in this *Workbook*.

Standards: Claim Productivity Measurement

Time: ______________________ minutes

Accuracy: ______________________

(Note: The time element and accuracy criteria may be given by your instructor.)

Directions:

1. Complete the CMS-1500 (08-05) claim form, using Medicare/Medigap OCR guidelines. If your instructor wants you to direct it to your local fiscal intermediary, obtain the name and address by going to the Evolve website listed in Internet Resources at the end of Chapter 12 in the *Handbook*. This case involves a patient who has a Medigap supplemental policy that is a secondary payer. Refer to Jeremiah W. Diffenderffer's patient record and financial statement for information. See Medicare participating provider fees in Appendix A in this *Workbook* to locate the fees to be recorded on the claim and posted to the financial statement. Fees in the participating column are also the approved amounts. Date the claim June 13. Dr. Coccidioides is accepting assignment in this case. Mr. Diffenderffer has met his deductible for the year, owing to previous care by Dr. Coccidioides.

2. Refer to Chapter 7 and Figure 7-8 of the *Handbook* for instructions on how to complete the CMS-1500 (08-05) claim form.

3. Use your CPT code book or Appendix A in this *Workbook* to determine the correct five-digit code number and modifiers for each professional service rendered. Refer to your HCPCS Level II code book or Appendix B in this *Workbook* for HCPCS procedure codes and modifiers. If your instructor tells you to also find the ICD-10-CM codes, a draft version may be downloaded from the following website: http://www.cdc.gov/nchs/icd/icd10cm.htm#10update.

4. Record all transactions on the financial record, and indicate the proper information when you have billed Medicare and Medigap.

5. On August 3, Medicare check number 654821 was received in the amount of $270.05, paying 80% of the approved amount for all services except the medication charge, of which they allowed $10. Post this payment to the patient's financial account, and calculate and post the courtesy adjustment. On August 15, United American Insurance Company check number 3254 was received in the amount of $67.51, paying 20% of the approved amount for all services, including the $10 allowed amount determined by Medicare for the medication. Post this payment to the patient's financial statement, and indicate the balance due from the patient.

6. A Performance Evaluation Checklist may be reproduced from the "Instruction Guide to the Workbook" chapter if your instructor wishes to submit it to assist with scoring and comments.

After the instructor has returned your work to you, either make the necessary corrections and place your work in a three-ring notebook for future reference or, if you received a high score, place it in your portfolio for reference when applying for a job.

Abbreviations pertinent to this record:

Est	________	hx	________
oft	________	exam	________
p.m.	________	HC	________
SOB	________	MDM	________
adv	________	imp	________
AP	________	RTO	________
lat	________	wk	________
tech	________	c/o	________
CXR	________	HCN	________
ABG	________	PF	________
PFT	________	SF	________
a.m.	________	IV	________
RTO	________	ml	________
CPX	________	appt	________
C	________		

Additional Coding

1. Refer to Mr. Diffenderffer's medical record, abstract information, and code procedures that would be billed by outside providers.

Site	*Description of Service*	*Code*
a. College Hospital Laboratory	________	________
b. College Hospital Respiratory Department	________	________

PATIENT RECORD NO. 12-8

LAST NAME	FIRST NAME	MIDDLE NAME	BIRTH DATE	SEX	HOME PHONE
Diffenderffer	Jeremiah	W	08-24-31	M	555-471 9930

ADDRESS	CITY	STATE	ZIP CODE
120 Elm Street	Woodland Hills	XY	12345

CELL PHONE	PAGER NO.	FAX NO.	E-MAIL ADDRESS
555-218-0087		555-471-9930	Diffenderffer@wb.net

PATIENT'S SOC. SEC. NO.	DRIVER'S LICENSE
731-XX-7401	none

PATIENT'S OCCUPATION	NAME OF COMPANY
retired painter	

ADDRESS OF EMPLOYER	PHONE

SPOUSE OR PARENT	OCCUPATION
deceased	

NAME OF INSURANCE	MEDICARE NO
Medicare	731-XX-7401T

NAME OF OTHER INSURANCE	ADDRESS	PHONE
United American Insurance Company	P.O. Box 810, Dallas, TX 75221	555-328-2841

POLICY/CERTIFICATE NO.	PAYERID NO.
007559715	UNITXY003

REFERRED BY: John M. Diffenderffer (brother)

DATE	PROGRESS NOTES
6-1-xx	Est pt telephoned ofc this p.m. stating he has been involved in a long painting project in
	his home and when he breathed paint fumes in his kitchen today he experienced
	SOB & coughing. Dr. Coccidioides is out of the ofc this p.m. and was paged. Physician
	adv pt to come into ofc for AP & lat chest x-ray and bilateral bronchogram this afternoon.
	Chest x-ray and bronchogram taken by x-ray tech.
	RH/llf Rene Holmes, CMA
6-2-xx	CXR and bronchogram showed pulmonary emphysema. Adv pt by phone to have ABG for
	direct O_2 saturation and PFT (spirometry) at College Hospital this a.m. and RTO for CPX
	this afternoon.
	BC/llf Brady Coccidioides, MD
6-2-xx	Pt returns for C hx/exam HC MDM. Imp: emphysema, bronchitis and pneumonitis due to
	inhalation of fumes and vapors. Adv no more painting; bed rest. RTO 1 wk.
	BC/llf Brady Coccidioides, MD
6-5-xx	Pt calls as ofc is closing c/o difficulty breathing; he has been ambulating and climbing
	stairs. HCN PF hx/exam SF MDM. Administered Coramine (nikethamide) medication IV
	(unclassified drug, 1.5 ml two ampules @ 12.50 each). Imp: recurrent bronchitis and pneumonitis,
	exertional dyspnea. Adv complete bed rest. RTO for appt on 6-9-xx.
	BC/llf Brady Coccidioides, MD

Figure 12-9

Acct. No. 12-8

STATEMENT
Financial Account
COLLEGE CLINIC
4567 Broad Avenue
Woodland Hills, XY 12345-0001
Tel. 555-486-9002
Fax No. 555-487-8976

Jeremiah W. Diffenderffer
120 Elm Street
Woodland Hills, XY 12345

Phone No. (H) (555) 471-9930 (W)

Birthdate 08-24-31

Insurance Co. Medicare/United American Insurance Co.

Policy/Group No. 007559715
Medicare No. 731-XX-7401T

	REFERENCE	DESCRIPTION	CHARGES		CREDITS PYMNTS.		CREDITS ADJ.		BALANCE	
20XX								BALANCE FORWARD →	20	00
06-01-xx		Chest x-ray								
06-01-xx		Bronchogram								
06-02-xx		OV								
06-05-xx		HC								
06-05-xx		IV administration								
06-05-xx		Medication								

PLEASE PAY LAST AMOUNT IN BALANCE COLUMN

THIS IS A COPY OF YOUR FINANCIAL ACCOUNT AS IT APPEARS ON OUR RECORDS

Figure 12-10

ASSIGNMENT 12-9 ▶ COMPLETE A CLAIM FORM FOR A MEDICARE CASE WITH AN ADVANCE BENEFICIARY NOTICE OF NONCOVERAGE

Performance Objective

Task: Complete a CMS-1500 (08-05) claim form for a Medicare case and an advance beneficiary notice of noncoverage, post transactions to the financial accounting record, and define patient record abbreviations.

Conditions: Use the patient's record (Figure 12-11) and financial statement (Figure 12-12), an advance beneficiary notice of noncoverage form (Figure 12-13), two health insurance claim forms (print from Evolve website), a computer, procedural and diagnostic code books, and Appendixes A and B in this *Workbook*.

Standards: Claim Productivity Measurement

Time: ____________________ minutes

Accuracy: ____________________

(Note: The time element and accuracy criteria may be given by your instructor.)

Directions:

1. Complete a CMS-1500 (08-05) claim form for a Medicare case, using OCR guidelines. If your instructor wants you to direct it to your local Medicare Railroad fiscal intermediary, obtain the name and address by going to the Evolve website listed in Internet Resources at the end of Chapter 12 in the *Handbook*. This assignment requires two claim forms, so make a photocopy for the second claim. Refer to Raymond D. Fay's patient record for information. Refer to Appendix A in this *Workbook* to locate the fees to be recorded on the claim and posted to the financial statement. Date the claim December 31. Dr. Antrum is a participating physician and is accepting assignment in this case.

2. Refer to Figure 7-6 in the *Handbook* for instructions on how to complete the CMS-1500 (08-05) claim form.

3. The nystagmus service is disallowed by Medicare, and an advance beneficiary notice of noncoverage needs to be completed. Refer to Figure 12-9 in the *Handbook* for a completed example of this form. Note: When a noncovered service is provided, a fee will not be listed in the Medicare fee schedule; therefore, list the regular (mock) fee.

4. Use your CPT code book or Appendix A in this *Workbook* to determine the correct five-digit code number and modifiers for each professional service rendered. Use your HCPCS Level II code book or refer to Appendix B in this *Workbook* for HCPCS procedure codes and modifiers. The patient has met $71 of the $162 deductible for 2011. If your instructor tells you to also find the ICD-10-CM codes, a draft version may be downloaded from the following website: http://www.cdc.gov/nchs/icd/icd10cm.htm#10update.

5. Record all transactions on the financial accounting record, and indicate the proper information when you have billed Medicare.

6. A Performance Evaluation Checklist may be reproduced from the "Instruction Guide to the Workbook" chapter if your instructor wishes you to submit it to assist with scoring and comments.

After the instructor has returned your work to you, either make the necessary corrections and place your work in a three-ring notebook for future reference or, if you received a high score, place it in your portfolio for reference when applying for a job.

Abbreviations pertinent to this record:

Pt	______	RTO	______
D	______	rtn	______
hx	______	OV	______
exam	______	appt(s)	______
retn	______	wk	______
R/O	______	inj.	______
LC	______	Dx	______
MDM	______	PF	______
N	______	SF	______
X	______	sx	______
incl	______	disc	______

Additional Fee Calculations

1. Medicare sent payment on this claim, allowing 80% of the approved amount after the partial deductible was met, which was subtracted from the amount of this claim. Note: For this case, the approved amount will be the limiting charge. Medicare denied payment on code 92531 as a noncovered service.

   a. What is the amount of the Medicare check? ______

   b. What is the amount of the patient responsibility? ______

   c. Is there a courtesy adjustment? ______

PATIENT RECORD NO. 12-9

LAST NAME	FIRST NAME	MIDDLE NAME	BIRTH DATE	SEX	HOME PHONE
Fay	Raymond		02-03-32	M	555-788-9090

ADDRESS	CITY	STATE	ZIP CODE
33 North Pencil Avenue	Woodland Hills	XY	12345

CELL PHONE	PAGER NO.	FAX NO.	E-MAIL ADDRESS
	555-250-4890	555-788-9090	fay@wb.net

PATIENT'S SOC. SEC. NO.	DRIVER'S LICENSE
887-66-1235	R8966543

PATIENT'S OCCUPATION	NAME OF COMPANY
retired railroad engineer	

ADDRESS OF EMPLOYER	PHONE

SPOUSE OR PARENT	OCCUPATION
Marilyn B. Fay	homemaker

EMPLOYER	ADDRESS	PHONE

NAME OF INSURANCE	INSURED OR SUB SCRIBER
Medicare Railroad	self

MEDICARE NO.
A 887-XX-1235A

REFERRED BY: George Gentle, MD, 1000 N. Main St., Woodland Hills, XY 12345 NPI# 402131102XX

DATE	PROGRESS NOTES
10-31-xx	New pt presents, a D hx was taken. Pt complains of skin rash and dizziness for 3 days.
	A detailed exam reveals rash on chest and arms. Retn in 4 days for tests to R/O eye/ear
	causes for dizziness and food allergies (LC MDM).
	CA/llf Concha Antrum, MD
11-4-xx	Comprehensive audiometric threshold evaluation (with speech)—N. 10 intradermal
	allergy tests; delayed reaction. Bilateral mastoid X (complete)—N. Spontaneous nystagmus
	test, incl. gaze—N. RTO in 3 days for skin test results.
	CA/llf Concha Antrum, MD
11-7-xx	Rtn OV for allergy skin test results—positive for 3 substances. Pt to purchase allergen
	extract and make sequential appts next wk for daily immunotherapy inj. Dx: food allergies.
	CA/llf Concha Antrum, MD
11-14-xx thru	Immunotherapy; 3 inj. per/day
11-18-xx	CA/llf Concha Antrum, MD
11-21-xx thru	Immunotherapy; 3 inj. per/day
11-25-xx	CA/llf Concha Antrum, MD
11-28-xx thru	Immunotherapy; 3 inj. per/day
12-2-xx	CA/llf Concha Antrum, MD
12-5-xx thru	Immunotherapy; 3 inj. per/day
12-8-xx	CA/llf Concha Antrum, MD
12-9-xx	OV (PF hx/exam SF MDM) Pt. sx improved. Received final inj and evaluated for disch.
	CA/llf Concha Antrum, MD

Figure 12-11

Acct No. 12-9

STATEMENT
Financial Account
COLLEGE CLINIC
4567 Broad Avenue
Woodland Hills, XY 12345-0001
Tel. 555-486-9002
Fax No. 555-487-8976

Raymond Fay
33 North Pencil Avenue
Woodland Hills, XY 12345

Phone No. (H) (555) 788-9090 (W) ______ Birthdate 02-03-32

Primary Insurance Co. Medicare Railroad Policy/Group No. A 887-XX 1235A

Secondary Insurance Co. N/A Policy/Group No. ______

DATE	REFERENCE	DESCRIPTION	CHARGES	CREDITS PYMNTS.	CREDITS ADJ.	BALANCE
20xx		BALANCE FORWARD →				
10-31-xx		OV				
11-4-xx		Audiometry evaluation				
11-4-xx		Intradermal allergy tests				
11-4-xx		Bilateral mastoid x-rays				
11-4-xx		Spontaneous nystagmus test				
11-7-xx		Allergy test results				
11-14 to 11-18-xx		Immunotherapy inj. (3/day X 5)				
11-21 to 11-25-xx		Immunotherapy inj. (3/day X 5)				
11-28 to 12-2-xx		Immunotherapy inj. (3/day X 5)				
12-5 to 12-9-xx		Immunotherapy inj. (3/day X 5)				
12-9-xx		OV				

PLEASE PAY LAST AMOUNT IN BALANCE COLUMN

THIS IS A COPY OF YOUR FINANCIAL ACCOUNT AS IT APPEARS ON OUR RECORDS

Figure 12-12

A. Notifier:

B. Patient Name: **C. Identification Number:**

Advance Beneficiary Notice of Noncoverage (ABN)

NOTE: If Medicare doesn't pay for **D.** ____________ below, you may have to pay.

Medicare does not pay for everything, even some care that you or your health care provider have good reason to think you need. We expect Medicare may not pay for the **D.** ____________ below.

D.	E. Reason Medicare May Not Pay:	F. Estimated Cost

WHAT YOU NEED TO DO NOW:

- Read this notice, so you can make an informed decision about your care.
- Ask us any questions that you may have after you finish reading.
- Choose an option below about whether to receive the **D.** ____________ listed above.

  Note: If you choose Option 1 or 2, we may help you to use any other insurance that you might have, but Medicare cannot require us to do this.

G. OPTIONS: Check only one box. We cannot choose a box for you.

☐ **OPTION 1.** I want the **D.** ____________ listed above. You may ask to be paid now, but I also want Medicare billed for an official decision on payment, which is sent to me on a Medicare Summary Notice (MSN). I understand that if Medicare doesn't pay, I am responsible for payment, but **I can appeal to Medicare** by following the directions on the MSN. If Medicare does pay, you will refund any payments I made to you, less co-pays or deductibles.

☐ **OPTION 2.** I want the **D.** ____________ listed above, but do not bill Medicare. You may ask to be paid now as I am responsible for payment. **I cannot appeal if Medicare is not billed.**

☐ **OPTION 3.** I don't want the **D.** ____________ listed above. I understand with this choice I am **not** responsible for payment, and **I cannot appeal to see if Medicare would pay.**

H. Additional Information:

This notice gives our opinion, not an official Medicare decision. If you have other questions on this notice or Medicare billing, call **1-800-MEDICARE** (1-800-633-4227/**TTY:** 1-877-486-2048).

Signing below means that you have received and understand this notice. You also receive a copy.

I. Signature:	J. Date:

According to the Paperwork Reduction Act of 1995, no persons are required to respond to a collection of information unless it displays a valid OMB control number. The valid OMB control number for this information collection is 0938-0566. The time required to complete this information collection is estimated to average 7 minutes per response, including the time to review instructions, search existing data resources, gather the data needed, and complete and review the information collection. If you have comments concerning the accuracy of the time estimate or suggestions for improving this form, please write to: CMS, 7500 Security Boulevard, Attn: PRA Reports Clearance Officer, Baltimore, Maryland 21244-1850.

Form CMS-R-131 (03/11) Form Approved OMB No. 0938-0566

Figure 12-13

ASSIGNMENT 12-10 ▶ COMPLETE A CLAIM FORM FOR A MEDICARE/MEDICAID CASE

Performance Objective

Task: Complete a CMS-1500 (08-05) claim form for a Medicare/Medicaid case, post transactions to the financial accounting record, and define patient record abbreviations.

Conditions: Use the patient's medical record (Figure 12-14) and financial statement (Figure 12-15), one health insurance claim form (print from Evolve website), a computer, procedural and diagnostic code books, and Appendixes A and B in this *Workbook*.

Standards: Claim Productivity Measurement

Time: ____________________ minutes

Accuracy: ____________________

(Note: The time element and accuracy criteria may be given by your instructor.)

Directions:

1. Complete the CMS-1500 (08-05) claim form, using OCR guidelines for a Medicare/Medicaid case. If your instructor wants you to direct it to your local Medicare fiscal intermediary, obtain the name and address by going to the Evolve website listed in Internet Resources at the end of Chapter 12 in the *Handbook*. Refer to Mr. Harris Fremont's patient record for information. Refer to Appendix A in this *Workbook* to locate the fees to be recorded on the claim and posted to the financial statement. Date the claim October 31.

2. Refer to Chapter 7 and Figure 7-7 of the *Handbook* for instructions on how to complete the CMS-1500 (08-05) claim form.

3. Use your CPT code book or Appendix A in this *Workbook* to determine the correct five-digit code number and modifiers for each professional service rendered. Use your HCPCS Level II code book or refer to Appendix B in this *Workbook* for HCPCS procedure codes and modifiers. If your instructor tells you to also find the ICD-10-CM codes, a draft version may be downloaded from the following website: http://www.cdc.gov/nchs/icd/icd10cm.htm#10update.

4. Record all transactions on the financial account and indicate the proper information when you have billed Medicare/Medicaid.

5. On December 12, Medicare paid $125 (check number 281362) on this claim. Post this payment to the patient's financial account. On December 29, you receive a voucher number 7234 from Medicaid for $45. Post this payment to the patient's financial account and show the courtesy adjustment.

6. A Performance Evaluation Checklist may be reproduced from the "Instruction Guide to the Workbook" chapter if your instructor wishes you to submit it to assist with scoring and comments.

After the instructor has returned your work to you, either make the necessary corrections and place your work in a three-ring notebook for future reference or, if you received a high score, place it in your portfolio for reference when applying for a job.

Abbreviations pertinent to this record:

NP	____________	pt	____________
c/o	____________	lab	____________
hx	____________	CBC	____________
R	____________	auto	____________
L	____________	diff	____________
N	____________	ESR	____________
Rx	____________	R/O	____________
adv	____________	PF	____________
rtn	____________	SF	____________
LC	____________	prn	____________
MDM	____________	imp	____________

Additional Coding

1. Refer to Mr. Fremont's medical record, abstract information, and code procedures that would be billed by outside providers.

Site	*Description of Service*	*Code*
a. ABC Laboratory	____________	____________
b. ABC Laboratory	____________	____________
c. ABC Laboratory	____________	____________
d. ABC Laboratory	____________	____________

2. Use your diagnostic code book and code the symptoms of which the patient complained.

Symptom	*ICD-9-CM Code*	*ICD-10-CM Code*
a. ____________	____________	____________
b. ____________	____________	____________

PATIENT RECORD NO. 12-10

LAST NAME	FIRST NAME	MIDDLE NAME	BIRTH DATE	SEX	HOME PHONE
Fremont	Harris		07-10-23	M	555-899-0109

ADDRESS	CITY	STATE	ZIP CODE
735 North Center Street	Woodland Hills,	XY	12345

CELL PHONE	PAGER NO.	FAX NO.	E-MAIL ADDRESS

PATIENT'S SOC. SEC. NO.	DRIVER'S LICENSE
454-XX-9569	none

PATIENT'S OCCUPATION	NAME OF COMPANY
retired baseball coach	

ADDRESS OF EMPLOYER	PHONE

SPOUSE OR PARENT	OCCUPATION
Emily B. Fremont	homemaker

EMPLOYER	ADDRESS	PHONE

NAME OF INSURANCE	INSURED OR SUBSCRIBER
Medicare/Medicaid	

MEDICARE NO.	MEDICAID NO.
454-XX-9569A	56-10-0020205-0-XX

REFERRED BY: Raymond Skeleton, MD

DATE	PROGRESS NOTES
10-2-xx	NP referred by Dr. Skeleton. He comes in c/o discomfort around toes of both feet and
	has difficulty walking. Pt states he dropped shelf on feet about a month ago. A detailed
	hx reveals gout and mycotic nails. X-ray R and L feet (2 views) N. Detailed exam reveals
	bilateral mycotic nails & ingrown nail on great R toe. Rx: Electrically débride and trimmed
	overgrowth of all nails and adv to rtn if pain continues in great R toe (LC MDM). Gave pt
	order to have lab work done at ABC Laboratory (CBC w/auto diff., ESR (automated), uric acid level)
	R/O gout. Imp: Mycotic nails; difficulty walking.
	NP/llf Nick Pedro, DPM
10-18-xx	Pt returns c/o ingrown nail on R great toe (PF hx/exam SF MDM). Lab work done on
	10/2/xx showed no signs of gout. Performed wedge excision of skin/nail fold.
	Rtn prn. Imp: Ingrown nail – great R toe; toe pain.
	NP/llf Nick Pedro, DPM

Figure 12-14

Acct No. 12-10

STATEMENT
Financial Account
COLLEGE CLINIC
4567 Broad Avenue
Woodland Hills, XY 12345-0001
Tel. 555-486-9002
Fax No. 555-487-8976

Harris Fremont
735 North Center Street
Woodland Hills, XY 12345

Phone No. (H) 555-899-0109 (W) ____ Birthdate 7/10/23

Primary Insurance Co. Medicare Policy/Group No. 454XX9569A

Secondary Insurance Co. Medicaid Policy/Group No. 561000202050XX

DATE	REFERENCE	DESCRIPTION	CHARGES	CREDITS PYMNTS.	CREDITS ADJ.	BALANCE
20xx				BALANCE FORWARD →		
10-2-xx		NP OV				
10-2-xx		X-rays R/L feet				
10-2-xx		Débridement nails				
10-18-xx		OV				
10-18-xx		Wedge excision R. great toe				

PLEASE PAY LAST AMOUNT IN BALANCE COLUMN

THIS IS A COPY OF YOUR FINANCIAL ACCOUNT AS IT APPEARS ON OUR RECORDS

Figure 12-15

STUDENT SOFTWARE CHALLENGE

ASSIGNMENT 12-11 ▶ ASSIGNMENTS FOR MEDICARE CASES 8 THROUGH 10 ONSCREEN COMPLETION OF CMS-1500 (08-05) INSURANCE CLAIM FORMS

Performance Objective

Task: Enter transactions from patients' onscreen encounter forms (superbills) and complete block-by-block onscreen health insurance claim forms.

Conditions: Onscreen encounter forms (superbills) and computer.

Standards: Time: ______________________ minutes

Accuracy: ______________________

(Note: The time element and accuracy criteria may be given by your instructor.)

Directions: Log on to your Evolve account at http://evolve.elsevier.com and access the student resources for Fordney: *Insurance Handbook for the Medical Office*, 12th edition. Then choose Student Software Challenge.

1. For these assignments, follow the instructions for entering data into the onscreen CMS-1500 (08-05) health insurance claim form, completing blocks 1 through 33 for cases 8 through 10.

2. Use your CPT code book or Appendix A in this *Workbook* to determine the correct five-digit code number and modifiers for each professional service rendered. If your instructor tells you to also find the ICD-10-CM codes, a draft version may be downloaded from the following website: http://www.cdc.gov/nchs/icd/icd10cm.htm#10update.

3. A Performance Evaluation Checklist may be reproduced from the "Instruction Guide to the Workbook" chapter if your instructor wishes you to submit it to assist with scoring and comments.

4. Print a hard copy of the completed health insurance claim form for each case.

5. After the instructor has returned your work to you, either make the necessary corrections and place your work in a three-ring notebook for future reference or, if you received a high score, place it in your portfolio for reference when applying for a job.

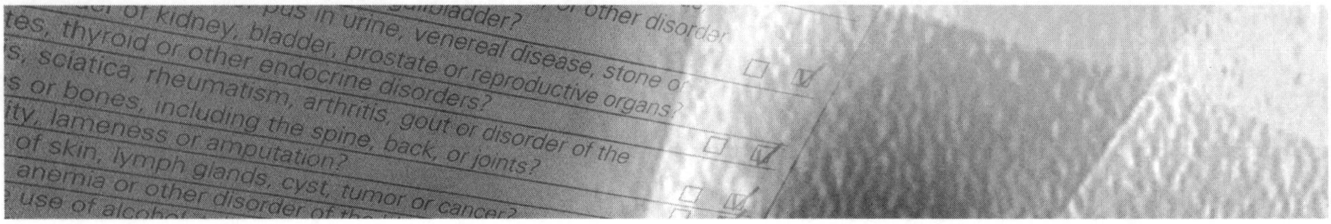

CHAPTER

13

Medicaid and Other State Programs

KEY TERMS

Your instructor may wish to select some words pertinent to this chapter for a test. For definitions of the terms, further study, and/or reference, the words, phrases, and abbreviations may be found in the glossary at the end of the Handbook. *Key terms for this chapter follow.*

categorically needy
coinsurance
copayment
covered services
Early and Periodic Screening, Diagnosis, and Treatment
fiscal agent
Maternal and Child Health Program
Medicaid
Medi-Cal
medically needy
prior approval
recipient
share of cost
State Children's Health Insurance Program
Supplemental Security Income

KEY ABBREVIATIONS

See how many abbreviations and acronyms you can translate and then use this as a handy reference list. Definitions for the key abbreviations are located near the back of the Handbook *in the glossary.*

DEFRA ____________________
EPSDT ____________________
FPL ____________________
MCHP ____________________
MN ____________________
MQMB ____________________
OBRA ____________________
OOY claims ____________________
POS machine ____________________
QI program ____________________
QMB ____________________
RA ____________________
SCHIP ____________________
SLMB ____________________
SSI ____________________
TANF ____________________
TEFRA ____________________

PERFORMANCE OBJECTIVES

The student will be able to:

- Define and spell the key terms and key abbreviations for this chapter, given the information from the *Handbook* glossary, within a reasonable time period and with enough accuracy to obtain a satisfactory evaluation.
- After reading the chapter, answer the fill-in-the-blank, multiple choice, and true/false review questions with enough accuracy to obtain a satisfactory evaluation.
- Fill in the correct meaning of each abbreviation, given a list of common medical abbreviations and symbols that appear in chart notes, within a reasonable time period and with enough accuracy to obtain a satisfactory evaluation.
- Given the patient's medical chart notes, ledger cards, and blank insurance claim forms, complete each CMS-1500 (08-05) Health Insurance Claim Form for billing within a reasonable time period and with enough accuracy to obtain a satisfactory evaluation.
- Correctly post payments, adjustments, and balances on the patient's ledger cards, using the Mock Fee Schedule in Appendix A in this *Workbook*, within a reasonable time period and with enough accuracy to obtain a satisfactory evaluation.

STUDY OUTLINE

History

Medicaid Programs

Maternal and Child Health Program
Low-Income Medicare Recipients

Medicaid Eligibility

Verifying Eligibility
Categorically Needy
Medically Needy
Maternal and Child Health Program Eligibility
Spousal Impoverishment Protection Law
New Freedom Initiative
Accepting Medicaid Patients

Medicaid Benefits

Covered Services
Disallowed Services

Medicaid Managed Care

Claim Procedures

Copayment
Prior Approval
Time Limit
Reciprocity
Claim Form

After Claim Submission

Remittance Advice
Appeals

Medicaid Fraud Control

ASSIGNMENT 13-1 ▶ REVIEW QUESTIONS

Part I Fill in the Blank

Review the objectives, key terms, glossary definitions of key terms, chapter information, and figures before completing the following review questions.

1. Medicaid is administered by ______________ with partial ______________ funding.

2. Medicaid is not an insurance program. It is a/an ______________________ program.

3. In all other states, the program is known as Medicaid, but in California the program is called ____

4. Because the federal government sets minimum requirements, states are free to enhance the Medicaid program. Name two ways in which Medicaid programs vary from state to state.

   a. ____

   b. ____

5. SCHIP means ______________________________ and MCHP means ______________________________ and covers children of what age group?

   ____

6. Name the three aid programs for low-income Medicare patients.

   a. ____

   b. ____

   c. ____

7. Name two broad classifications of people eligible for Medicaid assistance.

   a. ____

   b. ____

8. The name of the program for the prevention, early detection, and treatment of conditions of children receiving welfare is known as ______________________________.

   It is abbreviated as ____________________.

9. Your Medicaid patient seen today needs long-term hemodialysis services. You telephone for authorization to get verbal approval. Four important items to obtain are:

   a. ______________________________

   b. ______________________________

   c. ______________________________

   d. ______________________________

10. The time limit for submitting a Medicaid claim varies from ______________ to ______________ from the date the service is rendered. In your state, the time limit is ______________________________.

11. The insurance claim form for submitting Medicaid claims in all states is ______________________________.

12. Your Medicaid patient also has TRICARE. What billing procedure do you follow? Be exact in your steps for a dependent of an active military person.

   a. ______________________________

   b. ______________________________

13. Five categories of adjudicated claims that may appear on a Medicaid remittance advice document are:

   a. ______________________________

   b. ______________________________

   c. ______________________________

   d. ______________________________

   e. ______________________________

14. Name three levels of Medicaid appeals.

   a. ______________________________

   b. ______________________________

   c. ______________________________

Part II Multiple Choice

Choose the best answer.

15. When professional services are rendered, the Medicaid identification card or electronic verification must show eligibility for

    a. day of service

    b. year of service

    c. month of service

    d. week of service

16. When a Medicaid patient is injured in an automobile accident and the car has liability insurance, this involves a third-party payer so the insurance claim is sent to the

    a. patient

    b. automobile insurance carrier

    c. Medicaid fiscal agent

    d. none of the above

17. The only state without a Medicaid program that is similar to those existing in other states that has an alternative prepaid medical assistance program is

    a. Arizona

    b. California

    c. Colorado

    d. New Mexico

18. A patient's Medicaid eligibility may be verified by

    a. touch-tone telephone

    b. modem

    c. special Medicaid terminal equipment

    d. all of the above

19. When a Medicaid patient requires a piece of durable medical equipment, the physician must

    a. write a prescription

    b. obtain prior authorization, preferably written

    c. instruct the patient on how to use the equipment

    d. give name and address of where to purchase the equipment

20. Medicare beneficiaries who are disabled but have annual incomes below the federal poverty level may be eligible for

a. Medicaid Qualified Medicare Beneficiary Program

b. Qualifying Individuals Program

c. Specified Low-Income Medicare Beneficiary Program

d. all of the above.

Part III True/False

Write "T" or "F" in the blank to indicate whether you think the statement is true or false.

_______ 21. Cerebral palsy is a condition that qualifies a child for benefits under the Maternal and Child Health Program.

_______ 22. There is only one type of copayment requirement in the Medicaid program.

_______ 23. When filing a claim for a Medicaid managed care patient, transmit the claim to the managed care organization and not the Medicaid fiscal agent.

_______ 24. Providers must enroll for participation in the Medicaid program with the fiscal agent for their region.

_______ 25. A state agency that investigates complaints of mistreatment in long-term care facilities is the Medicaid Fraud Control Unit (MFCU).

ASSIGNMENT **13-2** ▸ **CRITICAL THINKING**

Performance Objective

Task: After reading the scenario, answer the following questions, using critical thinking skills.

Conditions: Use a pen or pencil.

Standards: Time: ____________________ minutes

Accuracy: ____________________

(Note: The time element and accuracy criteria may be given by your instructor.)

Directions: After reading the scenario, answer questions, using your critical thinking skills. Record your answers on the blank lines.

Scenario: Mrs. Ho suddenly experiences a pain in her right lower abdominal area and rushes to a local hospital for emergency care. Laboratory work verifies that she has a ruptured appendix, and immediate surgery is recommended. Is prior authorization required in a bona fide emergency situation like this?

1. ____

   Reason: ____

In referring to the instructions for completing a CMS-1500 (08-05) claim form for a Medicaid case, which two blocks on the CMS-1500 (08-05) claim form need to be completed for emergency services?

2. Block ____

   What data should be inserted? ____

3. Block ____

   What data should be inserted and/or document attached?

   ____

ASSIGNMENT 13-3 ▸ COMPLETE A CLAIM FORM FOR A MEDICAID CASE

Performance Objective

Task: Complete a CMS-1500 (08-05) claim form, post transactions to the financial accounting record, and define patient record abbreviations.

Conditions: Use the patient's record (Figure 13-1) and financial statement (Figure 13-2), one health insurance claim form (print from Evolve website), a computer, procedural and diagnostic code books, and Appendixes A and B in this *Workbook.*

Standards: Claim Productivity Measurement

Time: ______________________ minutes

Accuracy: ______________________

(Note: The time element and accuracy criteria may be given by your instructor.)

Directions:

1. Using OCR guidelines, complete the Health Insurance Claim Form and direct it to Medicaid for Rose Clarkson by referring to her patient record. Date the claim September 6. Refer to Appendix A in this *Workbook* to locate the fees to record on the claim and post them to the financial statement. If your instructor wants you to insert the name and address of your Medicaid fiscal agent on the claim, obtain the address by going to the Evolve website listed in Internet Resources at the end of Chapter 13 in the *Handbook*.

2. Refer to Chapter 7 (Figure 7-5) in the *Handbook* for instructions on how to complete this claim form and a Medicaid template.

3. Use your *Current Procedural Terminology* (CPT) code book or Appendix A in this *Workbook* to determine the correct five-digit code number and modifiers for each professional service rendered. Use your Healthcare Common Procedure Coding System (HCPCS) Level II code book or refer to Appendix B in this *Workbook* for HCPCS procedure codes and modifiers.

If your instructor tells you to also find the ICD-10-CM codes, a draft version may be downloaded from the following website: http://www.cdc.gov/nchs/icd/icd10cm.htm#10update.

4. Record all transactions on the financial account, and indicate the date when you have billed Medicaid.

5. Refer to Appendix A in this *Workbook* for the clinic and hospital provider numbers that are needed for completing Medicaid forms.

6. A Performance Evaluation Checklist may be reproduced from the "Instruction Guide to the Workbook" chapter if your instructor wishes you to submit it to assist with scoring and comments.

PATIENT RECORD NO. 13-3

LAST NAME	FIRST NAME	MIDDLE NAME	BIRTH DATE	SEX	HOME PHONE
Clarkson	Rose		03-09-54	F	555-487-2209

ADDRESS	CITY	STATE	ZIP CODE
3408 Jackson Street	Hempstead	XY	11551-0300

CELL PHONE	PAGER NO.	FAX NO.	E-MAIL ADDRESS
	555-340-2200		

PATIENT'S SOC. SEC. NO.	DRIVER'S LICENSE
030-XX-9543	R3207897

PATIENT'S OCCUPATION	NAME OF COMPANY
unemployed	

ADDRESS OF EMPLOYER	PHONE

SPOUSE OR PARENT	OCCUPATION

EMPLOYER	ADDRESS	PHONE

NAME OF INSURANCE	INSURED OR SUBSCRIBER
Medicaid	self

MEDICAID NO.	GROUP NO.
CC99756329346X	

REFERRED BY: James Jackson, MD, 100 North Main Street, Hempstead, XY 11551 NPI# 72011337XX

DATE	PROGRESS NOTES
9-4-xx	New pt presents complaining of cough & SOB. A detailed hx was taken which revealed
	mitral valve prolapse. A D exam was done indicating elevated cardiac and respiratory rates,
	diminished breath sounds, distended neck veins, and edema of both ankles. 12 lead ECG
	performed; normal sinus rhythm and elevated heart rate. Echocardiogram done
	(2D, complete with pulsed wave Doppler) to evaluate mitral valve, cardiac chamber size, and ventricular
	function; presence of mitral valve regurgitation. Single view chest x-ray indicated presence
	of fluid in lungs. Primary diagnosis: congestive heart disease and mitral valve prolapse
	(LC MDM). Pt given Rx for diuretic, digitalis, and vasodilator. Restrict fluid and sodium
	intake. Retn in 2 wks.
	PC/llf Perry Cardi, MD

Figure 13-1

Acct No. 13-3

STATEMENT
Financial Account
COLLEGE CLINIC
4567 Broad Avenue
Woodland Hills, XY 12345-0001
Tel. 555-486-9002
Fax No. 555-487-8976

Rose Clarkson
3408 Jackson Street
Hempstead, XY 11551-0300

Phone No. (H) (555) 487-2209 (W) Birthdate 3-9-54

Primary Insurance Co. Medicaid Policy/Group No. C99756E

Secondary Insurance Co. None Policy/Group No.

DATE	REFERENCE	DESCRIPTION	CHARGES	CREDITS PYMNTS.	CREDITS ADJ.	BALANCE
20xx		BALANCE FORWARD →				
9-4-xx		OV NP				
9-4-xx		12 lead ECG				
9-4-xx		Echocardiogram c̄ Doppler				
9-4-xx		Chest x-ray				

PLEASE PAY LAST AMOUNT IN BALANCE COLUMN

THIS IS A COPY OF YOUR FINANCIAL ACCOUNT AS IT APPEARS ON OUR RECORDS

Figure 13-2

After the instructor has returned your work to you, either make the necessary corrections and place your work in a three-ring notebook for future reference or, if you received a high score, place it in your portfolio for reference when applying for a job.

Abbreviations pertinent to this record:

Pt	__________	LC	__________
SOB	__________	MDM	__________
hx	__________	Rx	__________
D	__________	retn	__________
ECG	__________	wks	__________

ASSIGNMENT 13-4 ▶ COMPLETE A CLAIM FORM FOR A MEDICAID CASE

Performance Objective

Task: Complete a CMS-1500 (08-05) claim form for a Medicaid case, post transactions to the financial accounting record, and define patient record abbreviations.

Conditions: Use the patient's record (Figure 13-3) and financial statement (Figure 13-4), one health insurance claim form (print from Evolve website), a computer, procedural and diagnostic code books, and Appendixes A and B in this *Workbook*.

Standards: Claim Productivity Measurement

Time: ______________________ minutes

Accuracy: ______________________

(Note: The time element and accuracy criteria may be given by your instructor.)

Directions:

1. Using OCR guidelines, complete the Health Insurance Claim Form and direct it to Medicaid for Stephen M. Drake by referring to his patient record. Refer to Appendix A in this *Workbook* to locate the fees to record on the claim, and post them to the financial statement. On May 1, the fee for the injection of Bicillin is $10. As learned in Chapter 6, injectable drugs and medications may be billed separately for Medicaid patients. Date the claim May 26. If your instructor wants you to insert the name and address of your Medicaid fiscal agent on the claim, obtain it by going to the Evolve website listed in Internet Resources at the end of Chapter 13 in the *Handbook*. Do not list services not charged for (NC) on the claim form; however, do list postoperative follow-up visits during the global period on the financial statement. Locate the correct code number in the CPT Medicine section.

Remember that the physician must always sign all forms on Medicaid cases; stamped signatures are not allowed.

2. Refer to Chapter 7 (Figure 7-5) in the *Handbook* for instructions on how to complete this claim form and a Medicaid template.

3. Use your CPT code book or Appendix A in this *Workbook* to determine the correct five-digit code number and modifiers for each professional service rendered. Use your HCPCS Level II code book or refer to Appendix B in this *Workbook* for HCPCS procedure codes and modifiers. If your instructor tells you to also find the ICD-10-CM codes, a draft version may be downloaded from the following website: http://www.cdc.gov/nchs/icd/icd10cm.htm#10update.

4. Record all transactions of the financial account and indicate the date when you have billed Medicaid.

5. Refer to Appendix A in this *Workbook* for the clinic and hospital provider numbers that are needed for completing Medicaid forms.

PATIENT RECORD NO. 13-4

LAST NAME	FIRST NAME	MIDDLE NAME	BIRTH DATE	SEX	HOME PHONE
Drake	Stephen	M	04-03-91	M	555-277-5831

ADDRESS	CITY	STATE	ZIP CODE
2317 Charnwood Avenue	Woodland Hills	XY	12345

CELL PHONE	PAGER NO.	FAX NO.	E-MAIL ADDRESS

PATIENT'S SOC. SEC. NO.	DRIVER'S LICENSE
566-XX-0081	

PATIENT'S OCCUPATION	NAME OF COMPANY
full time student	

ADDRESS OF EMPLOYER	PHONE

SPOUSE OR PARENT	OCCUPATION
Mrs. Virginia B. Drake (mother)	none—family on welfare

EMPLOYER	ADDRESS	PHONE

NAME OF INSURANCE	INSURED OR SUBSCRIBER
Medicaid	

POLICY/CERTIFICATE NO.	GROUP NO.
Child's identification number	19-37-1524033-16X

REFERRED BY: James B. Jeffers, MD, 100 S. Broadway, Woodland Hills, XY 12345 Provider No. 12345069XX

DATE	PROGRESS NOTES
5-1-xx	NP comes in complaining of severe sore throat since April 4. A detailed hx was taken.
	Mother states Stephen has had many bouts of adenoid symptoms and tonsillitis since age 4. He has missed
	school on three occasions this year due to throat infections. Did complete phys exam (D)
	which showed enlargement & inflam of tonsils and adenoids. Temp 101.2. Strep culture done
	(screening) with a preliminary report; positive for strep. Administered penicillin G (Bicillin)
	1.2 million units IM and wrote Rx to start AB and continue x 10 d. Imp: Acute tonsillitis
	(LC MDM). RTO 1 week.
	GP/llf Gerald Practon, MD
5-8-xx	Pt returns; sore throat improved but still swollen. Tonsils are 4+ hypertrophic. Received
	medical records from past primary physician which indicated hx of 5 bouts of strep over
	last 3 yrs. Adv. tonsillectomy and adenoidectomy. Phoned for prior authorization 3 p.m.,
	Auth. No. 45042, given by Mrs. Jane Michaels. Pt to be admitted tomorrow for one day
	surgery (PF HX/PX SF MDM).
	GP/llf Gerald Practon, MD
5-9-xx	Admit to College Hospital. Tonsillectomy and adenoidectomy performed. Pt doing well,
	discharged 4:00 P.M. RTC 1 week.
	GP/llf Gerald Practon, MD
5-17-xx	PO visit. No complaints. Temp 98.1. Retn if necessary (PF HX/PX SF MDM).
	GP/llf Gerald Practon, MD

Figure 13-3

Acct No. 13-4

STATEMENT
Financial Account
COLLEGE CLINIC
4567 Broad Avenue
Woodland Hills, XY 12345-0001
Tel. 555-486-9002
Fax No. 555-487-8976

Stephen M. Drake
c/o Virginia B. Drake
2317 Charnwood Avenue
Woodland Hills, XY 12345

Phone No. (H) (555) 277-5831 (W)
Birthdate 4-3-91

Primary Insurance Co. Medicaid
Policy/Group No. 19-37-1524033-16X

Secondary Insurance Co. N/A
Policy/Group No.

DATE	REFERENCE	DESCRIPTION	CHARGES	CREDITS PYMNTS.	CREDITS ADJ.	BALANCE
20xx		BALANCE FORWARD →				
5-1-xx		NP OV				
5-1-xx		Strep culture				
5-1-xx		Injection AB				
5-1-xx		Bicillin				
5-8-xx		OV				
5-9-xx		T & A				
5-17-xx		PO OV				

PLEASE PAY LAST AMOUNT IN BALANCE COLUMN

THIS IS A COPY OF YOUR FINANCIAL ACCOUNT AS IT APPEARS ON OUR RECORDS

Figure 13-4

6. On July 1, Medicaid paid $200 on this claim. Post this payment (warrant number 766504) to the patient's financial account and adjust the balance, using the same line.

7. A Performance Evaluation Checklist may be reproduced from the "Instruction Guide to the Workbook" chapter if your instructor wishes you to submit it to assist with scoring and comments.

After the instructor has returned your work to you, either make the necessary corrections and place your work in a three-ring notebook for future reference or, if you received a high score, place it in your portfolio for reference when applying for a job.

Abbreviations pertinent to this record:

NP	______	imp	______
hx	______	LC	______
D	______	MDM	______
phys	______	RTO	______
inflam	______	yrs	______
temp	______	adv	______
strep	______	PF	______
IM	______	SF	______
Rx	______	RTC	______
AB	______	PO	______
X	______	retn	______
d	______		

Additional Coding

1. Using your diagnostic code book, code the symptoms that the patient presented with on May 1, 20xx.

	Symptom	*ICD-9-CM Code*	*ICD-10-CM Code*
a.	______	______	______
b.	______	______	______
c.	______	______	______

ASSIGNMENT 13-5 ▸ COMPLETE A CLAIM FORM FOR A MEDICAID CASE

Performance Objective

Task: Complete a CMS-1500 (08-05) claim form for a Medicaid case, post transactions to the financial accounting record, and define patient record abbreviations.

Conditions: Use the patient's record (Figure 13-5) and financial statement (Figure 13-6), one health insurance claim form (print from Evolve website), a computer, procedural and diagnostic code books, and Appendixes A and B in this *Workbook*.

Standards: Claim Productivity Measurement

Time: ____________________ minutes

Accuracy: ____________________

(Note: The time element and accuracy criteria may be given by your instructor.)

Directions:

1. Using OCR guidelines, complete the Health Insurance Claim Form and direct it to Medicaid for Barry L. Brooke by referring to his patient record. Refer to Appendix A in this *Workbook* to locate the fees to record on the claim, and post them to the financial statement. The financial statement should be sent in care of (c/o) the patient's parents because he is a minor. Date the claim June 10. If your instructor wants you to insert the name and address of your Medicaid fiscal agent on the claim, obtain it by going to the Evolve website listed in Internet Resources at the end of Chapter 13 in the *Handbook*.

2. Refer to Chapter 7 (Figure 7-5) in the *Handbook* for instructions on how to complete this claim form and a Medicaid template.

3. Use your CPT code book or Appendix A in this *Workbook* to determine the diagnostic codes and the correct five-digit code number and modifiers for each professional service rendered. Use your HCPCS Level II code book or refer to Appendix B in this *Workbook* for HCPCS procedure codes and modifiers.

   If your instructor tells you to also find the ICD-10-CM codes, a draft version may be downloaded from the following website: http://www.cdc.gov/nchs/icd/icd10cm.htm#10update.

4. Record all transactions on the financial account and indicate the date when you have billed Medicaid.

5. Refer to Appendix A in this *Workbook* for the clinic and hospital provider numbers that are needed for completing Medicaid forms.

6. On July 1, Medicaid paid $75 (warrant number 329670) on this claim. Post this payment to the patient's financial statement and adjust the balance.

7. A Performance Evaluation Checklist may be reproduced from the "Instruction Guide to the Workbook" chapter if your instructor wishes you to submit it to assist with scoring and comments.

PATIENT RECORD NO. 13-5

Brooke	Barry	L	02-03-90	M	555-487-9770
LAST NAME	FIRST NAME	MIDDLE NAME	BIRTH DATE	SEX	HOME PHONE

3821 Ocean Drive	Woodland Hills	XY	12345
ADDRESS	CITY	STATE	ZIP CODE

			brooke@wb.net
CELL PHONE	PAGER NO.	FAX NO.	E-MAIL ADDRESS

776-XX-1931	
PATIENT'S SOC. SEC. NO.	DRIVER'S LICENSE

child—full time student	
PATIENT'S OCCUPATION	NAME OF COMPANY

ADDRESS OF EMPLOYER	PHONE

Robert D. Brooke (father)	none—family on welfare (father totally disabled)
SPOUSE OR PARENT	OCCUPATION

EMPLOYER	ADDRESS	PHONE

Medicaid	Barry
NAME OF INSURANCE	INSURED OR SUB SCRIBER

54-32-7681533-10X
MEDICAID NO.

REFERRED BY: Virginia B. Drake (friend)

DATE	PROGRESS NOTES
5-28-xx	Sunday evening, new pt seen in ER at College Hospital. Pt twisted L knee while playing
	baseball at Grove Park. X-rays (3 views of L knee) were ordered –N for fx. Imp: effusion
	and ligament strain lt knee. Tx: aspirated lt knee and removed 5 cc bloody fluid.
	Discussion is held with mother and son; bracing versus casting. Mother insists on a cast
	because she states he is noncompliant and thinks he will remove the brace and injure his
	leg further. Barry agrees to have cast. Applied long leg fiberglass walking cast. Pt to be
	seen in office in 2 wks (D HX/PX M MDM).
	RS/llf Raymond Skeleton, MD
6-10-xx	Pt returns c/o continued knee pain and wants cast removed. He is in tears and says he
	has been miserable. Mother agrees to have cast removed; leg examined. Fitted pt with
	orthotic device for his knee (straight-leg canvas immobilizer, longitudinal, prefabricated $85).
	Ordered MRI without contrast of L knee to be done at College Hospital Radiology. Pt given directions and
	precautions regarding ambulation with brace (EPF HX/PX LC MDM). RTO 2 wks.
	RS/llf Raymond Skeleton, MD

Figure 13-5

Acct No. 13-5

STATEMENT
Financial Account
COLLEGE CLINIC
4567 Broad Avenue
Woodland Hills, XY 12345-0001
Tel. 555-486-9002
Fax No. 555-487-8976

Barry L Brooke
c/o Robert D. Brooke
3821 Ocean Drive
Woodland Hills, XY 12345

Phone No. (H) (555) 487-9770 (W) Birthdate 2-3-90

Primary Insurance Co. Medicaid Policy/Group No. 5432768153310X

Secondary Insurance Co. Policy/Group No.

DATE	REFERENCE	DESCRIPTION	CHARGES	CREDITS PYMNTS.	CREDITS ADJ.	BALANCE
20xx		BALANCE FORWARD →				
5-28-xx		ER				
5-28-xx		Aspiration L knee				
5-28-xx		Cast application				
6-10-xx		OV				
6-10-xx		L Knee immobilizer				

PLEASE PAY LAST AMOUNT IN BALANCE COLUMN

THIS IS A COPY OF YOUR FINANCIAL ACCOUNT AS IT APPEARS ON OUR RECORDS

Figure 13-6

After the instructor has returned your work to you, either make the necessary corrections and place your work in a three-ring notebook for future reference or, if you received a high score, place it in your portfolio for reference when applying for a job.

Abbreviations pertinent to this record:

Pt	______	lt	______
ER	______	tx	______
L	______	cc	______
N	______	MRI	______
fx	______	RTO	______
imp	______	wks	______

Additional Coding

1. Refer to Barry Brooke's medical record, abstract information, and code procedures that would be billed by outside providers.

Site	*Description of Service*	*Code*
a. College Hospital Radiology	______	______
b. College Hospital Central Supply	______	______
c. College Hospital Radiology	______	______

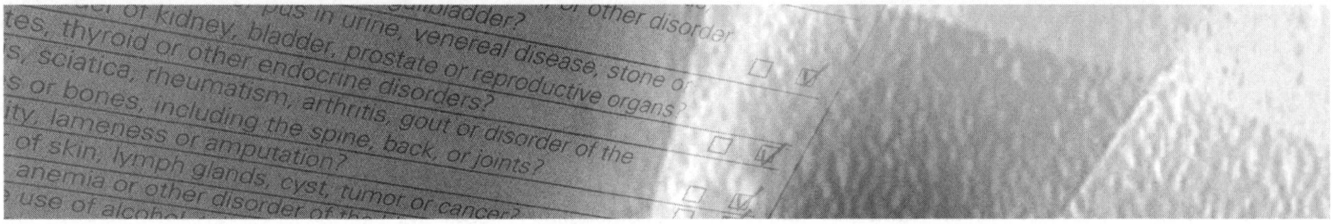

CHAPTER

14

TRICARE and CHAMPVA

KEY TERMS

Your instructor may wish to select some words pertinent to this chapter for a test. For definitions of the terms, further study, and/or reference, the words, phrases, and abbreviations may be found in the glossary at the end of the Handbook. *Key terms for this chapter follow.*

active duty service member
allowable charge
authorized provider
beneficiary
catastrophic cap
catchment area
Civilian Health and Medical Program of the Department of Veterans Affairs
cooperative care
coordination of benefits
cost share
Defense Enrollment Eligibility Reporting System
emergency
health benefits advisor
health care finder
medically (or psychologically) necessary
military treatment facility
nonparticipating provider
other health insurance
participating provider
partnership program
point-of-service option
preauthorization
primary care manager
quality assurance program
regional contractor
service benefit program
service-connected injury
service retiree (military retiree)
sponsor
summary payment voucher
total, permanent, service-connected disability
TRICARE Extra
TRICARE for Life
TRICARE Prime
TRICARE service center
urgent care
veteran

KEY ABBREVIATIONS

See how many abbreviations and acronyms you can translate and then use this as a handy reference list. Definitions for the key abbreviations are located near the back of the Handbook *in the glossary.*

ADSM ____________________
CHAMPVA ____________________
DEERS ____________________
FTM ____________________
HAC ____________________
HBA ____________________
HCF ____________________
MHS ____________________
MTF ____________________
NAS ____________________
nonpar ____________________
OHI ____________________
par ____________________
PCM ____________________
POS option ____________________
SHCP ____________________
TFL ____________________
TMA ____________________
TPR ____________________
TPRADFM ____________________
TSC ____________________
USFHP ____________________
VA ____________________

PERFORMANCE OBJECTIVES

The student will be able to:

- Define and spell the key terms and key abbreviations for this chapter, given the information from the *Handbook* glossary, within a reasonable time period and with enough accuracy to obtain a satisfactory evaluation.
- After reading the chapter, answer the fill-in-the-blank, multiple choice, and true/false review questions with enough accuracy to obtain a satisfactory evaluation.
- Fill in the correct meaning of each abbreviation, given a list of common medical abbreviations and symbols that appear in chart notes, within a reasonable time period and with enough accuracy to obtain a satisfactory evaluation.
- Given the patient's medical chart notes, ledger cards, and blank insurance claim forms, complete each CMS-1500 (08-05) Health Insurance Claim Form for billing within a reasonable time period and with enough accuracy to obtain a satisfactory evaluation.
- Using the Mock Fee Schedule in Appendix A in this *Workbook*, correctly post payments, adjustments, and balances on the patients' ledger cards within a reasonable time period and with enough accuracy to obtain a satisfactory evaluation.
- Compute mathematical calculations, given TRICARE problem situations, within a reasonable time period and with enough accuracy to obtain a satisfactory evaluation.

STUDY OUTLINE

History of TRICARE

TRICARE Programs
- Eligibility
- Nonavailability Statement

TRICARE Standard
- Enrollment
- Identification Card
- Benefits
- Fiscal Year
- Authorized Providers of Health Care
- Preauthorization
- Payment

TRICARE Extra
- Enrollment
- Identification Card
- Benefits
- Network Provider
- Preauthorization
- Payments

TRICARE Prime
- Enrollment
- Identification Card
- Benefits
- Primary Care Manager
- Preauthorization
- Payments

TRICARE Reserve Select

TRICARE for Life
- Enrollment
- Identification Card
- Benefits
- Referral and Preauthorization
- Payment

TRICARE Plus
- Enrollment
- Identification Card
- Benefits
- Payment

TRICARE Prime Remote Program
- Enrollment
- Identification Card
- Benefits
- Referral and Preauthorization
- Payments

Supplemental Health Care Program
- Enrollment
- Identification Card
- Benefits
- Referral and Preauthorization
- Payments

TRICARE Hospice Program

TRICARE and HMO Coverage

CHAMPVA Program
- Eligibility
- Enrollment
- Identification Card
- Benefits
- Provider
- Preauthorization

Medical Record Access
- Privacy Act of 1974
- Computer Matching and Privacy Protection Act of 1988

Claims Procedure
- Regional Contractor
- TRICARE Standard and CHAMPVA
- TRICARE Extra and TRICARE Prime
- TRICARE Prime Remote and Supplemental Health Care Program
- TRICARE for Life
- TRICARE/CHAMPVA and Other Insurance
- Medicare and TRICARE
- Medicare and CHAMPVA
- Dual or Double Coverage
- Third-Party Liability
- Workers' Compensation

After Claim Submission
- TRICARE Summary Payment Voucher
- CHAMPVA Explanation of Benefits Document
- Quality Assurance
- Claims Inquiries and Appeals

Procedure: Completing a CHAMPVA Claim Form

ASSIGNMENT 14-1 ▸ REVIEW QUESTIONS

Part I Fill in the Blank

Review the objectives, key terms, glossary definitions of key terms, chapter information, and figures before completing the following review questions.

1. CHAMPUS, the acronym for Civilian Health and Medical Program of the Uniformed Services, is now called ______________________________ and was organized to control escalating medical costs and to standardize benefits for active duty families and military retirees.

2. An active duty service member is known as a/an ________________________; once retired, this former member is called a/an ______________________________.

3. An individual who qualifies for TRICARE is known as a/an ________________________.

4. A system for verifying an individual's TRICARE eligibility is called
____.

5. Mrs. Hancock, a TRICARE beneficiary, lives 2 miles from a Uniformed Services Medical Treatment Facility but needs to be hospitalized for mental health care services at Orlando Medical Center, a civilian hospital. What type of authorization does she require?
____

6. TRICARE Standard and CHAMPVA beneficiary identification cards are issued to ________________ and ______________________. Information must be obtained from ______________________ and ____________________________ of the card and placed on the health insurance claim form.

7. Programs that allow TRICARE Standard beneficiaries to receive treatment, services, or supplies from civilian providers are called ________________________ and ________________________.

8. For patients whose sponsor is a rank of E4 and below, the TRICARE Standard deductible for outpatient care is how much per patient? ______________________________

   Per family? ____

9. For patients whose sponsor is a rank of E5 and above, the TRICARE Standard deductible for outpatient care is how much per patient? ______________________________

   Per family? ____

10. For TRICARE Standard, dependents of active duty members pay what percentage for outpatient services after the deductible has been met? ______________________________

    What percentage does TRICARE pay? ______________________________________

11. For retired members or their dependents on TRICARE Standard, what is their deductible responsibility for outpatient services? Per person? ____________________

    Per family? ____________________

12. For TRICARE Standard, retired members or their dependents pay what percentage for outpatient services after the deductible has been met? ____________________

    What percentage does TRICARE pay? ____________________

13. A voluntary TRICARE health maintenance organization type of option is known as ____________________.

14. CHAMPVA is the acronym for ____________________, now known as the ____________________.

15. Those individuals who serve in the United States Armed Forces, finish their service, and are honorably discharged are known as ____________________.

16. CHAMPVA is not an insurance program but is considered as a/an ____________________ program.

17. Which individuals are entitled to CHAMPVA medical benefits?

    a. ____________________

    b. ____________________

    c. ____________________

18. The public law establishing a person's right to review and contest inaccuracies in personal medical records is known as the ____________________.

19. An organization that contracts with the government to process TRICARE and CHAMPVA health insurance claims is known as a/an ____________________.

20. The time limit for submitting a TRICARE Standard or CHAMPVA claim for outpatient service is ____________________; for inpatient service, it is ____________________.

Part II Multiple Choice

Choose the best answer.

21. The TRICARE fiscal year

    a. begins January 1 and ends December 31

    b. begins April 1 and ends March 30

    c. begins June 1 and ends May 30

    d. begins October 1 and ends September 30

22. A health care professional who helps a patient who is under the TRICARE Standard program obtain preauthorization for care is called a/an

    a. primary care physician (PCP)

    b. health care finder (HCF)

    c. health benefits advisor (HBA)

    d. participating provider

23. TRICARE standard beneficiaries pay a certain amount each year for the cost share and annual deductible, which is known as

    a. catastrophic cap

    b. limiting charge

    c. coinsurance

    d. payment limitation

24. To qualify for TRICARE for Life (TFL), a beneficiary must be

    a. a TRICARE beneficiary

    b. eligible for Medicare Part A

    c. enrolled in Medicare Part B

    d. all of the above

25. The time limit for filing a TRICARE Standard claim is

    a. the end of the calendar year after the fiscal year in which services were furnished

    b. within 1 year from the date a service is provided

    c. within 1 year from the month of service

    d. within 2 years from when service is provided

Part III True/False

Write "T" or "F" in the blank to indicate whether you think the statement is true or false.

_______ 26. Medically necessary treatment needed for immediate illness or injury that would not result in further disability or death if not treated immediately is known as urgent care.

_______ 27. TRICARE beneficiaries who use nonauthorized providers and receive medical services may be responsible for their entire bill.

_______ 28. When an individual on TRICARE Prime shows you their identification card, it guarantees TRICARE eligibility.

_______ 29. TRICARE Prime Remote (TPR) is a program designed for military retirees and their families.

_______ 30. Beneficiaries of the CHAMPVA program have complete freedom of choice in selecting their civilian health care providers.

ASSIGNMENT 14-2 ▶ CRITICAL THINKING

Performance Objective

Task: After reading the scenarios, answer the following questions, using critical thinking skills.

Conditions: Use a pen or pencil.

Standards: Time: ____________________ minutes

Accuracy: ____________________

(Note: The time element and accuracy criteria may be given by your instructor.)

Directions: After reading the scenarios, answer the following questions, using your critical thinking skills. Record your answers on the blank lines.

1. If Bertha Evans is seen for an office visit and has other insurance besides TRICARE, and she is the dependent of an active military person, whom do you bill first?

   ____

   Reason: ____

2. If Jason Williams, a TRICARE beneficiary who became disabled at age 10 years and who is also receiving Medicare Part A and Medicare Part B benefits, is seen for a consultation, whom do you bill first?

   ____

   Reason: ____

3. If Tanner Vine, a CHAMPVA and Medicaid beneficiary, is seen on an emergency basis in the office, whom do you bill first?

   ____

   Reason: ____

ASSIGNMENT 14-3 ▶ CALCULATE MATHEMATICAL PROBLEMS

Performance Objective

Task: Calculate and insert the correct amounts for three TRICARE scenarios.

Conditions: Use a pen or pencil, the description of the problem, and calculation formulas.

Standards: Time: ________________ minutes

Accuracy: ________________

(Note: The time element and accuracy criteria may be given by your instructor.)

Directions: Calculate and insert the correct amounts for the following scenarios using these formulas.

Basic calculation formulas

TRICARE

$	TRICARE allowed amount
− ________	Minus deductible
$	Balance on which pmt calculated
× ______ %	Multiply TRICARE plan %
$	TRICARE payment

PATIENT

$	Allowed amount after deductible
× ______ %	Multiply TRICARE plan %
$	
+ ________	Add any deductible amt owed
$	Amount patient pays

ADJUSTED AMOUNT

$	Billed amount
− ________	Minus allowable amount
$	Adjusted amount

Problem 1: On October 1, in consultation, Dr. Caesar sees the wife of a Navy man who is stationed at Port Hueneme. Dr. Caesar orders her to the hospital because of a suspected ectopic pregnancy. She undergoes a laparotomy and salpingectomy. Her husband is a rank of E5. Here are her bills. Indicate what TRICARE Standard will pay.

Outpatient Services:	*TRICARE Standard*		
	Bill/Allowable	**TRICARE Payment**	**Patient Owes**
Consultation	$75	$________	$________
Inpatient services:			
Salpingectomy	$600		
Assistant surgeon	$120		
Anesthesiologist	$400		
3-day stay (drugs, laboratory tests, operating room)	$2500		
Total	$________		$________

Mathematical computations:

Problem 2: This is the same situation as in Problem 1, except that the patient is the wife of a retired military man and has TRICARE Standard.

Outpatient Services:	*TRICARE Standard*		
	Bill/Allowable	**TRICARE Payment**	**Patient Owes**
Consultation	$75	$________	$________
Inpatient services with separately billed professional charges			
	Bill/Allowable	**TRICARE Payment**	**Patient Owes**
Salpingectomy	$600	$________	$________
Assistant surgeon	$120	$________	$________
Anesthesiologist	$400	$________	$________
Inpatient services billed by hospital			
3-day stay (drugs, laboratory tests, operating room)	$2500	$________	
Total payment owed by patient to Dr. Caesar			$________

Mathematical computations:

Problem 3: A TRICARE patient whose sponsor is a rank of E5 asks Dr. Caesar to accept assignment on her medical care, and Dr. Caesar agrees. She has not met her deductible. She is the wife of an active duty man. She has TRICARE Extra.

Dr. Caesar's bill:

Consultation	$50	Allowable: $50
Complete blood cell count	20	20
Urinalysis	5	5
Blood serology and complement fixation	25	25
Posteroanterior and lateral chest radiograph	40	40
Electrocardiogram	35	30
Spirometry	40	40
Total	$215	$210

How much is Dr. Caesar's check from TRICARE Extra? $ ______________________. The patient owes the doctor $ ______________________. Dr. Caesar's courtesy adjustment is $ ______________________.

Mathematical computations:

ASSIGNMENT 14-4 ▶ COMPLETE A CLAIM FORM FOR A TRICARE STANDARD CASE

Performance Objective

Task: Complete a CMS-1500 (08-05) claim form for a TRICARE Standard case, post transactions to the financial accounting record, and define patient record abbreviations.

Conditions: Use the patient's record (Figure 14-1) and financial statement (Figure 14-2), one health insurance claim form (print from Evolve website), a computer, procedural and diagnostic code books, and Appendixes A and B in this *Workbook*.

Standards: Claim Productivity Measurement

Time: ______________________ minutes

Accuracy: ______________________

(Note: The time element and accuracy criteria may be given by your instructor.)

Directions:

1. Using optical character reader (OCR) guidelines, complete the CMS-1500 (08-05) claim form. If your instructor wants you to direct it to your local TRICARE fiscal intermediary, go to website http://www.tricare.osd.mil. On the map, click on the area where you reside and then choose a state to access claims information for that state. Refer to Miss Rosa M. Sandoval's patient record for information and Appendix A to locate the fees to record on the claim and post to the financial statement. Date the claim May 31. Dr. Atrics is not accepting assignment on this TRICARE Standard case but is completing the claim for the patient's convenience. The family of this patient has not previously met its deductible.

2. Refer to Chapter 7 (Figure 7-10) of the *Handbook* for instructions on how to complete this claim form and to view a TRICARE template.

3. Use your *Current Procedural Terminology* (CPT) code book or Appendix A in this *Workbook* to determine the correct five-digit code number and modifiers for each professional service rendered. Use your Healthcare Common Procedure Coding System (HCPCS) Level II code book or refer to Appendix B in this *Workbook* for HCPCS procedure codes and modifiers. If your instructor tells you to also find the ICD-10-CM codes, a draft version may be downloaded from the following website: http://www.cdc.gov/nchs/icd/icd10cm.htm#10update.

4. On May 8, Miss Sandoval makes a partial payment of $20 by check (No. 4013). Record the proper information on the financial record but not on the claim form, and note the date you have billed TRICARE (May 31).

5. A Performance Evaluation Checklist may be reproduced from the "Instruction Guide to the Workbook" chapter if your instructor wishes you to submit it to assist with scoring and comments.

After the instructor has returned your work to you, either make the necessary corrections and place your work in a three-ring notebook for future reference or, if you received a high score, place it in your portfolio for reference when applying for a job.

Abbreviations pertinent to this record:

pt	______	ofc	______
rt	______	FU	______
EPF	______	retn	______
yr(s)	______	PO	______
temp	______	PF	______
adv	______	HX	______
SF	______	PX	______
MDM	______	wk	______
c̄	______	T	______

PATIENT RECORD NO. 14-4

LAST NAME	FIRST NAME	MIDDLE NAME	BIRTH DATE	SEX	HOME PHONE
Sandoval	Rosa	M	11-01-91	F	555-456-3322

ADDRESS	CITY	STATE	ZIP CODE
209 West Maple Street	Woodland Hills	XY	12345

CELL PHONE	PAGER NO.	FAX NO.	E-MAIL ADDRESS

PATIENT'S SOC. SEC. NO.	DRIVER'S LICENSE
994-XX-1164	

PATIENT'S OCCUPATION	NAME OF COMPANY
Child—full time student (lives with mother)	

ADDRESS OF EMPLOYER	PHONE

SPOUSE OR PARENT	OCCUPATION
Hernan J. Sandoval (father)	Staff Sargeant—Grade 9 (active duty)

EMPLOYER	ADDRESS	PHONE
United States Army	HHC 3rd Batt, 25th Infantry, APO New York, New York, 10030	

NAME OF INSURANCE	INSURED OR SUBSCRIBER
TRICARE Standard	father (DOB 2/10/70)

POLICY/CERTIFICATE NO.	GROUP NO.
886-XX-0999	

REFERRED BY: Maria Sandoval (mother)

DATE	PROGRESS NOTES
5-1-xx	New pt comes in complaining of pain in rt ear for 3 days. An EPF history was taken which
	revealed several ear infections (suppurative) over the past 3 yrs. An EPF exam revealed
	fluid and pus in rt ear. Temp 101°. Adv mother a myringotomy was necessary. Scheduled
	outpatient surg at College Hospital this afternoon. Imp: Acute rt suppurative otitis media
	(SF MDM). The prior authorization number is 2076500781.
	PA/llf Pedro Atrics, MD
5-1-xx	Pt admitted to outpatient surgery (College Hospital). Rt myringotomy c̄ aspiration
	performed. Pt did well. To be seen in ofc for FU in 2 days.
	PA/llf Pedro Atrics, MD
5-3-xx	Pt retns PO (PF HX/PX SF MDM). No pain rt ear. Pt progressing well. Retn in 1 wk.
	PA/llf Pedro Atrics, MD
5-8-xx	Pt retns PO (PF HX/PX SF MDM). T 98°, no fluid or pus in rt ear. No pain. Pt discharged,
	retn prn.
	PA/llf Pedro Atrics, MD

Figure 14-1

Acct No. 14-4

STATEMENT

Financial Account

COLLEGE CLINIC
4567 Broad Avenue
Woodland Hills, XY 12345-0001
Tel. 555-486-9002
Fax No. 555-487-8976

Rosa M. Sandoval
c/o Maria Sandoval
209 West Maple Street
Woodland Hills, XY 12345-0001

Phone No. (H) (555) 456-3322 (W) ______ Birthdate 11-9-91

Primary Insurance Co. TRICARE Standard Policy/Group No. 886-XX-0999

Secondary Insurance Co. ______ Policy/Group No. ______

DATE	REFERENCE	DESCRIPTION	CHARGES	CREDITS PYMNTS.	CREDITS ADJ.	BALANCE
20xx		BALANCE FORWARD →				
5-1-xx		NP OV				
5-1-xx		Myringotomy				
5-3-xx		PO OV				
5-8-xx		PO OV				

PLEASE PAY LAST AMOUNT IN BALANCE COLUMN

THIS IS A COPY OF YOUR FINANCIAL ACCOUNT AS IT APPEARS ON OUR RECORDS

Figure 14-2

ASSIGNMENT 14-5 ▶ COMPLETE A CLAIM FORM FOR A TRICARE EXTRA CASE

Performance Objective

Task: Complete a CMS-1500 (08-05) claim form for a TRICARE Extra case, post transactions to the financial accounting record, and define patient record abbreviations.

Conditions: Use the patient's record (Figure 14-3) and financial statement (Figure 14-4), one health insurance claim form (print from Evolve website), a computer, procedural and diagnostic code books, and Appendixes A and B in this *Workbook*.

Standards: Claim Productivity Measurement

Time: ______________________ minutes

Accuracy: ______________________

(Note: The time element and accuracy criteria may be given by your instructor.)

Directions:

1. Using OCR guidelines, complete the CMS-1500 (08-05) claim form. If your instructor wants you to direct it to your local TRICARE fiscal intermediary, go to website http://www.tricare.osd.mil. On the map, click on the area where you reside and then choose a state to access claims information for that state. Refer to Mrs. Darlene B. Drew's patient record for information and Appendix A to locate the fees to record on the claim and post to the financial statement. Date the claim February 3. Assume that the Nonavailability Statement (NAS) has been transmitted electronically so that the physician can treat the patient at College Hospital. Dr. Ulibarri is accepting assignment on this TRICARE Extra case. This patient met her deductible last November when seen by a previous physician.

2. Refer to Chapter 7 (Figure 7-10) of the *Handbook* for instructions on how to complete this claim form and to view a TRICARE template.

3. Use your CPT code book or Appendix A in this *Workbook* to determine the correct five-digit code number and modifiers for each professional service rendered. Use your HCPCS Level II code book or refer to Appendix B in this *Workbook* for HCPCS procedure codes and modifiers. If your instructor tells you to also find the ICD-10-CM codes, a draft version may be downloaded from the following website: http://www.cdc.gov/nchs/icd/icd10cm.htm#10update.

4. Record the proper information on the financial record and claim form and note the date when you have billed TRICARE Extra.

5. A Performance Evaluation Checklist may be reproduced from the "Instruction Guide to the Workbook" chapter if your instructor wishes you to submit it to assist with scoring and comments.

After the instructor has returned your work to you, either make the necessary corrections and place your work in a three-ring notebook for future reference, or, if you received a high score, place it in your portfolio for reference when applying for a job.

Abbreviations pertinent to this record:

Pt	______	LC	______
D	______	MDM	______
HX	______	PF	______
PX	______	rec	______
UA	______	SF	______
WBC	______	C	______
RBC	______	M	______
cc	______	surg	______
lab	______	ofc	______
Rx	______	PO	______
caps	______	OV	______
t.i.d	______	rtn	______
Retn	______	PRN	______
Dx	______		

PATIENT RECORD NO. 14-5

Drew	Darlene	B	12-22-51	F	555-466-1002
LAST NAME	FIRST NAME	MIDDLE NAME	BIRTH DATE	SEX	HOME PHONE

720 Ganley Street,	Woodland Hills,	XY	12345
ADDRESS	CITY	STATE	ZIP CODE

555-320-9988	555-210-9400	555-466-1002	drew@wb.net
CELL PHONE	PAGER NO.	FAX NO.	E-MAIL ADDRESS

450-XX-3762	H0492188
PATIENT'S SOC. SEC. NO.	DRIVER'S LICENSE

Seamstress	J. B. Talon Company
PATIENT'S OCCUPATION	NAME OF COMPANY

2111 Ventura Road, Merck, XY 12346	555-733-0156
ADDRESS OF EMPLOYER	PHONE

Harry M. Drew	U.S. Navy Lieutenant Commander (L/C), Active Status
SPOUSE OR PARENT	OCCUPATION

Service #221-XX-0711 Social Security No. 221-XX-0711 Grade12 4-15-37
BIRTH DATE

P.O. Box 2927, A.P.O., New York, New York 09194
ADDRESS

TRICARE Extra	67531	01-01-80
NAME OF INSURANCE	TRICARE EXTRA I.D. CARD NO.	EFFECTIVE DATE

REFERRED BY: James B. Jeffers, MD, 100 S. Broadway, Woodland Hills, XY 12345 Tax ID#77621074X

DATE	PROGRESS NOTES
1-13-xx	New pt comes in complaining of large sore in vagina causing extreme pain. Performed a
	D HX/PX. UA (non-automated with microscopy) loaded with WBCs and RBCs. Upon pelvic
	examination, a very tender mass is located in the paraurethral area (Skene's gland).
	I incised and drained the abscess and obtained 10 cc greenish pus; took culture and sent
	to lab. Pt feels much better. Rx Terramycin 30 caps 1 t.i.d. Retn in 5 days. Dx: Paraurethral
	abscess (LC/MDM).
	GU/llf Gene Ulibarri, MD
1-18-xx	Pt returns and a PF HX/PX performed. Abscess is filled with fluid again, opened, and a
	wick of Iodoform gauze placed to help with drainage. Rec daily sitz baths and outpatient
	hospitalization to remove gland. Culture results show pseudomonas organism.
	Arrangements made for surgery on the 24th, admit at 5:30 a.m., surgery at 7:30 a.m.
	(SF MDM).
	GU/llf Gene Ulibarri, MD
1-24-xx	Admit to College Hospital outpatient facility (C HX/PX M MDM). Surg: Excision of Skene's
	gland. To be seen in ofc next week for PO exam. Renewed Rx Terramycin.
	GU/llf Gene Ulibarri, MD
1-27-xx	PO OV (PF HX/PX SF/MDM). Pt doing well. No pain, urethral tissue and perineum looks
	healthy, healing well. Rtn PRN.
	GU/llf Gene Ulibarri, MD

Figure 14-3

Acct No. 14-5

STATEMENT
Financial Account
COLLEGE CLINIC
4567 Broad Avenue
Woodland Hills, XY 12345-0001
Tel. 555-486-9002
Fax No. 555-487-8976

Darlene B. Drew
720 Ganley Street
Woodland Hills, XY 12345

Phone No. (H) 555-466-1002 (W) 555-733-0156 Birthdate 12-22-51

Primary Insurance Co. TRICARE Extra Policy/Group No. 221-XX-0711

Secondary Insurance Co. ______ Policy/Group No. ______

DATE	REFERENCE	DESCRIPTION	CHARGES	CREDITS		BALANCE
				PYMNTS.	ADJ.	
20xx		BALANCE FORWARD →				
1-13-xx		NP OV				
1-13-xx		UA				
1-13-xx		Drainage of Skene's gland abscess				
1-13-xx		Handling/Transport culture specimen				
1-18-xx		OV				
1-24-xx		Excision Skene's gland				
1-27-xx		PO OV				

PLEASE PAY LAST AMOUNT IN BALANCE COLUMN

THIS IS A COPY OF YOUR FINANCIAL ACCOUNT AS IT APPEARS ON OUR RECORDS

Figure 14-4

ASSIGNMENT 14-6 ▸ COMPLETE THREE CLAIM FORMS FOR A TRICARE STANDARD CASE

Performance Objective

Task: Complete three CMS-1500 (08-05) claim forms for a TRICARE Standard case, post transactions to the financial accounting record, and define patient record abbreviations.

Conditions: Use the patient's record (Figure 14-5) and financial statement (Figure 14-6), health insurance claim forms (print from Evolve website), a computer, procedural and diagnostic code books, and Appendixes A and B in this *Workbook*.

Standards: Claim Productivity Measurement

Time: ______________________ minutes

Accuracy: ______________________

(Note: The time element and accuracy criteria may be given by your instructor.)

Directions:

1. This case requires three claim forms. Make photocopies of a CMS-1500 (08-05) claim form or print from Evolve website. Using OCR guidelines, complete the CMS-1500 (08-05) claim forms. If your instructor wants you to direct them to your local TRICARE fiscal intermediary, go to website http://www.tricare.osd.mil. On the map, click on the area where you reside and then choose a state to access claims information for that state. Refer to Mrs. Mae I. Abbreviate's patient record for information and Appendix A in this *Workbook* to locate the fees to record on the claim, and post them to the financial statement. Date the claims January 31. Dr. Coccidioides is not accepting assignment on this TRICARE Standard case but is completing the claim for the patient's convenience.

2. Refer to Chapter 7 (Figure 7-10) of the *Handbook* for instructions on how to complete these claim forms and to view a TRICARE template.

3. Use your CPT code book or Appendix A in this *Workbook* to determine the correct five-digit code number and modifiers for each professional service rendered. Use your HCPCS Level II code book or refer to Appendix B in this *Workbook* for HCPCS procedure codes and modifiers. If your instructor tells you to also find the ICD-10-CM codes, a draft version may be downloaded from the following website: http://www.cdc.gov/nchs/icd/icd10cm.htm#10update.

4. Record the proper information on the financial record and note the date when you have billed TRICARE.

5. A Performance Evaluation Checklist may be reproduced from the "Instruction Guide to the Workbook" chapter if your instructor wishes you to submit it to assist with scoring and comments.

After the instructor has returned your work to you, either make the necessary corrections and place your work in a three-ring notebook for future reference, or, if you received a high score, place it in your portfolio for reference when applying for a job.

Abbreviations pertinent to this record:

NP	______	F	______
W	______	P	______
PE	______	R	______
CC	______	EENT	______
wk	______	GGE	______
X	______	HC	______
pt	______	MDM	______
PH	______	STAT	______
UCHD	______	CBC	______
T & A	______	diff	______
aet	______	WBC	______
Grav	______	RTO	______
Para1	______	RTW	______
D & C	______	CT	______
DUB	______	dx	______
LMP	______	a.m.	______
surg	______	D	______
OS	______	MC	______
yr	______	cm	______
FH	______	lt	______
CA	______	C & S	______
L & W	______	gm	______
GB	______	mg	______
SH	______	IM	______
PX	______	retn	______

ht	______________________	ofc	______________________
wt	______________________	OV	______________________
lbs	______________________	PF	______________________
BP	______________________	SF	______________________
T	______________________	HC	______________________

Additional Coding

1. Refer to Mrs. Abbreviate's medical record, abstract information, and code procedures that would be billed by outside providers.

Site	*Description of Service*	*Code*
a. College Hospital Radiology	______________	______________
b. College Hospital Laboratory	______________	______________
c. College Hospital Laboratory	______________	______________
d. College Hospital Radiology	______________	______________
e. College Hospital Microbiology	______________	______________
f. College Hospital Radiology	______________	______________

2. Use your diagnostic code book and code the symptoms that the patient complained of on January 14, 20xx.

Symptom	*ICD-9-CM Code*	*ICD-10-CM Code*
a. ______________	______________	______________
b. ______________	______________	______________
c. ______________	______________	______________
d. ______________	______________	______________

PATIENT RECORD NO. 14-6

LAST NAME	FIRST NAME	MIDDLE NAME	BIRTH DATE	SEX	HOME PHONE
Abbreviate	Mae	I	01-02-52	F	555-986-7667

ADDRESS	CITY	STATE	ZIP CODE
4667 Symbol Road	Woodland Hills	XY	12345

CELL PHONE	PAGER NO.	FAX NO.	E-MAIL ADDRESS
555-740-3300		555-986-7667	abbreviate@wb.net

PATIENT'S SOC. SEC. NO.	DRIVER'S LICENSE
865-XX-2311	E0598247

PATIENT'S OCCUPATION	NAME OF COMPANY
administrative assistant	U. R. Wright Company

ADDRESS OF EMPLOYER	PHONE
6789 Abridge Road, Woodland Hills, XY 12346	555-988-7540

SPOUSE OR PARENT	OCCUPATION
Shorty S. Abbreviate	Staff Sargeant, Grade 12 (Active Duty)

EMPLOYER	ADDRESS	PHONE
United States Army	HHC, 2nd Batt., 27th Infantry, APO New York, New York, 10030	

NAME OF INSURANCE	INSURED OR SUBSCRIBER
TRICARE Standard	husband (DOB 3/25/40)

POLICY/CERTIFICATE NO.	GROUP NO.
023-XX-7866	

REFERRED BY: Jane B. Accurate (friend)

Figure 14-5a

DATE	PROGRESS NOTES No. 14-6
1-14-xx	NP, 45-year-old W F in for complete PE. CC: Recent onset of flu-like symptoms of
	approximate 2 wk duration, including cough; chest pain X 2 days. Pt states beginning to
	cough up moderate amounts of greenish sputum with blood streaks, fatigue, fever, and chills.
	Comprehensive history includes PH: UCHD, T & A aet 6, Grav 1 Para 1, D & C aet 41 for
	DUB, LMP 12-18-XX, surg on OS after accident last yr. FH: Father expired of kidney CA aet
	63; mother L & W after GB surg in 1999; no siblings. SH: Pt admits to past alcohol abuse,
	denies alcohol use in last 6 months. No smoking, denies drug abuse. Comprehensive PX:
	Ht 5' 7", wt 150 lbs, BP 150/80, T 100.5 F, P 88, R 18; EENT o¯ except OS opaque;
	chest, rales scattered bilaterally, pt is dyspneic. Abdomen soft, nontender.
	GGE (HC MDM). Pt would like to avoid hospitalization if at all possible. Sent to College
	Hospital for STAT chest x-ray (2 views) and laboratory tests (electrolyte panel and complete
	CBC, automated with diff WBC. RTO tomorrow morning for test results. Disability from work began Jan. 13
	Completed disability form for work; estimated RTW, 2 weeks.
	BC/llf Brady Coccicioides, MD
1-14-xx	Call received from hospital radiology department: Chest x-rays revealed probable lung
	abscess in left lower lobe; inconclusive. Ordered STAT CT of thorax without contrast for
	more definitive dx. Contacted pt and recommended she have CT done this evening.
	RTO tomorrow a.m.
	BC/llf Brady Coccicioides, MD
1-15-xx	Pt returns to office for test results (D HX/PX MC/MDM). CT reveals lung abscess of
	3.0 cm in lt lower lobe. Pt able to produce sputum for C & S (Gram stain smear), sent to
	College Hospital laboratory, microbiology department. Rocephin (Ceftriaxone sodium)
	1 gm ($5 per 250 mg and 1000 mg = 1 gm) given IM in office, instructed pt to retn to ofc daily
	for Rocephin injections; reevaluate on Friday.
	BC/llf Brady Coccicioides, MD
1-16-xx	Rocephin 1 gm IM ordered by Dr. Coccicioides; administered by medical assistant in left
	gluteus maximus.
	BC/llf Ali Marie Hobkins, CMA
1-17-xx	Rocephin 1 gm IM ordered by Dr. Coccicioides; administered by medical assistant in right
	gluteus maximus.
	BC/llf Ali Marie Hobkins, CMA
1-18-xx	Pt returns for reevaluation (OV PF HX/PX SF MDM). Culture revealed streptococcal
	pneumoniae. Administered Rocephin 1 gm IM. Will continue daily injections.
	Arrangements made for house call over weekend.
	BC/llf Brady Coccicioides, MD
1-19-xx	HC Saturday (PF HX/PX SF MDM). Rocephin 1 gm IM. Pt states she is feeling much
	better, fatigue gone, cough decreased, afebrile. Ordered repeat chest x-ray (2 views) at
	College Hospital Monday. RTO Monday afternoon.
	BC/llf Brady Coccicioides, MD
1-21-xx	OV (PF HX/PX SF MDM). Repeat chest x-ray negative except few residual shadows.
	No injection today, start oral antibiotics. Pt to return in 1 wk for f/u or call sooner if
	symptoms reappear. Estimated RTW, 1/28/XX.
	BC/llf Brady Coccicioides, MD

Figure 14-5b

Acct No. 14-6

STATEMENT
Financial Account
COLLEGE CLINIC
4567 Broad Avenue
Woodland Hills, XY 12345-0001
Tel. 555-486-9002
Fax No. 555-487-8976

Mae I. Abbreviate
4667 Symbol Road
Woodland Hills, XY 12345

Phone No. (H) 555-986-7667 (W) 555-988-7540 Birthdate 01/02/52

Primary Insurance Co. TRICARE Standard Policy/Group No. 023-XX-7866

Secondary Insurance Co. ______ Policy/Group No. ______

DATE	REFERENCE	DESCRIPTION	CHARGES	CREDITS PYMNTS.	CREDITS ADJ.	BALANCE
20xx		BALANCE FORWARD →				
1-14-xx		NP OV				
1-15-xx		OV				
1-15-xx		Injection AB				
1-15-xx		Rocefin 1 gm				
1-16-xx		Injection AB				
1-16-xx		Rocefin 1 gm				
1-17-xx		Injection AB				
1-17-xx		Rocefin 1 gm				
1-18-xx		OV				
1-18-xx		Injection AB				
1-18-xx		Rocefin 1 gm				
1-19-xx		HC				
1-19-xx		Injection AB				
1-19-xx		Rocefin 1 gm				
1-21-xx		OV				

PLEASE PAY LAST AMOUNT IN BALANCE COLUMN

THIS IS A COPY OF YOUR FINANCIAL ACCOUNT AS IT APPEARS ON OUR RECORDS

Figure 14-6

ASSIGNMENT 14-7 ▶ FOR TRICARE CASE 7 ONSCREEN COMPLETION OF CMS-1500 (08-05) INSURANCE CLAIM FORM

Performance Objective

Task: Enter transactions from patient's onscreen encounter form (superbill) and complete block-by-block onscreen health insurance claim form.

Conditions: Onscreen encounter form (superbill) and computer

Standards: Time: ______________________ minutes

Accuracy: ______________________

(Note: The time element and accuracy criteria may be given by your instructor.

Directions: Log on to your Evolve account at http://evolve.elsevier.com and access the student resources for Fordney: *Insurance Handbook for the Medical Office*, 12th edition. Then choose Student Software Challenge.

1. For this assignment, follow the instructions for entering data into the onscreen CMS-1500 (08-05) health insurance claim form, completing blocks 1 through 33 for Case 7.
2. Use your CPT code book or Appendix A in this *Workbook* to determine the correct five-digit code number and modifiers for each professional service rendered. If your instructor tells you to also find the ICD-10-CM codes, a draft version may be downloaded from the following website: http://www.cdc.gov/nchs/icd/icd10cm.htm#10update.
3. A Performance Evaluation Checklist may be reproduced from the "Instruction Guide to the Workbook" chapter if your instructor wishes you to submit it to assist with scoring and comments.
4. Print a hard copy of the completed health insurance claim form.
5. After the instructor has returned your work to you, either make the necessary corrections and place your work in a three-ring notebook for future reference, or, if you received a high score, place it in your portfolio for reference when applying for a job.

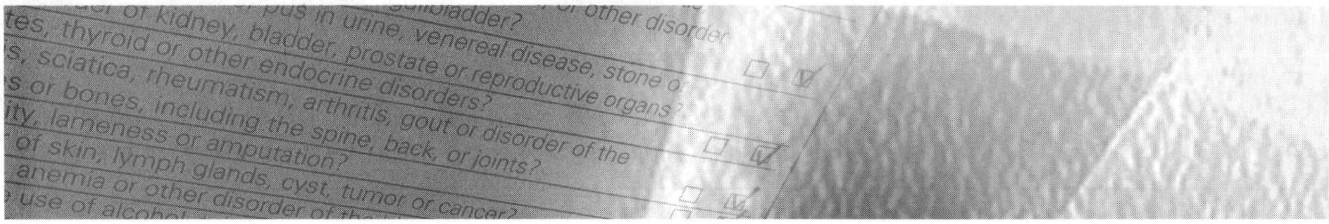

CHAPTER

15

Workers' Compensation

KEY TERMS

Your instructor may wish to select some words pertinent to this chapter for a test. For definitions of the terms, further study, and/or reference, the words, phrases, and abbreviations may be found in the glossary at the end of the Handbook. *Key terms for this chapter follow.*

accident
adjudication
by report
claims examiner
compromise and release
deposition
ergonomic
extraterritorial
Federal Employees' Compensation Act
fee schedule
injury
insurance adjuster
lien
medical service order
nondisability claim
occupational illness (or disease)
Occupational Safety and Health Administration
permanent and stationary
permanent disability
petition
second-injury fund
sequelae
sub rosa films
subsequent-injury fund
temporary disability
third-party liability
third-party subrogation
waiting period
work hardening
Workers' Compensation Appeals Board
workers' compensation insurance

KEY ABBREVIATIONS

See how many abbreviations and acronyms you can translate and then use this as a handy reference list. Definitions for the key abbreviations are located near the back of the Handbook *in the glossary.*

AME ____________________
BR ____________________
C and R ____________________
ERISA ____________________
FECA ____________________
IAIABC ____________________
IME ____________________
LHWCA ____________________
MSDS ____________________
ND claim ____________________
OSHA ____________________
P and S ____________________
PD ____________________
QME ____________________
ROM ____________________
SIF ____________________
TD ____________________
WC ____________________
WCAB ____________________
WP ____________________

PERFORMANCE OBJECTIVES

The student will be able to:

- Define and spell the key terms and key abbreviations for this chapter, given the information from the *Handbook* glossary, within a reasonable time period and with enough accuracy to obtain a satisfactory evaluation.
- After reading the chapter, answer the fill-in-the-blank, multiple choice, and true/false review questions with enough accuracy to obtain a satisfactory evaluation.
- Given a list of common medical abbreviations and symbols that appear in chart notes, fill in the correct meaning of each abbreviation within a reasonable time period and with enough accuracy to obtain a satisfactory evaluation.
- Given the patients' medical chart notes, ledger cards, and blank insurance forms, complete each workers' compensation form for billing, within a reasonable time period and with enough accuracy to obtain a satisfactory evaluation.
- Given the patients' medical chart notes, ledger cards, and blank insurance claim forms, complete each CMS-1500 (08-05) Health Insurance Claim Form for submission to a workers' compensation insurance company within a reasonable time period and with enough accuracy to obtain a satisfactory evaluation.
- Using the Mock Fee Schedule in Appendix A in this *Workbook*, correctly post payments, adjustments, and balances on the patients' ledger cards within a reasonable time period and with enough accuracy to obtain a satisfactory evaluation.

STUDY OUTLINE

History
- Workers' Compensation Statutes
- Workers' Compensation Reform

Workers' Compensation Laws and Insurance
- Purposes of Workers' Compensation Laws
- Self-Insurance
- Managed Care

Eligibility
- Industrial Accident
- Occupational Illness

Coverage
- Federal Laws
- State Laws
- State Disability and Workers' Compensation

Benefits

Types of State Claims
- Nondisability Claim
- Temporary Disability Claim
- Permanent Disability Claim

Fraud and Abuse

Occupational Safety and Health Administration Act of 1970
- Background
- Coverage
- Regulations
- Filing a Complaint
- Inspection
- Record Keeping and Reporting

Legal Situations
- Medical Evaluator
- Depositions
- Medical Testimony
- Liens
- Third-Party Subrogation

Medical Reports
- Privacy and Confidentiality
- Documentation
- Health Information Record Keeping
- Terminology

Reporting Requirements
- Employer's Report
- Medical Service Order
- Physician's First Report
- Progress or Supplemental Report
- Final Report

Claim Submission
- Financial Responsibility
- Fee Schedules
- Helpful Billing Tips
- Billing Claims
- Out-of-State Claims
- Delinquent or Slow Pay Claims

Procedure: Completing the Doctor's First Report of Occupational Injury or Illness

ASSIGNMENT 15-1 ▶ REVIEW QUESTIONS

Part I Fill in the Blank

Review the objectives, key terms, glossary definitions of key terms, chapter information, and figures before completing the following review questions.

1. Name two kinds of statutes under workers' compensation.

   a. ______________________________

   b. ______________________________

2. An unexpected, unintended event that occurs at a particular time and place, causing injury to an individual not of his or her own making, is called a/an

   ______________________________.

3. Maria Cardoza works in a plastics manufacturing company and inhales some fumes that cause bronchitis. Because this condition is associated with her employment, it is called a/an

   ______________________________.

4. Name the federal workers' compensation acts that cover workers.

   a. ______________________________

   b. ______________________________

   c. ______________________________

   d. ______________________________

5. State compensation laws that require each employer to accept its provisions and provide for specialized benefits for employees who are injured at work are called

   ______________________________.

6. State compensation laws that may be accepted or rejected by the employer are known as

   ______________________________.

7. State five methods used for funding workers' compensation.

   a. ______________________________

   b. ______________________________

   c. ______________________________

   d. ______________________________

   e. ______________________________

8. Who pays the workers' compensation insurance premiums?

   ____

9. What is the time limit in your state for submitting the employers' and/or physicians' report on an industrial accident?

____.

10. When an employee with a preexisting condition is injured at work and the injury produces a disability greater than what would have been caused by the second injury alone, the benefits are derived from a/an

____.

11. Name jobs that may not be covered by workers' compensation insurance.

a. ____

b. ____

c. ____

d. ____

e. ____

f. ____

12. What is the minimum number of employees per business needed in your state for workers' compensation statutes to become effective? ____

13. What waiting period must elapse in your state before workers' compensation payments begin?

____

14. List five types of workers' compensation benefits.

a. ____

b. ____

c. ____

d. ____

e. ____

15. Who can treat an industrial injury?

____

____

16. What are three types of workers' compensation claims and the differences among them?

a. ____

____

b. ______________________________

____

c. ______________________________

____

17. Weekly temporary disability payments are based on

______________________________.

18. After suffering an industrial injury, Mr. Fields is in a treatment program in which he is given real work tasks for building strength and endurance. This form of therapy is called ______________________________.

19. When an industrial case reaches the time for rating the disability, this is accomplished by what state agency? ______________________________

20. May an injured person appeal his or her case if he or she is not satisfied with the rating? ______________ If so, to whom does he or she appeal? ______________ or ______________________________.

21. When fraud or abuse is suspected in a workers' compensation case, the physician should report the situation to ______________________________.

22. Explain third-party subrogation.

____

____

23. When an individual suffers a work-related injury or illness, the employer must complete and send a form called a/an ______________________________ to the insurance company and workers' compensation state offices, and if the employee is sent to a physician's office for medical care, the employer must complete a form called a/an ______________________________, which authorizes the physician to treat the employee.

Part II Multiple Choice

Choose the best answer.

24. Employers are required to meet health and safety standards for their employees under federal and state statutes known as
    a. Occupational Safety and Health Administration (OSHA) Act of 1970
    b. Health Insurance Portability and Accountability Act (HIPAA)
    c. Clinical Laboratory Improvement Amendment (CLIA)
    d. Employee Retirement Income Security Act (ERISA)

25. The process of carrying on a lawsuit is called
   a. lien
   b. litigation
   c. deposition
   d. adjudication

26. A proceeding during which an attorney questions a witness who answers under oath but not in open court is called a/an
   a. subpoena
   b. subrogation
   c. petition
   d. deposition

27. The legal promise of a patient to satisfy a debt to the physician from proceeds received from a litigated case is termed a/an
   a. medical service order
   b. subpoena
   c. lien
   d. promissory note

28. When a physician treats an industrial injury, he or she must complete a First Treatment Medical Report or Doctor's First Report of Occupational Injury or Illness and send it to the following:
   a. insurance carrier
   b. employer
   c. state workers' compensation office
   d. all of the above

Part III True/False

Write "T" or "F" in the blank to indicate whether you think the statement is true or false.

_______ 29. The first thing an employee should do after he or she is injured on the job is to notify his or her employer or immediate supervisor.

_______ 30. A roofer takes his girlfriend to a roofing job and she is injured. She is covered under workers' compensation insurance.

_______ 31. A stamped physician's signature is acceptable on the Doctor's First Report of Occupational Injury or Illness form.

_______ 32. In a workers' compensation case, bills should be submitted monthly or at the time of termination of treatment, and a claim becomes delinquent after a time frame of 45 days.

_______ 33. If an individual seeks medical care for a workers' compensation injury from another state, the state's regulations are followed in which the injured person's claim was originally filed.

_______ 34. When a patient arrives at a medical office and says he or she was hurt at work, you should verify insurance information with the benefits coordinator for the employer.

ASSIGNMENT 15-2 ▶ COMPLETE A DOCTOR'S FIRST REPORT OF OCCUPATIONAL INJURY OR ILLNESS FORM FOR A WORKERS' COMPENSATION CASE

Performance Objective

Task: Complete a Doctor's First Report of Occupational Injury or Illness form and define patient record abbreviations.

Conditions: Use the patient's record (Figure 15-1), a Doctor's First Report of Occupational Injury or Illness form (Figure 15-2), and a computer.

Standards: Claim Productivity Measurement

Time: ____________________ minutes

Accuracy: ____________________

(Note: The time element and accuracy criteria may be given by your instructor.)

Directions:

1. Complete the Doctor's First Report of Occupational Injury or Illness form (see Figure 15-2) for this nondisability type of claim.

2. Define abbreviations found in the patient's medical record.

After the instructor has returned your work to you, either make the necessary corrections and place your work in a three-ring notebook for future reference or, if you received a high score, place it in your portfolio for reference when applying for a job.

Abbreviations pertinent to this record:

Apt	____________	CT	____________
Lt	____________	Neg	____________
pt	____________	MC	____________
ED	____________	MDM	____________
Hosp	____________	DC	____________
ER	____________	PD	____________
C	____________	FU	____________
HX	____________	Wks	____________
PX	____________	Approx	____________
c/o	____________	RTW	____________
L	____________	WC	____________

PATIENT RECORD NO. 15-2-3

LAST NAME	FIRST NAME	MIDDLE NAME	BIRTH DATE	SEX	HOME PHONE
Hiranuma	Glen	M	12-24-55	M	555-467-3383

ADDRESS	CITY	STATE	ZIP CODE
4372 Hanley Avenue	Woodland Hills	XY	12345

CELL PHONE	PAGER NO.	FAX NO.	E-MAIL ADDRESS
555-908-3433		555-467-3383	hiranuma@wb.net

PATIENT'S SOC. SEC. NO.	DRIVER'S LICENSE
558-XX-9960	U3402189

PATIENT'S OCCUPATION	NAME OF COMPANY
house painter	Pittsburgh Paint Company (commercial painting company)

ADDRESS OF EMPLOYER	PHONE
3725 Bonfeld Avenue, Woodland Hills, XY 12345	555-486-9070

SPOUSE OR PARENT	OCCUPATION
Esme M. Hiranuma	homemaker

EMPLOYER	ADDRESS	PHONE

NAME OF INSURANCE: State Compensation Insurance Fund, 14156 Magnolia Boulevard, Torres, XY 12349

POLICY/CERTIFICATE NO.	GROUP NO.
016-2432-211	

REFERRED BY: Pittsburgh Paint Company

DATE	PROGRESS NOTES
5-22-xx	At 9:30 a.m. this ♂ house painter was painting an apt ceiling (apt located at 3540 W. 87th Street, Woodland Hills, XY 12345, County of Woodland Hills) when he slipped and fell from a tall ladder landing on his head and lt side of body; brief unconsciousness for approximately 15 minutes. Employer was notified by coworker and pt was sent to College Hosp ED. I was called to the hosp at request of employer and saw pt in ER at 5 p.m. (performed a C HX/PX). Pt c/o L shoulder pain and swelling; L leg and hip pain; neck and head pain. X-rays were taken of lt hip (complete), lt femur (2 views), and cervical spine (3 views) as well as CT of brain (without contrast)—all neg. I admitted pt for overnight stay in hosp for concussion. Applied sling for L shoulder sprain. Cleaned and dressed L hip and leg abrasions (MC/MDM). Plan to DC 5/23/xx. No PD expected. Pt to FU in 2 wks. Approx. RTW 6/6 xx. Prepared WC report.
	GP/llf Gerald Practon, MD
5-23-xx	Pt's HA gone. Vital signs normal. Discharged home. RTO 1 wk.
	GP/llf Gerald Practon, MD

Figure 15-1

DOCTOR'S FIRST REPORT OF OCCUPATIONAL INJURY OR ILLNESS

Within 5 days of initial examination, for every occupational injury or illness, send 2 copies of this report to the employers' workers' compensation insurance carrier or the self-insured employer. Failure to file a timely doctor's report may result in assessment of a civil penalty. In the case of diagnosed or suspected pesticide poisoning, send a copy of this report to Division of Labor Statistics and Research.

1. INSURER NAME AND ADDRESS

2. EMPLOYER NAME Policy No.

3. Address No. and Street City Zip

4. Nature of business (e.g., food manufacturing, building construction, retailer of women's clothes)

5. PATIENT NAME (first, middle initial, last name) | 6. Sex ☐Male ☐Female | 7. Date of Birth Mo. Day Yr.

8. Address No. and Street City Zip | 9. Telephone Number

10. Occupation (Specific job title) | 11. Social Security Number

12. Injured at: No. and Street City County

13. Date and hour of injury or onset or illness Mo. Day Yr. Hour ____a.m____p.m | 14. Date last worked Mo. Day Yr.

15. Date and hour of first examination or treatment Mo. Day Yr. Hour ____a.m____p.m | 16. Have you (or your office) previously treated patient? ☐Yes ☐No

Patient please complete this portion, if able to do so. Otherwise, doctor please complete immediately. Inability or failure of a patient to complete this portion shall not affect his/her rights to workers' compensation under the Labor Code.
17. DESCRIBE HOW THE ACCIDENT OR EXPOSURE HAPPENED (Give specific object, machinery or chemical.)

18. SUBJECTIVE COMPLAINTS (Describe fully.)

19. OBJECTIVE FINDINGS
A. Physical examination

B. X-ray and laboratory results (State if none or pending.)

20. DIAGNOSIS (If occupational illness specify etiologic agent and duration of exposure.) Chemical or toxic compound involved? ICD-9 Code ☐Yes ☐No

21. Are your findings and diagnosis consistent with patient's account of injury or onset of illness? ☐Yes ☐No If "no" please explain

22. Is there any other current condition that will impede or delay patient's recovery? ☐ Yes ☐ No If "yes" please explain

23. TREATMENT REQUIRED

24. If further treatment required, specify treatment plan/estimated duration.

25. If hospitalized as inpatient, give hospital name and location Date admitted Mo. Day Yr. Estimated stay

26. WORK STATUS –Is patient able to perfom usual work? ☐ Yes ☐ No
If "no," date when patient can return to: Regular work____/____/
Modified work____/____/ Specify restrictions

Doctor's Signature ________ License Number ________
Doctor's Name and Degree ________ IRS Number ________
Address ________ Telephone Number ________

Figure 15-2

ASSIGNMENT 15-3 ▶ COMPLETE A CLAIM FORM FOR A WORKERS' COMPENSATION CASE

Performance Objectives

Task: Complete a CMS-1500 (08-05) claim form for a workers' compensation case and post transactions to the financial accounting record.

Conditions: Use the patient's record (see Figure 15-1) and financial statement (Figure 15-3), a CMS-1500 claim form (print from Evolve website), a computer, procedural and diagnostic code books, and Appendix A in this *Workbook*.

Standards: Claim Productivity Measurement

Time: ____________________ minutes

Accuracy: ____________________

(Note: The time element and accuracy criteria may be given by your instructor.)

Directions:

1. Using optical character reader (OCR) guidelines, complete a CMS-1500 (08-05) claim form and direct it to the proper workers' compensation carrier. Refer to Mr. Glen M. Hiranuma's patient record for information and Appendix A in this *Workbook* to locate the fees to record on the claim, and post them to the financial statement. Date the claim May 24 of the current year.
2. Refer to Chapter 7 (Figure 7-12) of the *Handbook* for instructions on how to complete this claim form and a workers' compensation template.
3. Use your CPT code book or Appendix A in this *Workbook* to determine the correct five-digit code number and modifiers for each professional service rendered. Use your HCPCS Level II code book or refer to Appendix B in this Workbook for HCPCS procedure codes and modifiers. Note: In your state, a workers' compensation fee schedule may be available with this information. If your instructor tells you to also find the ICD-10-CM codes, a draft version may be downloaded from the following website: http://www.cdc.gov/nchs/icd/icd10cm.htm#10update.
4. Record the proper information on the financial record and claim form, and note the date you have billed the workers' compensation carrier.
5. A Performance Evaluation Checklist may be reproduced from the "Instruction Guide to the Workbook" chapter if your instructor wishes you to submit it to assist with scoring and comments.

After the instructor has returned your work to you, either make the necessary corrections and place your work in a three-ring notebook for future reference or, if you received a high score, place it in your portfolio for reference when applying for a job.

Additional Coding

1. Refer to Mr. Glen M. Hiranuma's medical record, abstract information, and code procedures that would be billed by outside providers.

Site	*Description of Service*	*Code*
a. College Hospital Radiology	____________	____________
b. College Hospital Radiology	____________	____________
c. College Hospital Radiology	____________	____________
d. College Hospital Radiology	____________	____________

Acct No. 15-2-3

STATEMENT
Financial Account
COLLEGE CLINIC
4567 Broad Avenue
Woodland Hills, XY 12345-0001
Tel. 555-486-9002
Fax No. 555-487-8976

Workers' Compensation

State Compensation Insurance Fund
14156 Magnolia Boulevard
Torres, CY 12349-0218

Patient's Name Glen M. Hiranuma
Social Security No. 558-XX-9960
Date of Injury 5-22-xx Employer Pittsburgh Paint Company
Policy No. 016-2432-211
Phone No. (H) 555-467-3383 Phone No. (W) 555-486-9070
Claim No. unassigned

DATE	REFERENCE	DESCRIPTION	CHARGES	CREDITS PYMNTS.	CREDITS ADJ.	BALANCE
20xx		BALANCE FORWARD →				
5-22-xx		Hospital Admit				
5-22-xx		WC Report				
5-23-xx		Discharge				

PLEASE PAY LAST AMOUNT IN BALANCE COLUMN

THIS IS A COPY OF YOUR FINANCIAL ACCOUNT AS IT APPEARS ON OUR RECORDS

Figure 15-3

ASSIGNMENT 15-4 ▶ COMPLETE A DOCTOR'S FIRST REPORT OF OCCUPATIONAL INJURY OR ILLNESS FORM FOR A WORKERS' COMPENSATION CASE

Performance Objective

Task: Complete a Doctor's First Report of Occupational Injury or Illness form and define patient record abbreviations.

Conditions: Use the patient's record (Figure 15-4), a Doctor's First Report of Occupational Injury or Illness form (Figure 15-5), and a computer.

Standards: Claim Productivity Measurement

Time: ____________________ minutes

Accuracy: ____________________

(Note: The time element and accuracy criteria may be given by your instructor.)

Directions:

1. Complete the Doctor's First Report of Occupational Injury or Illness form for this temporary disability type of claim. Refer to Carlos A. Giovanni's patient record for November 11 through November 15.

2. Define abbreviations found in the patient's medical record.

After the instructor has returned your work to you, either make the necessary corrections and place your work in a three-ring notebook for future reference or, if you received a high score, place it in your portfolio for reference when applying for a job.

Abbreviations pertinent to this record:

pt	____________________	H	____________________
ER	____________________	MDM	____________________
C	____________________	TD	____________________
HX	____________________	RTW	____________________
PX	____________________	approx	____________________
CT	____________________	HV	____________________
R	____________________	EPF	____________________
tr	____________________	M	____________________
adm	____________________	PO	____________________

DC	______	PF	______
Hosp	______	SF	______
OV	______	X	______
LC	______	adv	______
HA	______	trt	______
BP	______	reg	______
RTO	______	W	______
Wks	______	Cons	______

PATIENT RECORD NO. 15-4-5

LAST NAME	FIRST NAME	MIDDLE NAME	BIRTH DATE	SEX	HOME PHONE
Giovanni	Carlos	A	10-24-55	M	555-677-3485

ADDRESS	CITY	STATE	ZIP CODE
89 Beaumont Court	Woodland Hills	XY	12345

CELL PHONE	PAGER NO.	FAX NO.	E-MAIL ADDRESS
	555-230-7788	555-677-3485	giovannic@wb.net

PATIENT'S SOC. SEC. NO.	DRIVER'S LICENSE
556-XX-9699	Y0394876

PATIENT'S OCCUPATION	NAME OF COMPANY
TV repairman	Giant Television Co. (TV repair company)

ADDRESS OF EMPLOYER	PHONE
8764 Ocean Avenue, Woodland Hills, XY 12345	555-647-8851

SPOUSE OR PARENT	OCCUPATION
Maria B. Giovanni	homemaker

EMPLOYER	ADDRESS	PHONE

NAME OF INSURANCE
State Compensation Insurance Fund, 600 S. Lafayette Park Place, Ehrlich, XY 12350

POLICY/CERTIFICATE NO.	GROUP NO.
57780	

REFERRED BY: Giant Television Company

Figure 15-4

Patient: Giovanni, Carlos A. Patient Record No. 15-04-05

DATE	PROGRESS NOTES
11-11-xx	Pt referred to College Hospital ER by employer for workers' compensation injury. I was called in as on-call neurosurgeon to evaluate the pt. Pt states that today at 2 p.m. he fell from the roof of a private home while installing an antenna at 2231 Duarte St., Woodland Hills, XY 12345 in Woodland Hills County. He describes the incident as follows: "When I was attaching the base of an antenna, the weight of the antenna shifted and knocked me off the roof." Pt complains of head pain and indicates brief loss of consciousness. I performed a C HX/PX. Complete skull x-rays showed fractured skull. CT of head/brain (without contrast) indicates well-defined R. subdural hematoma. Pt suffering from cerebral concussion; no open wound. Tr plan: Adm pt to College Hospital (5 p.m.) and schedule R infratentorial craniotomy to evacuate hematoma. (H/MDM). Obtained authorization and prepared Dr.'s First Report.
	AP/llf Astro Parkinson, MD
11-12-xx	Performed R infratentorial craniotomy and evacuated subdural hematoma. Pt stable and returned to room; will be seen daily. TD: Estimated RTW 1-15-xx. Possible cranial defect & head disfigurement resulting. Pt to be hospitalized for approx 2 weeks.
	AP/llf Astro Parkinson, MD
11-13-xx	HV (EPF HX/PX M/MDM). Pt improving; recommend consult with Dr. Graff for cranial defect. Authorization obtained from adjuster (Steve Burroughs) at State Comp.
	AP/llf Astro Parkinson, MD
11-14-xx	Pt seen in cons by Dr. Cosmo Graff who stated he does not recommend correcting PO cranial defect. Both Dr. Graff and I explained how the defect resulted from the injury; there may be some improvement over time. Pt states he is grateful to be alive (EPF HX/PX M/MDM).
	AP/llf Astro Parkinson, MD
11-15-xx	Daily HV (EPF HX/PX M/MDM). Pt progressing appropriately; no complications have occurred.
thru	
11-29-xx	AP/llf Astro Parkinson, MD
11-30-xx	DC from hosp. Permanent cranial defect resulting from fracture and surgery. RTO 1 wk.
	AP/llf Astro Parkinson, MD
12-7-xx	OV (EPF HX/PX LC/MDM) Pt doing very well. No HA or visual disturbances, BP 120/80, alert and oriented. He is anxious to return to work. Pt cautioned about maintaining low activity level until released. RTO 2 wks.
	AP/llf Astro Parkinson, MD
12-21-xx	OV (PF HX/PX SF/MDM). Pt continues to improve. Suggested he start a walking program 3 x wk and monitor symptoms. May do light activity and lifting (10 lbs). Adv to call if any symptoms return. RTO 10 days.
	AP/llf Astro Parkinson, MD
12-29-xx	OV (PF HX/PX SF/MDM). Pt did not experience any symptoms with increased activity. No further trt necessary. Pt will increase activity and call if any problems occur. Pt scheduled to resume reg W on 1-15-xx. Final report submitted to workers' compensation carrier.
	AP/llf Astro Parkinson, MD

Figure 15-4, cont'd

DOCTOR'S FIRST REPORT OF OCCUPATIONAL INJURY OR ILLNESS

Within 5 days of initial examination, for every occupational injury or illness, send 2 copies of this report to the employers' workers' compensation insurance carrier or the self-insured employer. Failure to file a timely doctor's report may result in assessment of a civil penalty. In the case of diagnosed or suspected pesticide poisoning, send a copy of this report to Division of Labor Statistics and Research.

1. **INSURER NAME AND ADDRESS**

2. **EMPLOYER NAME** Policy No.

3. Address No. and Street City Zip

4. Nature of business (e.g., food manufacturing, building construction, retailer of woman's clothes)

5. **PATIENT NAME** (first, middle initial, last name)	6. Sex ☐Male ☐Female	7. Date of Birth mo. Day Yr.
8. Address No. and Street City Zip		9. Telephone Number
10. Occupation (Specific job title)		11. Social Security Number
12. Injured at: No. and Street City		County
13. Date and hour of injury or onset or illness Mo. Day Yr. Hour ____a.m____p.m		14. Date last worked Mo. Day Yr.
15. Date and hour of first examination or treatment Mo. Day Yr. Hour ____a.m____p.m		16. Have you (or your office) previously treated patient? ☐ Yes ☐ No

Patient please complete this portion, if able to do so. Otherwise, doctor please complete immediately. Inability or failure of a patient to complete this portion shall not affect his/her rights to workers' compensation under the Labor Code.

17. DESCRIBE HOW THE ACCIDENT OR EXPOSURE HAPPENED (Give specific object, machinery or chemical.)

18. SUBJECTIVE COMPLAINTS (Describe fully.)

19. OBJECTIVE FINDINGS

A. Physical examination

B. X-ray and laboratory results (State if none or pending.)

20. DIAGNOSIS (if occupational illness specify etiologic agent and duration of exposure.) Chemical or toxic compound involved? ICD-9 Code ☐Yes ☐No

21. Are your findings and diagnosis consistent with patient's account of injury or onset of illness? ☐Yes ☐No If "no" please explain

22. Is there any other current condition that will impede or delay patient's recovery? ☐ Yes ☐ No If "yes" please explain

23. TREATMENT REQUIRED

24. If further treatment required, specify treatment plan/estimated duration.

25. If hospitalized as inpatient, give hospital name and location Date admitted Mo. Day Yr. Estimated stay

26. WORK STATUS –is patient able to perfom usual work? ☐ Yes ☐ No

If "no," date when patient can return to: Regular work____/____/

Modified work____/____/ Specify restrictions

Doctor's Signature ____________ License Number ____________

Doctor's Name and Degree ____________ IRS Number ____________

Address ____________ Telephone Number ____________

Figure 15-5

ASSIGNMENT 15-5 ▶ COMPLETE A CLAIM FORM FOR A WORKERS' COMPENSATION CASE

Performance Objective

Task:	Complete a CMS-1500 (08-05) claim form for a workers' compensation case and post transactions to the financial accounting record.
Conditions:	Use the patient's record (see Figure 15-4) and financial statement (Figure 15-6), a CMS-1500 (08-05) claim form (print from Evolve website), a computer, procedural and diagnostic code books, and Appendix A in this *Workbook*.
Standards:	Claim Productivity Measurement
	Time: ______________________ minutes
	Accuracy: ______________________
	(Note: The time element and accuracy criteria may be given by your instructor.)

Directions:

1. Using OCR guidelines, complete a CMS-1500 (08-05) claim form for November dates of service and direct it to the correct workers' compensation carrier for this temporary disability workers' compensation claim. Refer to Mr. Carlos A. Giovanni's patient record for information and Appendix A in this *Workbook* to locate the fees to record on the claim and post to the financial statement. Date the claim November 30 of the current year.

   Note: A progress report is being submitted with this claim; services for December will be billed on a separate claim (see Assignment 15-6).

2. Refer to Chapter 7 (Figure 7-12) of the *Handbook* for instructions on how to complete this claim form and a workers' compensation template.

3. Use your CPT code book or Appendix A in this *Workbook* to determine the correct five-digit code number and modifiers for each professional service rendered. Use your HCPCS Level II code book or refer to Appendix B in this *Workbook* for HCPCS procedure codes and modifiers. If your instructor tells you to also find the ICD-10-CM codes, a draft version may be downloaded from the following website: http://www.cdc.gov/nchs/icd/icd10cm.htm#10update.

4. Record the proper information on the financial record and claim form, and note the date you have billed the workers' compensation insurance carrier.

5. A Performance Evaluation Checklist may be reproduced from the "Instruction Guide to the Workbook" chapter if your instructor wishes you to submit it to assist with scoring and comments.

After the instructor has returned your work to you, either make the necessary corrections and place your work in a three-ring notebook for future reference or, if you received a high score, place it in your portfolio for reference when applying for a job.

Additional Coding

1. Refer to Mr. Giovanni's medical record, abstract information, and code procedures that would be billed by outside providers.

Site	*Description of Service*	*Code*
a. College Hospital Radiology	____________________	____________________
b. College Hospital Radiology	____________________	____________________

Acct No. 15-5

STATEMENT
Financial Account
COLLEGE CLINIC
4567 Broad Avenue
Woodland Hills, XY 12345-0001
Tel. 555-486-9002
Fax No. 555-487-8976

Workers' Compensation

State Compensation Insurance Fund
14156 Magnolia Boulevard
Torres, CY 12349-0218

Patient's Name Carlos A. Giovanni — Social Security No. 556-XX9699

Date of Injury 11-11-20xx Employer Giant Television Company — Policy No. 57780

Phone No. (H) 555-677-3485 Phone No. (W) 555-647-8851 — Claim No. unassigned

DATE	REFERENCE	DESCRIPTION	CHARGES	CREDITS PYMNTS.	CREDITS ADJ.	BALANCE
20xx		BALANCE FORWARD →				
11-11-xx		Hospital admit				
11-11-xx		WC Report				
11-12-xx		Craniotomy				
11-13 to 11-29-xx		HV				
11-30-xx		Discharge				
12-7-xx		OV				
12-21-xx		OV				
12-29-xx		OV				
12-29-xx		Medical Report				

PLEASE PAY LAST AMOUNT IN BALANCE COLUMN

THIS IS A COPY OF YOUR FINANCIAL ACCOUNT AS IT APPEARS ON OUR RECORDS

Figure 15-6

ASSIGNMENT 15-6 ▶ COMPLETE A CLAIM FORM FOR A WORKERS' COMPENSATION CASE

Performance Objective

Task: Complete a CMS-1500 (08-05) claim form for a workers' compensation case and post transactions to the financial accounting record.

Conditions: Use the patient's record (see Figure 15-4) and financial statement (Figure 15-6), a CMS-1500 (08-05) claim form (print from Evolve website), a computer, procedural and diagnostic code books, and Appendix A in this *Workbook*.

Standards: Claim Productivity Measurement

Time: ______________________ minutes

Accuracy: ______________________

(Note: The time element and accuracy criteria may be given by your instructor.)

Directions:

1. Using OCR guidelines, complete a CMS-1500 (08-05) claim form for December services and direct it to the correct workers' compensation carrier for this temporary disability workers' compensation claim. Refer to Mr. Carlos A. Giovanni's patient record for information and Appendix A in this *Workbook* to locate the fees to record on the claim, and post them to the financial statement. Date the claim December 29 of the current year.

2. Refer to Chapter 7 (Figure 7-12) of the *Handbook* for instructions on how to complete this claim form and a workers' compensation template.

3. Use your CPT code book or Appendix A in this *Workbook* to determine the correct five-digit code number and modifiers for each professional service rendered. Use your HCPCS Level II code book or refer to Appendix B in this *Workbook* for HCPCS procedure codes and modifiers. If your instructor tells you to also find the ICD-10-CM codes, a draft version may be downloaded from the following website: http://www.cdc.gov/nchs/icd/icd10cm.htm#10update.

4. Record the proper information on the financial record and claim form, and note the date you have billed the workers' compensation insurance carrier.

5. A Performance Evaluation Checklist may be reproduced from the "Instruction Guide to the Workbook" chapter if your instructor wishes you to submit it to assist with scoring and comments.

After the instructor has returned your work to you, either make the necessary corrections and place your work in a three-ring notebook for future reference or, if you received a high score, place it in your portfolio for reference when applying for a job.

6. Ledger lines: Insert date of service (DOS), reference (CPT code number, check number, or dates of service for posting adjustments or when insurance was billed), description of the transaction, charge amounts, payments, adjustments, and running current balance. The posting date is the actual date the transaction is recorded. If the DOS differs from the posting date, list the DOS in the reference or description column.

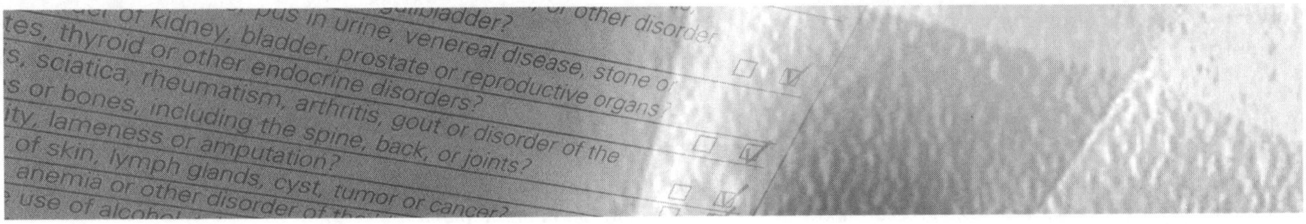

CHAPTER

16

Disability Income Insurance and Disability Benefit Programs

KEY TERMS

Your instructor may wish to select some words pertinent to this chapter for a test. For definitions of the terms, further study, and/or reference, the words, phrases, and abbreviations may be found in the glossary at the end of the Handbook.

Some of the insurance terms presented in this chapter are shown marked with an asterisk (*) and may seem familiar from previous chapters. However, their meanings may or may not have a slightly different connotation when referring to disability income insurance. Key terms for this chapter follow.

accidental death and dismemberment
Armed Services Disability
benefit period*
Civil Service Retirement System
consultative examiner
cost-of-living adjustment
Disability Determination Services
disability income insurance
double indemnity
exclusions*
Federal Employees Retirement System
future purchase option
guaranteed renewable*
hearing
long-term disability insurance
noncancelable clause*
partial disability*
reconsideration
regional office
residual benefits*
residual disability
short-term disability insurance
Social Security Administration
Social Security Disability Insurance program
State Disability Insurance
supplemental benefits
Supplemental Security Income
temporary disability*
temporary disability insurance
total disability*
unemployment compensation disability
Veterans Affairs disability program
Veterans Affairs outpatient clinic card
voluntary disability insurance
waiting period*
waiver of premium*

KEY ABBREVIATIONS

See how many abbreviations and acronyms you can translate and then use this as a handy reference list. Definitions for the key abbreviations are located near the back of the Handbook *in the glossary.*

AIDS ____________________
CE ____________________
CSRS ____________________
DDS ____________________
FERS ____________________
HIV ____________________
OASDHI ____________________
RO ____________________
SDI ____________________
SSA ____________________
SSDI program ____________________
SSI ____________________
TDI ____________________
UCD ____________________
VA ____________________

PERFORMANCE OBJECTIVES

The student will be able to:

- Define and spell the key terms and key abbreviations for this chapter, given the information from the *Handbook* glossary, within a reasonable time period, and with enough accuracy to obtain a satisfactory evaluation.
- After reading the chapter, answer the fill-in-the-blank, multiple choice, and true/false review questions with enough accuracy to obtain a satisfactory evaluation.
- Fill in the correct meaning of each abbreviation, given a list of common medical abbreviations and symbols that appear in chart notes, within a reasonable time period and with enough accuracy to obtain a satisfactory evaluation.
- Complete each state disability form, given the patients' medical chart notes and blank state disability forms, within a reasonable time period and with enough accuracy to obtain a satisfactory evaluation.

STUDY OUTLINE

Disability Claims
History
Disability Income Insurance
- Individual
- Group

Federal Disability Programs
- Workers' Compensation
- Disability Benefit Programs

State Disability Insurance
- Background
- State Programs
- Funding
- Eligibility
- Benefits
- Time Limits
- Medical Examinations
- Restrictions

Voluntary Disability Insurance
Claims Submission Guidelines
- Disability Income Claims

Conclusion

29. When the purchase of insurance is investigated, the word/words to look for in the insurance contract that mean the premium cannot be increased at renewal time is/are

    a. guaranteed renewable

    b. conditional provision

    c. noncancelable clause

    d. optional provision

30. Provisions that limit the scope of insurance coverage are known as

    a. clauses

    b. deductibles

    c. conditions

    d. exclusions

31. A Social Security Administration division that determines an individual's eligibility to be placed under the federal disability program is called

    a. Disability Determination Services

    b. Social Security Disability

    c. Supplemental Security Income

    d. none of the above

32. The time period from the beginning of disability to receiving the first payment of benefits is called a/an

    a. exclusion period

    b. waiting period

    c. insurance period

    d. elimination phase

Part III True/False

Write "T" or "F" in the blank to indicate whether you think the statement is true or false.

_______ 33. When a person insured under a disability income insurance policy cannot, for a limited period of time, perform all functions of his or her regular job duties, this is known as permanent disability.

_______ 34. To be eligible to apply for disability benefits under Social Security, an individual must be unable to perform any type of work for a period of not less than 12 months.

_______ 35. Hospital benefits may be paid for nonoccupational illness or injury under state temporary disability benefits.

_______ 36. If a woman has an abnormal condition that arises from her pregnancy (e.g., diabetes or varicose veins) and is unable to work because of the condition, she may not receive state disability benefits.

_______ 37. When a claim form is submitted for a patient applying for state disability benefits, the most important item required on the form is the claimant's Social Security number.

ASSIGNMENT 16-2 ▸ COMPLETE TWO STATE DISABILITY INSURANCE FORMS

Performance Objective

Task: Complete two state disability insurance forms and define patient record abbreviations.

Conditions: Use the patient's record (Figure 16-1), a Claim Statement of Employee form (Figure 16-2), a Doctor's Certificate form (Figure 16-3), and a computer.

Standards: Time: ____________________ minutes

Accuracy: ____________________

(Note: The time element and accuracy criteria may be given by your instructor.)

Directions:

1. To familiarize you with what information the employee must furnish, this assignment will encompass completing both the Claim Statement of Employee (see Figure 16-2) and the Doctor's Certificate (see Figure 16-3).
2. Mr. Broussard (see Figure 16-1) is applying for state disability benefits, and he does not receive sick leave pay from his employer. The language he prefers is English. He does not want any disclosure of benefit payment information to his employer. During his disability, he was not in the custody of law enforcement authorities for any violation and he has no alcoholic tendencies.
3. Date the Claim Statement of Employee November 5, and date the Doctor's Certificate November 10. Remember that this is not a claim for payment to the physician, and so no financial accounting record (ledger card) has been furnished for this patient.
4. Refer to Chapter 16 and Figures 16-3 and 16-4 of the *Handbook* to assist you in completing this form.

After the instructor has returned your work to you, either make the necessary corrections and place your work in a three-ring notebook for future reference or, if you received a high score, place it in your portfolio for reference when applying for a job.

Abbreviations pertinent to this record:

NP ____________________ c/o ____________________

LBP ____________________ pt ____________________

lt ____________________ wk ____________________

reg ____________________ exam ____________________

SLR ____________________ rt ____________________

WNL ____________________ STAT ____________________

MRI ____________________ RTO ____________________

imp ____________________ retn ____________________

PATIENT RECORD NO. 16-2

LAST NAME	FIRST NAME	MIDDLE NAME	BIRTH DATE	SEX	HOME PHONE
Broussard	Jeff	L	03-09-52	M	555-466-2490

ADDRESS	CITY	STATE	ZIP CODE
3577 Plain Street	Woodland Hills	XY	12345

CELL PHONE	PAGER NO.	FAX NO.	E-MAIL ADDRESS
555-667-7654	555-399-5903	555-466-2490	broussard@wb.net

PATIENT'S SOC. SEC. NO.	DRIVER'S LICENSE
566-XX-0090	F0394588

PATIENT'S OCCUPATION	NAME OF COMPANY
carpenter Payroll #2156	Ace Construction Company

ADDRESS OF EMPLOYER	PHONE
4556 West Eighth Street, Dorland, XY 12347	555-447-8900

SPOUSE OR PARENT	OCCUPATION
Harriet M. Broussard	secretary

EMPLOYER	ADDRESS	PHONE
Merit Accounting Company,	6743 Main Street, Woodland Hills, XY 12345	555-478-0980

NAME OF INSURANCE	INSURED OR SUBSCRIBER
Blue Cross	Jeff L. Broussard

POLICY/CERTIFICATE NO.	GROUP NO.
466-XX-9979	6131

REFERRED BY: Harold B. Hartburn (friend)

DATE	PROGRESS NOTES
10-21-xx	8:30 a.m. NP seen c/o ongoing LBP. On 8-15-XX after swinging a golf club, pt had sudden onset of severe
	pain in low back with radiation to lt side. Pt unable to work 8-16 but resumed wk on 8-17 and has been working
	full time but doing no lifting while working. Pain is exacerbating affecting his work and reg duties. Exam
	showed SLR strongly positive on lt, on rt causes pain into lt side. Neurological exam WNL. Ordered STAT
	MRI. Off work. RTO.
	RS/mtf Raymond Skeleton, MD
10-23-xx	Pt returns for test results. MRI showed huge defect of L4-5. Imp: acute herniated disc L4-5 with spinal stenosis.
	Recommended laminotomy, foraminotomy, and diskectomy L4-5.
	RS/mtf Raymond Skeleton, MD
11-1-xx	Admit to College Hospital. Operation: Lumbar laminotomy with exploration and decompression of spinal
	cord with diskectomy L4-5; lumbar anteriorarthrodesis.
	RS/mtf Raymond Skeleton, MD
11-5-xx	Pt seen daily in hosp. At 3 p.m. pt discharged to home. Will retn to wk 12-15-XX.
	RS/mtf Raymond Skeleton, MD

Figure 16-1

EDD Employment Development Department State of California

Claim for Disability Insurance Benefits – Claim Statement of Employee

TYPE or PRINT with BLACK INK.

1A. YOUR SOCIAL SECURITY NUMBER

1B. IF YOU HAVE EVER USED OTHER SOCIAL SECURITY NUMBERS, SHOW THOSE NUMBERS BELOW

2. STATE GOVERNMENT EMPLOYEE (IF YES, INDICATE BARGAINING UNIT #.)
☐ YES ____ (UNIT #) ☐ NO

3. DATE YOUR DISABILITY BEGAN
MM DD YY

4. LAST DATE YOU WORKED
MM DD YY

5. HAVE YOU WORKED ANY FULL OR PARTIAL DAYS SINCE YOUR DISABILITY BEGAN?
☐ YES ☐ NO

6. DATE YOU RECOVERED OR RETURNED TO WORK (IF ANY)
MM DD YY

7. GENDER
☐ MALE ☐ FEMALE

8. YOUR LEGAL NAME
FIRST NAME MIDDLE NAME OR INITIAL LAST NAME

9. YOUR DATE OF BIRTH
MM DD YY

10. OTHER NAMES, IF ANY, UNDER WHICH YOU HAVE WORKED

11. LANGUAGE YOU PREFER TO USE
☐ ENGLISH ☐ ESPAÑOL ☐ OTHER ____

12. YOUR MAILING ADDRESS (IF YOU WISH TO RECEIVE MAIL AT A PRIVATE MAIL BOX—NOT A US POSTAL SERVICE BOX—YOU MUST SHOW THE NUMBER IN THE "PMB#" SPACE.)
NUMBER / STREET / P.O. BOX / APARTMENT OR SPACE # | PMB # (PRIVATE MAIL BOX #)
CITY | STATE | COUNTRY (IF NOT UNITED STATES OF AMERICA) | ZIP CODE

13. YOUR AREA CODE AND TELEPHONE NUMBER
(   )

14. YOUR RESIDENCE ADDRESS, IF DIFFERENT FROM YOUR MAILING ADDRESS
NUMBER / STREET / APARTMENT OR SPACE #
CITY | STATE | COUNTRY (IF NOT UNITED STATES OF AMERICA) | ZIP CODE

15. WHY DID YOU STOP WORKING?

16. YOUR LAST OR CURRENT EMPLOYER – IF YOUR LAST OR CURRENT EMPLOYMENT WAS SELF-EMPLOYMENT, ENTER "SELF"
EMPLOYER 'S AREA CODE AND TELEPHONE NUMBER (   ) | NAME OF EMPLOYER [STATE GOVERNMENT EMPLOYEES: PROVIDE THE AGENCY OR DEPARTMENT NAME (FOR EXAMPLE: CALTRANS)]
NUMBER / STREET / SUITE # (STATE GOVERNMENT EMPLOYEES: PLEASE PROVIDE THE ADDRESS OF YOUR PERSONNEL OFFICE)
CITY | STATE | COUNTRY (IF NOT UNITED STATES OF AMERICA) | ZIP CODE

17. YOUR REGULAR OCCUPATION

18. IF YOUR EMPLOYER CONTINUED TO PAY YOU, INDICATE TYPE OF PAY
☐ SICK ☐ VACATION ☐ OTHER ____

19. MAY WE DISCLOSE BENEFIT PAYMENT INFORMATION TO YOUR EMPLOYER?
☐ YES ☐ NO

20. SECOND EMPLOYER (IF YOU HAVE MORE THAN ONE EMPLOYER)
EMPLOYER'S AREA CODE AND TELEPHONE NUMBER (   ) | NAME OF EMPLOYER
NUMBER / STREET / SUITE #
CITY | STATE | COUNTRY (IF NOT UNITED STATES OF AMERICA) | ZIP CODE

21. AT ANY TIME DURING YOUR DISABILITY WERE YOU IN THE CUSTODY OF LAW ENFORCEMENT AUTHORITIES BECAUSE YOU WERE CONVICTED OF VIOLATING A LAW OR ORDINANCE?
☐ YES ☐ NO IF "YES," INDICATE NAME OF FACILITY: ____

DE 2501 Rev. 77 (3-06) **(INTERNET)**

Figure 16-2

Claim Statement of Employee - continued

22. PLEASE RE-ENTER YOUR SOCIAL SECURITY NUMBER..

23. IF YOU ARE A RESIDENT OF AN ALCOHOLIC RECOVERY HOME OR A DRUG-FREE RESIDENTIAL FACILITY, SHOW THE NAME, TELEPHONE NUMBER, AND ADDRESS

NAME OF FACILITY	FACILITY AREA CODE AND TELEPHONE NUMBER ( )
ADDRESS OF FACILITY (NUMBER AND STREET / CITY / STATE / ZIP CODE)	

24. HAVE YOU FILED OR DO YOU INTEND TO FILE FOR WORKERS' COMPENSATION BENEFITS?	25. WAS THIS DISABILITY CAUSED BY YOUR JOB?	26. DATE(S) OF INJURY SHOWN ON YOUR WORKERS' COMPENSATION CLAIM
☐ YES–COMPLETE ITEMS 25 THROUGH 32 ☐ NO– COMPLETE ITEMS 25, 31 AND 32	☐ YES ☐ NO	

27. WORKERS' COMPENSATION INSURANCE COMPANY

COMPANY NAME			COMPANY AREA CODE AND TELEPHONE NUMBER ( )
NUMBER / STREET / SUITE #			
CITY	STATE	ZIP CODE	YOUR WORKERS' COMPENSATION CLAIM NUMBER

28. WORKERS' COMPENSATION ADJUSTER

ADJUSTER NAME	ADJUSTER AREA CODE AND TELEPHONE NUMBER ( )

29. EMPLOYER SHOWN ON YOUR WORKERS' COMPENSATION CLAIM

EMPLOYER NAME	EMPLOYER AREA CODE AND TELEPHONE NUMBER ( )

30. YOUR ATTORNEY (IF ANY) FOR YOUR WORKERS' COMPENSATION CASE

ATTORNEY NAME			ATTORNEY AREA CODE AND TELEPHONE NUMBER ( )
NUMBER / STREET / SUITE #			
CITY	STATE	ZIP CODE	WORKERS' COMPENSATION APPEALS BOARD CASE NUMBER

PLEASE REVIEW, SIGN, AND DATE BOTH NO. 31 AND NO. 32.

31. Health Insurance Portability and Accountability Act Authorization. I authorize any physician, practitioner, hospital, vocational rehabilitation counselor, or workers' compensation insurance carrier to furnish and disclose to employees of California Employment Development Department (EDD) all facts concerning my disability that are within their knowledge and to allow inspection of and provide copies of any medical, vocational rehabilitation, and billing records concerning my disability that are under their control. I understand that EDD may disclose information as authorized by the California Unemployment Insurance Code and that such redisclosed information may no longer be protected by this rule. I agree that photocopies of this authorization shall be as valid as the original. I understand that, unless revoked by me in writing, this authorization is valid for fifteen years from the date received by EDD or the effective date of the claim, whichever is later. I understand that I may not revoke this authorization to avoid prosecution or to prevent EDD's recovery of monies to which it is legally entitled.

Claimant's Signature (DO NOT PRINT)	Date Signed

32. Declaration and Signature. By my signature on this claim statement, I claim benefits and certify that for the period covered by this claim I was unemployed and disabled. I understand that willfully making a false statement or concealing a material fact in order to obtain payment of benefits is a violation of California law and that such violation is punishable by imprisonment or fine or both. I declare under penalty of perjury that the foregoing statement, including any accompanying statements, is to the best of my knowledge and belief true, correct, and complete. By my signature on this claim statement, I authorize the California Department of Industrial Relations and my employer to furnish and disclose to State Disability Insurance all facts concerning my disability, wages or earnings, and benefit payments that are within their knowledge. By my signature on this claim statement, I authorize release and use of information as stated in the "Information Collection and Access" portion of this form. I agree that photocopies of this authorization shall be as valid as the original, and I understand that authorizations contained in this claim statement are granted for a period of fifteen years from the date of my signature or the effective date of the claim, whichever is later.

Claimant's Signature (DO NOT PRINT)	Date Signed

If your signature is made by mark (X), it must be attested by two witnesses with their addresses

1st Witness Signature and Address	2nd Witness Signature and Address

33. Personal Representative signing on behalf of claimant must complete the following: I,______________________, represent the claimant in this matter as authorized by ☐ power of attorney (attach copy) ☐ Declaration of Individual Claiming Disability Insurance Benefits Due an Incapacitated or Deceased Claimant, DE 2522 (see pg. A,#4)

Personal Representative's Signature (DO NOT PRINT)	Date Signed

DE 2501 Rev. 77 (3-06) **(INTERNET)**

Figure 16-2, cont'd

EDD Employment Development Department State of California

Claim for Disability Insurance Benefits – Doctor's Certificate

TYPE or PRINT with BLACK INK.

34. PATIENT'S FILE NUMBER	35. PATIENT'S SOCIAL SECURITY NO.	36. PATIENT'S LAST NAME
37. DOCTOR'S NAME AS SHOWN ON LICENSE	38. DOCTOR'S TELEPHONE NUMBER ( )	39. DOCTOR'S STATE LICENSE NO.

40. DOCTOR'S ADDRESS – NUMBER AND STREET, CITY, STATE, COUNTRY (IF NOT USA), ZIP CODE. POST OFFICE BOX NUMBER IS NOT ACCEPTED AS THE SOLE ADDRESS

41. THIS PATIENT HAS BEEN UNDER MY CARE AND TREATMENT FOR THIS MEDICAL PROBLEM
FROM ____/____/____ TO ____/____/____ AT INTERVALS OF ☐ DAILY ☐ WEEKLY ☐ MONTHLY ☐ AS NEEDED

42. AT ANY TIME DURING YOUR ATTENDANCE FOR THIS MEDICAL PROBLEM, HAS THE PATIENT BEEN INCAPABLE OF PERFORMING HIS/HER REGULAR OR CUSTOMARY WORK? ☐ NO – SKIP TO THE DOCTOR'S CERTIFICATION SECTION ☐ YES – ENTER DATE DISABILITY BEGAN: ____/____/____	43. DATE YOU RELEASED OR ANTICIPATE RELEASING PATIENT TO RETURN TO HIS/HER REGULAR / CUSTOMARY WORK ("UNKNOWN," "INDEFINITE," ETC., NOT ACCEPTED.) ____/____/____
44. ICD9 DISEASE CODE, PRIMARY (REQUIRED UNLESS DIAGNOSIS NOT YET OBTAINED) ____.____	45. ICD9 DISEASE CODE(S), SECONDARY ____.____, ____.____, ____.____

46. DIAGNOSIS (REQUIRED) – IF NO DIAGNOSIS HAS BEEN DETERMINED, ENTER OBJECTIVE FINDINGS OR A DETAILED STATEMENT OF SYMPTOMS

47. FINDINGS – STATE NATURE, SEVERITY, AND EXTENT OF THE INCAPACITATING DISEASE OR INJURY. INCLUDE ANY OTHER DISABLING CONDITIONS

48. TYPE OF TREATMENT / MEDICATION RENDERED TO PATIENT	49. IF PATIENT WAS HOSPITALIZED, PROVIDE DATES OF ENTRY AND DISCHARGE ____/____/____ TO ____/____/____
50. DATE AND TYPE OF SURGERY / PROCEDURE PERFORMED OR TO BE PERFORMED ____/____/____	ICD9 PROCEDURE CODE(S)
51. IF PATIENT IS NOW PREGNANT OR HAS BEEN PREGNANT, WHAT DATE DID PREGNANCY TERMINATE OR WHAT DATE DO YOU EXPECT DELIVERY? ____/____/____	52. IF PREGNANCY IS / WAS ABNORMAL, STATE THE ABNORMAL AND INVOLUNTARY COMPLICATION CAUSING MATERNAL DISABILITY

53. BASED ON YOUR EXAMINATION OF PATIENT, IS THIS DISABILITY THE RESULT OF "OCCUPATION," EITHER AS AN "INDUSTRIAL ACCIDENT" OR AS AN "OCCUPATIONAL DISEASE"? (INCLUDE SITUATIONS WHERE PATIENT'S OCCUPATION HAS AGGRAVATED PRE-EXISTING CONDITIONS.) ☐ YES ☐ NO	54. ARE YOU COMPLETING THIS FORM FOR THE SOLE PURPOSE OF REFERRAL / RECOMMENDATION TO AN ALCOHOLIC RECOVERY HOME OR DRUG-FREE RESIDENTIAL FACILITY AS INDICATED BY THE PATIENT IN QUESTION 23? ☐ YES ☐ NO	55. WOULD DISCLOSURE OF THIS INFORMATION TO YOUR PATIENT BE MEDICALLY OR PSYCHOLOGICALLY DETRIMENTAL? ☐ YES ☐ NO

Doctor's Certification and Signature (REQUIRED): Having considered the patient's regular or customary work, I certify under penalty of perjury that, based on my examination, this Doctor's Certificate truly describes the patient's disability (if any) and the estimated duration thereof.

I further certify that I am a ____________ (TYPE OF DOCTOR) ____________ (SPECIALTY, IF ANY) licensed to practice in the State of ____________.

► ________________________________ ORIGINAL SIGNATURE OF ATTENDING DOCTOR – RUBBER STAMP IS NOT ACCEPTABLE

► ________________________________ DATE SIGNED

Under sections 2116 and 2122 of the California Unemployment Insurance Code, it is a violation for any individual who, with intent to defraud, falsely certifies the medical condition of any person in order to obtain disability insurance benefits, whether for the maker or for any other person, and is punishable by imprisonment and/or a fine not exceeding $20,000. Section 1143 requires additional administrative penalties.

DE 2501 Rev. 77 (3-06) **(INTERNET)**

Figure 16-3

ASSIGNMENT 16-3 ▶ COMPLETE TWO STATE DISABILITY INSURANCE FORMS

Performance Objective

Task: Complete two state disability insurance forms and define patient record abbreviations.

Conditions: Use the patient's record (Figure 16-4), a Doctor's Certificate form (Figure 16-5), a Physician's Supplementary Certificate form (Figure 16-6), and a computer.

Standards: Time: ____________________ minutes

Accuracy: ____________________

(Note: The time element and accuracy criteria may be given by your instructor.)

Directions:

1. Assume that the Claim Statement of Employee has been completed satisfactorily by Mr. Fred E. Thorndike (see Figure 16-4). Complete the Doctor's Certificate form (see Figure 16-5) and date it December 2. In completing this portion of the assignment, look at the first entry made by Dr. Practon on November 25 only.

2. Mr. Thorndike returns to see Dr. Practon on December 7, at which time his disability leave needs to be extended. Complete the Physician's Supplementary Certificate form (see Figure 16-6) by referring to the entry made during the second visit, and date the certificate December 7. Remember that this is not a claim for payment to the physician, and so no ledger card has been furnished for this patient.

3. Refer to Chapter 16 and Figures 16-4 and 16-5 of the *Handbook* to assist you in completing these forms.

After the instructor has returned your work to you, either make the necessary corrections and place your work in a three-ring notebook for future reference or, if you received a high score, place it in your portfolio for reference when applying for a job.

Abbreviations pertinent to this record:

pt ____________________ SDI ____________________

PE ____________________ wks ____________________

dx ____________________ Cont ____________________

RTO ____________________ wk ____________________

est ____________________ FU ____________________

c̄ ____________________ CXR ____________________

reg ____________________

PATIENT RECORD NO. 16-3

LAST NAME	FIRST NAME	MIDDLE NAME	BIRTH DATE	SEX	HOME PHONE
Thorndike	Fred	E	02-17-54	M	555-465-7820

ADDRESS	CITY	STATE	ZIP CODE
5784 Helen Street	Woodland Hills	XY	12345

CELL PHONE	PAGER NO.	FAX NO.	E-MAIL ADDRESS
555-432-7744	555-320-5500	555-466-7820	thorndike@wb.net

PATIENT'S SOC. SEC. NO.	DRIVER'S LICENSE
549-XX-8721	M00430548

PATIENT'S OCCUPATION	NAME OF COMPANY
salesman Payoll No. 6852	Easy on Paint Company

ADDRESS OF EMPLOYER	PHONE
4586 West 20th Street, Woodland Hills, XY 12345	555-467-8898

SPOUSE OR PARENT	OCCUPATION
Jennifer B. Thorndike	homemaker

EMPLOYER	ADDRESS	PHONE

NAME OF INSURANCE
Pacific Mutual Insurance Company,120 South Main Street, Merck, XY 12346

POLICY/CERTIFICATE NO.	GROUP NO.	INSURED OR SUBSCRIBER
	6709	Fred E. Thorndike

REFERRED BY: John Diehl (Friend)

DATE	PROGRESS NOTES
11-25-xx	On or about 11-3-xx, pt began to have chest pain and much coughing. On 11-24-xx, pt too ill to work and
	decided to file for SDI benefits. Pt states illness is not work connected and he does not receive sick pay.
	PE: Pt examined and complained of productive cough of 3 wks duration and chest pain. Chest x-rays
	confirmed dx-mucopurulent chronic bronchitis. Cont home rest and prescribed antibiotic medication. RTO
	12-7-xx. Pt will be capable of returning to wk 12-8-xx.
	GP/mtf Gerald Practon, MD
12-07-xx	Est pt returns for F/U c bronchitis. Chest pain improved. Still running low grade temp c̄ productive cough.
	F/U CXR shows clearing. Recommended bed rest x 7d. Will extend disability to 12-15-xx at which time pt
	can resume reg work. No complications anticipated.
	GP/mtf Gerald Practon, MD

Figure 16-4

EDD Employment Development Department State of California

Claim for Disability Insurance Benefits – Doctor's Certificate

TYPE or PRINT with BLACK INK.

34. PATIENT'S FILE NUMBER	35. PATIENT'S SOCIAL SECURITY NO.	36. PATIENT'S LAST NAME

37. DOCTOR'S NAME AS SHOWN ON LICENSE	38. DOCTOR'S TELEPHONE NUMBER ( )	39. DOCTOR'S STATE LICENSE NO.

40. DOCTOR'S ADDRESS – NUMBER AND STREET, CITY, STATE, COUNTRY (IF NOT USA), ZIP CODE. POST OFFICE BOX NUMBER IS NOT ACCEPTED AS THE SOLE ADDRESS

41. THIS PATIENT HAS BEEN UNDER MY CARE AND TREATMENT FOR THIS MEDICAL PROBLEM

FROM ____/____/____ TO ____/____/____ AT INTERVALS OF ☐ DAILY ☐ WEEKLY ☐ MONTHLY ☐ AS NEEDED

42. AT ANY TIME DURING YOUR ATTENDANCE FOR THIS MEDICAL PROBLEM, HAS THE PATIENT BEEN INCAPABLE OF PERFORMING HIS/HER REGULAR OR CUSTOMARY WORK?
☐ NO – SKIP TO THE DOCTOR'S CERTIFICATION SECTION ☐ YES – ENTER DATE DISABILITY BEGAN: ____/____/____

43. DATE YOU RELEASED OR ANTICIPATE RELEASING PATIENT TO RETURN TO HIS/HER REGULAR / CUSTOMARY WORK ("UNKNOWN," "INDEFINITE," ETC., NOT ACCEPTED.) ____/____/____

44. ICD9 DISEASE CODE, PRIMARY (REQUIRED UNLESS DIAGNOSIS NOT YET OBTAINED)
____ . ____

45. ICD9 DISEASE CODE(S), SECONDARY
____ . ____, ____ . ____, ____ . ____

46. DIAGNOSIS (REQUIRED) – IF NO DIAGNOSIS HAS BEEN DETERMINED, ENTER OBJECTIVE FINDINGS OR A DETAILED STATEMENT OF SYMPTOMS

47. FINDINGS – STATE NATURE, SEVERITY, AND EXTENT OF THE INCAPACITATING DISEASE OR INJURY. INCLUDE ANY OTHER DISABLING CONDITIONS

48. TYPE OF TREATMENT / MEDICATION RENDERED TO PATIENT

49. IF PATIENT WAS HOSPITALIZED, PROVIDE DATES OF ENTRY AND DISCHARGE
____/____/____ TO ____/____/____

50. DATE AND TYPE OF SURGERY / PROCEDURE PERFORMED OR TO BE PERFORMED
____/____/____

ICD9 PROCEDURE CODE(S)

51. IF PATIENT IS NOW PREGNANT OR HAS BEEN PREGNANT, WHAT DATE DID PREGNANCY TERMINATE OR WHAT DATE DO YOU EXPECT DELIVERY?
____/____/____

52. IF PREGNANCY IS / WAS ABNORMAL, STATE THE ABNORMAL AND INVOLUNTARY COMPLICATION CAUSING MATERNAL DISABILITY

53. BASED ON YOUR EXAMINATION OF PATIENT, IS THIS DISABILITY THE RESULT OF "OCCUPATION," EITHER AS AN "INDUSTRIAL ACCIDENT" OR AS AN "OCCUPATIONAL DISEASE"? (INCLUDE SITUATIONS WHERE PATIENT'S OCCUPATION HAS AGGRAVATED PRE-EXISTING CONDITIONS.)
☐ YES ☐ NO

54. ARE YOU COMPLETING THIS FORM FOR THE SOLE PURPOSE OF REFERRAL / RECOMMENDATION TO AN ALCOHOLIC RECOVERY HOME OR DRUG-FREE RESIDENTIAL FACILITY AS INDICATED BY THE PATIENT IN QUESTION 23?
☐ YES ☐ NO

55. WOULD DISCLOSURE OF THIS INFORMATION TO YOUR PATIENT BE MEDICALLY OR PSYCHOLOGICALLY DETRIMENTAL?
☐ YES ☐ NO

Doctor's Certification and Signature (REQUIRED): Having considered the patient's regular or customary work, I certify under penalty of perjury that, based on my examination, this Doctor's Certificate truly describes the patient's disability (if any) and the estimated duration thereof.

I further certify that I am a ____________ (TYPE OF DOCTOR) ____________ (SPECIALTY, IF ANY) licensed to practice in the State of ____________.

► ______________________________
ORIGINAL SIGNATURE OF ATTENDING DOCTOR – RUBBER STAMP IS NOT ACCEPTABLE

► ______________________________
DATE SIGNED

Under sections 2116 and 2122 of the California Unemployment Insurance Code, it is a violation for any individual who, with intent to defraud, falsely certifies the medical condition of any person in order to obtain disability insurance benefits, whether for the maker or for any other person, and is punishable by imprisonment and/or a fine not exceeding $20,000. Section 1143 requires additional administrative penalties.

DE 2501 Rev. 77 (3-06) **(INTERNET)**

Figure 16-5

NOTICE OF FINAL PAYMENT

The information contained in your claim for Disability Insurance indicates that you are now able to work, therefore, this is the final check that you will receive on this claim.

IF YOU ARE ***STILL*** DISABLED: You should complete the Claimant's Certification portion of this form and contact your doctor immediately to have him/her complete the Physician's Supplementary Certificate below.

IF YOU BECOME DISABLED ***AGAIN:*** File a new Disability Insurance claim form.

IF YOU ARE UNEMPLOYED AND AVAILABLE FOR WORK: Report to the nearest Unemployment Insurance office of the Department for assistance in finding work and to determine your entitlement to Unemployment Insurance Benefits.

This determination is final unless you file an appeal within twenty (20) days from the date of the mailing of this notification. You may appeal by giving a detailed statement as to why you believe the determination is in error. All communications regarding this Disability Insurance claim should include your Social Security Account Number and be addressed to the office shown.

CLAIMANT'S CERTIFICATION

I certify that I continue to be disabled and incapable of doing my regular work, and that I have reported all wages, Worker's Compensation benefits and other monies received during the claim period to the Employment Development Department.

ENTER YOUR SOCIAL SECURITY NUMBER 549 XX 8721

Sign Your Name ____________________ Fred E. Thorndike

Date Signed ____________________ December 6, 20XX

PHYSICIAN'S SUPPLEMENTARY CERTIFICATE

Department Use Only	

1. Are you still treating patient?________ Date of last treatment______________, 20___.
2. What present condition continues to make the patient disabled?

____

____

____

3. Date patient recovered, or will recover sufficiently (even if under treatment) to be able to perform his/her regular and customary work______________, 20______. Please enter a specific or estimated recovery date.
4. Would the disclosure of this information to your patient be medically or psychologically detrimental to the patient?
   Yes ☐ No ☐

I hereby certify that the above statements in my opinion truly describe the claimant's condition and the estimated duration thereof.

Doctor's Signature ____________________

______________, 20____
Date

Phone Number ____________________

DE 2525XX Rev. 13 (3-86) – Versión en español en el dorso –

Figure 16-6

ASSIGNMENT 16-4 ► COMPLETE A STATE DISABILITY INSURANCE FORM

Performance Objective

Task:	Complete a state disability insurance form and define patient record abbreviations.
Conditions:	Use the patient's record (Figure 16-7), a Doctor's Certificate form (Figure 16-8), and a computer.
Standards:	Time: ____________ minutes
	Accuracy: ____________
	(Note: The time element and accuracy criteria may be given by your instructor.)

Directions:

1. Assume that the Claim Statement of Employee has been completed satisfactorily by Mr. James T. Fujita (see Figure 16-7). Complete the Doctor's Certificate form (see Figure 16-8) and date it December 15. Remember that this is not a claim for payment to the physician, and so no ledger card has been furnished for this patient.

2. Refer to Chapter 16 and Figure 16-4 of the *Handbook* to assist you in completing this form.

After the instructor has returned your work to you, either make the necessary corrections and place your work in a three-ring notebook for future reference or, if you received a high score, place it in your portfolio for reference when applying for a job.

Abbreviations pertinent to this record:

pt	____________	exam	____________
hx	____________	neg	____________
WBC	____________	imp	____________
wk	____________	SDI	____________

PATIENT RECORD NO. 16-4

LAST NAME	FIRST NAME	MIDDLE NAME	BIRTH DATE	SEX	HOME PHONE
Fujita	James	T	03-27-54	M	555-677-2881

ADDRESS	CITY	STATE	ZIP CODE
3538 South A Street	Woodland Hills	XY	12345

CELL PHONE	PAGER NO.	FAX NO.	E-MAIL ADDRESS
555-499-6556	555-988-4100	555-677-2881	fujita@wb.net

PATIENT'S SOC. SEC. NO.	DRIVER'S LICENSE
567-XX-8898	M4387931

PATIENT'S OCCUPATION	NAME OF COMPANY
electrician Payoll No. 8834	Macy Electric Company

ADDRESS OF EMPLOYER	PHONE
2671 North C Street, Woodland Hills, XY 12345	555-677-2346

SPOUSE OR PARENT	OCCUPATION
Mary J. Fujita	homemaker

EMPLOYER	ADDRESS	PHONE

NAME OF INSURANCE
Atlantic Mutual Insurance Company, 111 South Main Street, Woodland Hills, XY 12345

POLICY/CERTIFICATE NO.	GROUP NO.	INSURED OR SUBSCRIBER
F20015		James T. Fujita

REFERRED BY: Cherry Hotta (aunt)

DATE	PROGRESS NOTES
12-07-XX	Today pt could not go to work and came for exam complaining of pain in abdomen, nausea, and no vomiting. Pt has hx of mesentery adenopathy. Exam neg except abdomen showed tenderness all over with voluntary guarding. WBC 10,000. Imp: Mesenteric adenitis. Advised strict bed rest at home and bland diet. To return in 1 wk. Will file for SDI benefits. Pt states illness is not work connected and he receives sick leave pay of $150/wk.
	GI/mtf Gaston Input, MD
12-15-xx	Exam showed normal nontender abdomen. No nausea. Pt tolerating food well. WBC 7,500. Pt will be capable of returning to work 12-22-xx.
	GI/mtf Gaston Input, MD

Figure 16-7

EDD Employment Development Department State of California

Claim for Disability Insurance Benefits – Doctor's Certificate

TYPE or PRINT with BLACK INK.

34. PATIENT'S FILE NUMBER	35. PATIENT'S SOCIAL SECURITY NO.	36. PATIENT'S LAST NAME	
37. DOCTOR'S NAME AS SHOWN ON LICENSE		38. DOCTOR'S TELEPHONE NUMBER ( )	39. DOCTOR'S STATE LICENSE NO.

40. DOCTOR'S ADDRESS – NUMBER AND STREET, CITY, STATE, COUNTRY (IF NOT USA), ZIP CODE. POST OFFICE BOX NUMBER IS NOT ACCEPTED AS THE SOLE ADDRESS

41. THIS PATIENT HAS BEEN UNDER MY CARE AND TREATMENT FOR THIS MEDICAL PROBLEM

FROM ____/____/____ TO ____/____/____ AT INTERVALS OF ☐ DAILY ☐ WEEKLY ☐ MONTHLY ☐ AS NEEDED

42. AT ANY TIME DURING YOUR ATTENDANCE FOR THIS MEDICAL PROBLEM, HAS THE PATIENT BEEN INCAPABLE OF PERFORMING HIS/HER REGULAR OR CUSTOMARY WORK?
☐ NO – SKIP TO THE DOCTOR'S CERTIFICATION SECTION ☐ YES – ENTER DATE DISABILITY BEGAN: ____/____/____

43. DATE YOU RELEASED OR ANTICIPATE RELEASING PATIENT TO RETURN TO HIS/HER REGULAR / CUSTOMARY WORK ("UNKNOWN," "INDEFINITE," ETC., NOT ACCEPTED.) ____/____/____

44. ICD9 DISEASE CODE, PRIMARY (REQUIRED UNLESS DIAGNOSIS NOT YET OBTAINED)
____.____

45. ICD9 DISEASE CODE(S), SECONDARY
____.____, ____.____, ____.____

46. DIAGNOSIS (REQUIRED) – IF NO DIAGNOSIS HAS BEEN DETERMINED, ENTER OBJECTIVE FINDINGS OR A DETAILED STATEMENT OF SYMPTOMS

47. FINDINGS – STATE NATURE, SEVERITY, AND EXTENT OF THE INCAPACITATING DISEASE OR INJURY. INCLUDE ANY OTHER DISABLING CONDITIONS

48. TYPE OF TREATMENT / MEDICATION RENDERED TO PATIENT

49. IF PATIENT WAS HOSPITALIZED, PROVIDE DATES OF ENTRY AND DISCHARGE
____/____/____ TO ____/____/____

50. DATE AND TYPE OF SURGERY / PROCEDURE PERFORMED OR TO BE PERFORMED
____/____/____

ICD9 PROCEDURE CODE(S)

51. IF PATIENT IS NOW PREGNANT OR HAS BEEN PREGNANT, WHAT DATE DID PREGNANCY TERMINATE OR WHAT DATE DO YOU EXPECT DELIVERY?
____/____/____

52. IF PREGNANCY IS / WAS ABNORMAL, STATE THE ABNORMAL AND INVOLUNTARY COMPLICATION CAUSING MATERNAL DISABILITY

53. BASED ON YOUR EXAMINATION OF PATIENT, IS THIS DISABILITY THE RESULT OF "OCCUPATION," EITHER AS AN "INDUSTRIAL ACCIDENT" OR AS AN "OCCUPATIONAL DISEASE"? (INCLUDE SITUATIONS WHERE PATIENT'S OCCUPATION HAS AGGRAVATED PRE-EXISTING CONDITIONS.)
☐ YES ☐ NO

54. ARE YOU COMPLETING THIS FORM FOR THE SOLE PURPOSE OF REFERRAL / RECOMMENDATION TO AN ALCOHOLIC RECOVERY HOME OR DRUG-FREE RESIDENTIAL FACILITY AS INDICATED BY THE PATIENT IN QUESTION 23?
☐ YES ☐ NO

55. WOULD DISCLOSURE OF THIS INFORMATION TO YOUR PATIENT BE MEDICALLY OR PSYCHOLOGICALLY DETRIMENTAL?
☐ YES ☐ NO

Doctor's Certification and Signature (REQUIRED): Having considered the patient's regular or customary work, I certify under penalty of perjury that, based on my examination, this Doctor's Certificate truly describes the patient's disability (if any) and the estimated duration thereof.

I further certify that I am a ____________ (TYPE OF DOCTOR) ____________ (SPECIALTY, IF ANY) licensed to practice in the State of ____________.

► ______________________________
ORIGINAL SIGNATURE OF ATTENDING DOCTOR – RUBBER STAMP IS NOT ACCEPTABLE

► ______________________________
DATE SIGNED

Under sections 2116 and 2122 of the California Unemployment Insurance Code, it is a violation for any individual who, with intent to defraud, falsely certifies the medical condition of any person in order to obtain disability insurance benefits, whether for the maker or for any other person, and is punishable by imprisonment and/or a fine not exceeding $20,000. Section 1143 requires additional administrative penalties.

DE 2501 Rev. 77 (3-06) **(INTERNET)**

Figure 16-8

ASSIGNMENT 16-5 ▸ COMPLETE TWO STATE DISABILITY INSURANCE FORMS

Performance Objective

Task:	Complete two state disability insurance forms and define patient record abbreviations.
Conditions:	Use the patient's record (Figure 16-9), a Doctor's Certificate form (Figure 16-10), a Request for Additional Medical Information form (Figure 16-11), and a computer.
Standards:	Time: __________ minutes
	Accuracy: __________
	(Note: The time element and accuracy criteria may be given by your instructor.)

Directions:

1. Mr. Jake J. Burrows (see Figure 16-9) has previously applied for state disability benefits. After 2 months, he is referred to another doctor for further care. Complete the form (see Figure 16-10) and date it June 25. You will notice that this form is almost identical to the Doctor's Certificate and is mailed to the claimant to secure the certification of a new physician or to clarify a specific claimed period of disability. In completing this part of the assignment, look at the first three entries on the patient record only.
2. Complete the Request for Additional Medical Information form (see Figure 16-11) by looking at the last entry on Mr. Burrows' record, and date the report July 15. Remember that this is not a claim for payment to the physician, and so no ledger card has been furnished for this patient.
3. Refer to Chapter 16 and Figure 16-6 of the *Handbook* to assist you in completing one of these forms.

After the instructor has returned your work to you, either make the necessary corrections and place your work in a three-ring notebook for future reference or, if you received a high score, place it in your portfolio for reference when applying for a job.

Abbreviations pertinent to this record:

pt	__________	$\bar{c}$	__________
C5/6	__________	imp	__________
adm	__________	hosp	__________
approx	__________	retn	__________
RTO	__________	wks	__________

PATIENT RECORD NO. 16-5

Burrows	Jake	J	04-26-50	M	555-478-9009
LAST NAME	FIRST NAME	MIDDLE NAME	BIRTH DATE	SEX	HOME PHONE

319 Barry Street	Woodland Hills	XY	12345
ADDRESS	CITY	STATE	ZIP CODE

555-765-9080	555-542-0979	555-478-9009	burrows@wb.net
CELL PHONE	PAGER NO.	FAX NO.	E-MAIL ADDRESS

457-XX-0801	D0453298
PATIENT'S SOC. SEC. NO.	DRIVER'S LICENSE

assembler	Convac Electronics Company
PATIENT'S OCCUPATION	NAME OF COMPANY

3440 West 7th Street, Woodland Hills, XY 12345	555-467-9008
ADDRESS OF EMPLOYER	PHONE

Jane B. Burrows	homemaker
SPOUSE OR PARENT	OCCUPATION

EMPLOYER	ADDRESS	PHONE

Blue Shield	Jake J. Burrows
NAME OF INSURANCE	INSURED OR SUBSCRIBER

T8471811A	53553AT
POLICY/CERTIFICATE NO.	GROUP NO.

REFERRED BY: Clarence Butler, MD, 300 Sixth Street, Woodland Hills, XY 12345 NPI# 620114352X

DATE	PROGRESS NOTES
6-02-xx	Pt. referred by Dr. Butler. Pt states on 4-19-xx was wrestling c̄ son and jerked his neck the wrong way.
	2 days later had much pain and muscle spasm in the cervical region. X-rays show degenerated disk C5/6.
	Exam: limited range of neck motion and limited abduction both arms. Imp: Degenerated cervical disk C5/6.
	Pt unable to work as of this date. Myelogram ordered. Return for test results.
	RS/mtf Raymond Skeleton, MD
6-24-xx	Myelogram positive at C5/6. Scheduled for surgery the following day.
	RS/mtf Raymond Skeleton, MD
6-25-xx	Pt adm to College Hospital at 9 AM for disk excision and anterior cervical fusion at C5/6. Pt will be discharged from
	hosp on 6-29-xx. Approx date of retn to work 8-15-xx.
	RS/mtf Raymond Skeleton, MD
6-26 to	Pt seen daily in hospital. Discharged 6-29. RTO 2 weeks.
6-29-xx	RS/mtf Raymond Skeleton, MD
7-15-xx	Pt has some restriction of cervical motion. No muscle spasm. Very little cervical pain. Pt to be seen in
	2 wks. To retn to work 8-15-xx.
	RS/mtf Raymond Skeleton, MD

Figure 16-9

In order that any disability insurance to which you may be entitled may be paid without undue delay, please have the physician who treats or treated you during the period indicated below complete this form and return it to us at his earliest convenience.

Para que cualquier beneficio del Segurdo de Incapacidad a que Ud. pueda tener derecho a recibir sea pagado sin demoras excesivas, haga el favor de hacer que el médicio que le atiende o atiendó, durante el período indicado abajo, complete este formulario y que lo regrese a nuestra oficina cuanto antes.

Henry B. Garcia
Disability Insurance Program Representative

6-2 thru 6-25-XX
Period Dates - Feches del Periodo

457-XX-0801
S.S.A. – No. Des S.S.

1. I attended the patient for the present medical problem from: Month Day Year To: Month Day Year At intervals of:

2. History:
State the nature, severity and the bodily extent of the incapacitating disease or injury.
Findings:
Diagnosis:
Type of treatment and/or medication rendered to patient:

3. Diagnosis confirmed by: (*Specify type of test or X-ray)*

4. Is this patient now pregnant or has she been pregnant since the date of treatment as reported above? Yes☐ No☐ If "Yes", date pregnancy terminated or future EDC:
Is the pregnancy normal? Yes☐ No☐ If "No", state the abnormal and involuntary complication causing maternal disability:

5. Operation: Date performed: ☐ Date to be performed: ☐ Type of Operation:

6. Has the patient at any time during your attendance for this medical problem been incapable of performing his/her regular work? Yes☐ No☐ If "Yes", the disability commenced on:

7. APPROXIMATE date, based on your examination of patient, disability (if any) should end or has ended sufficiently to permit the patient to resume regular or customary work. Even if considerable question exists, make *SOME* "estimate." This is a requirement of the Code, and the claim will be delayed if such date is not entered. Such answers as "indefinite" or "don't know" will not suffice. (ENTER DATE) ☐

8. Based on your examination of patient, is this disability the result of "occupation" either as an "industrial accident" or as an "occupational disease?"
(This should include aggravation of pre-existing conditions by occupation.) Yes☐ No☐

9. Have you reported this *OR A CONCURRENT DISABILITY* to any insurance carrier as a Workers' Compensation Claim?
Yes☐ No☐ If "Yes," to whom?

10. Was or is patient confined as a registered bed patient in a hospital? Yes☐ No☐
Was patient treated in the surgical unit of a hospital or surgical unit? Yes☐ No☐
If "Yes," please provide name and address:

11. Date and hour entered as a registered bed patient and discharged pursuant to your orders:

ENTERED	STILL CONFINED	DISCHARGED
on , 20 , at A.M. P.M.	on , 20	on , 20 , at A.M. P.M.

12. Would the disclosure of this information to your patient be medically or psychologically detrimental to the patient?
Yes☐ No☐

I hereby certify that, based on my examination, the above statements truly descibe the patient's disability (if any) and the estimated duration thereof, and that I am a ______________ licensed to practice by the State of______________
(TYPE OF DOCTOR)

PRINT OR TYPE DOCTOR'S NAME AS SHOWN ON LICENSE   SIGNATURE OF ATTENDING DOCTOR

NO. AND STREET   CITY   ZIP CODE   STATE LICENSE NUMBER   ( ) TELEPHONE NUMBER   DATE OF SIGNING THIS FORM

Certification may be made by a licensed physician and surgeon, osteopath, chiropractor, dentist, podiatrist, optometrist, designated psychologist, or an authorized medical officer of a United States Government facility. All items on this sheet must be completed.

Figure 16-10

STATE OF CALIFORNIA
EMPLOYMENT DEVELOPMENT DEPARTMENT

REQUEST FOR ADDITIONAL MEDICAL INFORMATION

457-XX-0801	– Our file No.
Jake J. Burrows	– Your patient
	– Regular or Customary Work

Raymond Skeleton, M.D.
4567 Broad Avenue
Woodland Hills, XY 12345

The original basic information and estimate of duration of your patient's disability have been carefully evaluated. At the present time, the following additional information based upon the progress and present condition of this patient is requested. This will assist the Department in determining eligibilty for further disability insurance benefits. Return of the completed form as soon as possible will be appreciated.

WM. C. SCHMIDT, M.D., MEDICAL DIRECTOR

CLAIMS EXAMINER *DOCTOR: Please complete either part A or B, date and sign.*

PART A IF YOUR PATIENT HAS RECOVERED SUFFICIENTLY TO BE ABLE TO RETURN TO HIS/HER REGULAR OR CUSTOMARY WORK LISTED ABOVE, PLEASE GIVE THE DATE, ______________ 20____

PART B THIS PART REFERS TO PATIENT WHO IS STILL DISABLED.

Are you still treating the patient? Yes ☐ No ☐ ______________ 20____.
DATE OF LAST TREATMENT

What are the medical circumstances which continue to make your patient disabled?

____

____

____

____

What is your present estimate of the date your patient will be able to perform his/her regular or customary work listed above? Date______________ 20____ .

Further comments:

____

____

____

Would the disclosure of this information to your patient be medically or physically detrimental to the patient? Yes ☐ No ☐

Date______________ 20____ ______________
DOCTOR'S SIGNATURE

ENCLOSED IS A STAMPED PREADDRESSED ENVELOPE FOR YOUR CONVENIENCE.

DE 2547 Rev. 17 (4-84)

Figure 16-11

ASSIGNMENT 16-6 ▶ COMPLETE A STATE DISABILITY INSURANCE FORM

Performance Objective

Task:	Complete a state disability insurance form and define patient record abbreviations.
Conditions:	Use the patient's record (Figure 16-12), a Doctor's Certificate form (Figure 16-13), and a computer.
Standards:	Time: ____________ minutes
	Accuracy: ____________
	(Note: The time element and accuracy criteria may be given by your instructor.)

Directions:

1. Mr. Vincent P. Michael (see Figure 16-12) is applying for state disability benefits. Complete the Doctor's Certificate form (see Figure 16-13) and date it September 21. Assume that the Claim Statement of Employee has been completed satisfactorily by Mr. Michael. Remember that this is not a claim for payment to the physician, and so no ledger card has been furnished for this patient.

2. Refer to Chapter 16 and Figure 16-4 of the *Handbook* to assist you in completing this form.

After the instructor has returned your work to you, either make the necessary corrections and place your work in a three-ring notebook for future reference or, if you received a high score, place it in your portfolio for reference when applying for a job.

Abbreviations pertinent to this record:

Pt	____________	exam	____________
ESR	____________	mm	____________
hr	____________	imp	____________
CVA	____________	adv	____________
retn	____________	wk	____________
approx	____________	L	____________

PATIENT RECORD NO. 16-6

LAST NAME	FIRST NAME	MIDDLE NAME	BIRTH DATE	SEX	HOME PHONE
Michael	Vincent	P	05-17-55	M	555-567-9001

ADDRESS	CITY	STATE	ZIP CODE
1529 1/2 Thompson Boulevard	Woodland Hills	XY	12345

CELL PHONE	PAGER NO.	FAX NO.	E-MAIL ADDRESS
555-398-5677	555-311-0098	555-567-9001	michael@wb.net

PATIENT'S SOC. SEC. NO.	DRIVER'S LICENSE
562-XX-8888	E0034578

PATIENT'S OCCUPATION	NAME OF COMPANY
assembler "A"	Burroughs Corporation

ADDRESS OF EMPLOYER	PHONE
5411 North Lindero Canyon Road, Woodland Hills, XY 12345	555-560-9008

SPOUSE OR PARENT	OCCUPATION
Helen J. Michael	homemaker

EMPLOYER	ADDRESS	PHONE

NAME OF INSURANCE	INSURED OR SUBSCRIBER
Blue Shield	Vincent P. Michael

POLICY/CERTIFICATE NO.	GROUP NO.
T8411981A	677899AT

REFERRED BY: Robert T. Smith (friend)

DATE	PROGRESS NOTES
9-20-xx	Pt complains of having had the flu, headache, dizziness, and of being tired. Pt unable to go to work today. Exam shows weakness of L hand. Pt exhibits light dysphasia and confusion. Chest x-ray shows cardiomegaly and slight pulmonary congestion. ESR 46 mm/hr. Imp: Post flu syndrome, transient ischemic attack, possible CVA. Prescribed medication for congestion and adv pt to take aspirin 1/day. Pt to stay off work and retn in 1 wk. Approx date of retn to work 10-16-xx.
	BC/mtf Brady Coccidioides, MD

Figure 16-12

EDD Employment Development Department State of California

Claim for Disability Insurance Benefits – Doctor's Certificate

TYPE or PRINT with BLACK INK.

34. PATIENT'S FILE NUMBER

35. PATIENT'S SOCIAL SECURITY NO.

36. PATIENT'S LAST NAME

37. DOCTOR'S NAME AS SHOWN ON LICENSE

38. DOCTOR'S TELEPHONE NUMBER ( )

39. DOCTOR'S STATE LICENSE NO.

40. DOCTOR'S ADDRESS – NUMBER AND STREET, CITY, STATE, COUNTRY (IF NOT USA), ZIP CODE. POST OFFICE BOX NUMBER IS NOT ACCEPTED AS THE SOLE ADDRESS

41. THIS PATIENT HAS BEEN UNDER MY CARE AND TREATMENT FOR THIS MEDICAL PROBLEM
FROM ___/___/___ TO ___/___/___ AT INTERVALS OF ☐ DAILY ☐ WEEKLY ☐ MONTHLY ☐ AS NEEDED

42. AT ANY TIME DURING YOUR ATTENDANCE FOR THIS MEDICAL PROBLEM, HAS THE PATIENT BEEN INCAPABLE OF PERFORMING HIS/HER REGULAR OR CUSTOMARY WORK?
☐ NO – SKIP TO THE DOCTOR'S CERTIFICATION SECTION ☐ YES – ENTER DATE DISABILITY BEGAN: ___/___/___

43. DATE YOU RELEASED OR ANTICIPATE RELEASING PATIENT TO RETURN TO HIS/HER REGULAR / CUSTOMARY WORK ("UNKNOWN," "INDEFINITE," ETC., NOT ACCEPTED.) ___/___/___

44. ICD9 DISEASE CODE, PRIMARY (REQUIRED UNLESS DIAGNOSIS NOT YET OBTAINED)
____ . __

45. ICD9 DISEASE CODE(S), SECONDARY
____ . __, ____ . __, ____ . __

46. DIAGNOSIS (REQUIRED) – IF NO DIAGNOSIS HAS BEEN DETERMINED, ENTER OBJECTIVE FINDINGS OR A DETAILED STATEMENT OF SYMPTOMS

47. FINDINGS – STATE NATURE, SEVERITY, AND EXTENT OF THE INCAPACITATING DISEASE OR INJURY. INCLUDE ANY OTHER DISABLING CONDITIONS

48. TYPE OF TREATMENT / MEDICATION RENDERED TO PATIENT

49. IF PATIENT WAS HOSPITALIZED, PROVIDE DATES OF ENTRY AND DISCHARGE
___/___/___ TO ___/___/___

50. DATE AND TYPE OF SURGERY / PROCEDURE PERFORMED OR TO BE PERFORMED
___/___/___

ICD9 PROCEDURE CODE(S)

51. IF PATIENT IS NOW PREGNANT OR HAS BEEN PREGNANT, WHAT DATE DID PREGNANCY TERMINATE OR WHAT DATE DO YOU EXPECT DELIVERY?
___/___/___

52. IF PREGNANCY IS / WAS ABNORMAL, STATE THE ABNORMAL AND INVOLUNTARY COMPLICATION CAUSING MATERNAL DISABILITY

53. BASED ON YOUR EXAMINATION OF PATIENT, IS THIS DISABILITY THE RESULT OF "OCCUPATION," EITHER AS AN "INDUSTRIAL ACCIDENT" OR AS AN "OCCUPATIONAL DISEASE"? (INCLUDE SITUATIONS WHERE PATIENT'S OCCUPATION HAS AGGRAVATED PRE-EXISTING CONDITIONS.)
☐ YES ☐ NO

54. ARE YOU COMPLETING THIS FORM FOR THE SOLE PURPOSE OF REFERRAL / RECOMMENDATION TO AN ALCOHOLIC RECOVERY HOME OR DRUG-FREE RESIDENTIAL FACILITY AS INDICATED BY THE PATIENT IN QUESTION 23?
☐ YES ☐ NO

55. WOULD DISCLOSURE OF THIS INFORMATION TO YOUR PATIENT BE MEDICALLY OR PSYCHOLOGICALLY DETRIMENTAL?
☐ YES ☐ NO

Doctor's Certification and Signature (REQUIRED): Having considered the patient's regular or customary work, I certify under penalty of perjury that, based on my examination, this Doctor's Certificate truly describes the patient's disability (if any) and the estimated duration thereof.

I further certify that I am a ________ (TYPE OF DOCTOR) ________ (SPECIALTY, IF ANY) licensed to practice in the State of ________.

► ________________
ORIGINAL SIGNATURE OF ATTENDING DOCTOR – RUBBER STAMP IS NOT ACCEPTABLE

► ________________
DATE SIGNED

Under sections 2116 and 2122 of the California Unemployment Insurance Code, it is a violation for any individual who, with intent to defraud, falsely certifies the medical condition of any person in order to obtain disability insurance benefits, whether for the maker or for any other person, and is punishable by imprisonment and/or a fine not exceeding $20,000. Section 1143 requires additional administrative penalties.

DE 2501 Rev. 77 (3-06) **(INTERNET)**

Figure 16-13

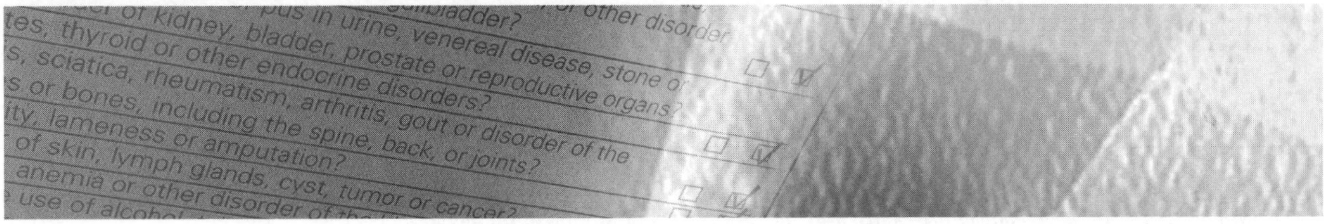

CHAPTER

17

Hospital Billing

KEY TERMS

Your instructor may wish to select some words pertinent to this chapter for a test. For definitions of the terms, further study, and/or reference, the words, phrases, and abbreviations may be found in the glossary at the end of the Handbook. *Key terms for this chapter follow.*

admission review
ambulatory payment classifications
appropriateness evaluation protocols
capitation
case rate
charge description master
charges
clinical outliers
code sequence
comorbidity
cost outlier
cost outlier review
day outlier review
diagnosis-related groups
DRG creep
DRG validation
elective surgery
grouper
inpatient
International Classification of Diseases, Ninth Revision, Clinical Modification
International Classification of Diseases, Tenth Revision, Procedure Classification System
looping
major diagnostic categories
outpatient
percentage of revenue
per diem
preadmission testing
principal diagnosis
procedure review
Quality Improvement Organization program
readmission review
scrubbing
stop loss
transfer review
Uniform Bill CMS-1450 paper or electronic claim form
utilization review

KEY ABBREVIATIONS

See how many abbreviations and acronyms you can translate and then use this as a handy reference list. Definitions for the key abbreviations are located near the back of the Handbook *in the glossary.*

AEPs ____________
APCs ____________
APGs ____________
ASCs ____________
AVGs ____________
CC ____________
CDM ____________
CMHCs ____________
CMS-1450 ____________
DRGs ____________
FL ____________
GAO ____________
HSI ____________
ICD-9-CM ____________
ICD-10-CM ____________
LOS ____________
MCC ____________
MDCs ____________
MCE ____________
MS-DRGs ____________
OCE ____________
OPPS ____________
PAT ____________
QIO program ____________
RHIA ____________
RHIT ____________
RN ____________
TJC ____________
UB-04 paper or electronic claim form ____________
UR ____________

PERFORMANCE OBJECTIVES

The student will be able to:

- Define and spell the key terms and key abbreviations for this chapter, given the information from the *Handbook* glossary, within a reasonable time period and with enough accuracy to obtain a satisfactory evaluation.
- Answer the fill-in-the-blank, mix and match, multiple choice, and true/false review questions after reading the chapter, with enough accuracy to obtain a satisfactory evaluation.
- Given computer-generated UB-04 claim forms, state the reasons why claims may be either rejected or delayed or why incorrect payment is received; state these reasons within a reasonable time period and with enough accuracy to obtain a satisfactory evaluation.
- Analyze, edit, and insert entries on computer-generated UB-04 claim forms so that payment will be accurate, within a reasonable time period and with enough accuracy to obtain a satisfactory evaluation.
- Answer questions about the UB-04 claim form to become familiar with the data it contains, within a reasonable time period and with enough accuracy to obtain a satisfactory evaluation.
- Answer questions about the UB-04 claim form to learn which hospital departments input data for different blocks on this form, within a reasonable time period and with enough accuracy to obtain a satisfactory evaluation.

ASSIGNMENT 17-2 ▶ LOCATE AND SEQUENCE DIAGNOSTIC CODES FOR CONDITIONS

Performance Objective

Task: Locate the correct diagnostic code for each diagnosis listed for five cases.

Conditions: Use a pen or pencil and the ICD-9-CM diagnostic code boo[illegible]

Standards: Time: ____________________ minutes

Accuracy: ____________________

(Note: The time element and accuracy criteria may be given by your instructor.)

Directions: These cases point out the value of proper versus improper coding with regard to correct sequence and inclusion of specific codes that indicate the variance of payment. Assign the correct ICD-9-CM code numbers. Note that the same case was assigned different DRG codes, thereby listing different principal and secondary hospital diagnoses, and that the DRG payment for each is substantially different. Also note the difference in the major diagnostic category (MDC).

CASE 1

Age: 12 Sex: Male

MDC: Four diseases and disorders of the respiratory system
DRG: Code 98: Bronchitis and asthma, age 0 to 17

Principal Diagnosis

Asthma unspecified ____________________

Secondary Diagnoses

Pneumonia, organism NOS ____________________

Otitis media NOS ____________________

DRG Payment: $2705

MDC: Four diseases and disorders of the respiratory system
DRG: Code 91: Simple [illegible]monia and pleurisy, age 0 to17

Principal Diagnosis

Pneumonia, organism not otherw[illegible]ied (NOS) ____________________

Secondary Diagnoses

Asthma unspecified ____________________

Otitis media NOS ____________________

DRG Payment: $3246

CASE 2

Age: 77 Sex: Male

MDC: Five diseases and disorders of the circulatory system

DRG: Code 138: Cardiac arrhythmia and conduction disorders, age >69 and/or chief complaint (CC)

MDC: Four diseases and disorders of the circulatory respiratory system

DRG: Code 83: Major chest trauma, age >69 and/or CC

Principal Diagnosis

Atrial fibrillation ____________________

Secondary Diagnoses

Fracture (Fx) six ribs—closed ____________________

Transient ischemia NOS ____________________

Syncope and collapse ____________________

Fx scapula NOS—closed ____________________

Fall not elsewhere classifiable

(NEC) and NOS ____________________

Principal Diagnosis

Fx six ribs—closed ____________________

Secondary Diagnoses

Atrial fibrillation ____________________

Transient ischemia NOS ____________________

Syncope and collapse ____________________

Fx scapula NOS—closed ____________________

Fall NEC and NOS ____________________

Procedures

Contrast cerebral arteriogram ____________________

Computed axial tomographic (CAT) scan of head ____________________

Diagnostic (Dx) ultrasonography—heart ____________________

Physical therapy NEC ____________________

DRG Payment: $5882

DRG Payment: $6206

Note: Because this is a hospital case, ICD-9-CM Volume 3 should be used to code the procedures. However, Volume 3 is not used in the medical office.

CASE 3

Age: 42 Sex: Male

MDC: Nineteen mental diseases and disorders
DRG: Code 426: Depressive neuroses

Principal Diagnosis

Neurotic depression ____________________

Secondary Diagnoses

Acute myocardial infarction anterior wall

Chest pain NOS ____________________

Heart disease NOS ____________________

Paranoid personality ____________________

MDC: Five diseases and disorders of the circulatory system
DRG: Code 122: Circulatory disorders with ami w/o cv comp disch alive

Principal Diagnosis

Acute myocardial infarction anterior

wall ____________________

Secondary Diagnoses

Neurotic depression ____________________

Chest pain NOS ____________________

Heart disease NOS ____________________

Paranoid personality ____________________

Procedures

Dx ultrasound—heart ____________________

Other resp procedures ____________________

DRG Payment: $6007

DRG Payment: $8637

Note: Because this is a hospital case, ICD-9-CM Volume 3 should be used to code the procedures. However, as mentioned, Volume 3 is not used in the medical office.

CASE 4

Age: 65 Sex: Male

MDC: Five diseases and disorders of the circulatory system
DRG: Code 468: Unrelated OR proc

Principal Diagnosis

Hypertensive heart disease NOS ____________________

Secondary Diagnoses

Hematuria ____________________

Hyperplasia of prostate ____________________

Hemiplegia NOS ____________________

Late eff cerebrovasc dis ____________________

Malig neopl prostate ____________________

MDC: Twelve diseases and disorders of the male reproductive system
DRG: Code 336: Transurethral prostatectomy, age >69 and/or CC

Principal Diagnosis

Malig neopl prostate ____________________

Secondary Diagnoses

Hematuria ____________________

Hypertensive heart disease NOS ____________________

Hemiplegia NOS ____________________

Late eff cerebrovasc dis ____________________

Hyperplasia of prostate ____________________

Procedures

Transurethral prostatect ____________________

Urethral dilation ____________________

Cystoscopy NEC ____________________

Intravenous pyelogram ____________________

Nephrotomogram NEC ____________________

DRG Payment: $13,311

DRG Payment: $6377

Note: Because this is a hospital case, ICD-9-CM Volume 3 should be used to code the procedures. However, as mentioned, Volume 3 is not used in the medical office.

CASE 5

Age: 62 Sex: Female

MDC: Six diseases and disorders of the digestive system
DRG: Code 188: Other digestive system diagnoses, age >69 and/or CC

Principal Diagnosis

Descending colon inj—closed ____________________

Secondary Diagnoses

Liver injury NOS—closed ____________________

Open wnd knee/leg—compl ____________________

Firearm accident NOS ____________________

No procedures performed

DRG Payment: $4710

MDC: Seven diseases and disorders of the hepatobiliary system and pancreas
DRG: Code 205: Disorders of the liver exc malig, cirr, alc hepa, age >69 and/or CC

Principal Diagnosis

Liver injury NOS—closed ____________________

Secondary Diagnoses

Atrial fibrillation ____________________

Urin tract infection NOS ____________________

Descending colon inj—closed ____________________

Open wnd knee/leg—compl ____________________

Firearm accident NOS ____________________

E. coli infect NOS ____________________

DRG Payment: $6847

ASSIGNMENT 17-3 ▶ IDENTIFY HOSPITAL DEPARTMENTS THAT INPUT DATA FOR THE UB-04 CLAIM FORM

Performance Objective

Task: Answer questions about the hospital departments that supply data for the UB-04 claim form.

Conditions: Use an ink pen.

Standards: Time: ________________ minutes

Accuracy: ________________

(Note: The time element and accuracy criteria may be given by your instructor.)

Directions: Depending on your instructor's preference, you may complete this exercise with or without notes or other material.

You have become familiar with the information in all 86 blocks of the UB-04 claim form. This assignment will help you learn which of six hospital departments input information into the computer system to be printed out in the various blocks.

This assignment will enhance your understanding of how multiple employees in a large facility take part in helping produce a completed UB-04 claim form. It will also increase your understanding of where errors and omissions originate so that you may amend them when you start the editing and correction process. Answer the following questions.

1. Which department is responsible for inputting the charges for a blood test?

____

2. Which department is responsible for inputting an insurance certificate or subscriber number?

____

3. Which department is responsible for inputting the procedure codes?

____

4. Which department is responsible for inputting the patient's name and address?

____

5. Which department is responsible for inputting the diagnostic codes?

____

ASSIGNMENT 17-4 ▶ STUDY UB-04 CLAIM FORM BLOCK OR FIELD FORM LOCATOR (FL) DATA

Performance Objective

Task: Answer questions about the UB-04 claim form blocks.

Conditions: Use an ink pen.

Standards: Time: ______________ minutes

Accuracy: ______________

(Note: The time element and accuracy criteria may be given by your instructor.)

Directions: Depending on your instructor's preference, you may complete this exercise with or without notes or other material.

You have learned about a number of reimbursement methods, confidentiality issues, evaluation protocols, and the utilization review process. This information is necessary for processing an insurance claim to obtain maximum reimbursement. To complete the UB-04 claim form, you must become familiar with the data it contains, including codes and the location of various types of information. Answer the following questions.

1. In FL 4, state the correct billing codes for

    a. Inpatient services ______________

    b. Outpatient services ______________

2. What is listed in FL 7? ______________

3. What insurance carriers or programs require FL 9 to be completed? ______________

4. What format is required in FL 10 for the patient's date of birth? ______________

5. If a patient was in the hospital for the delivery of a premature infant, what code would be used in FL 15?

6. If a patient was discharged from inpatient care at 2:15 PM, how would this be noted in FL 16?

7. What is the correct code to use in FL 17 if a patient was discharged to a home hospice situation?

8. If neither the patient nor spouse was employed, what code would be used to indicate this in FL 18 through 28?

____

9. State the reason for the codes used in FL 31 through 34.

____

____

10. What revenue code must be shown on all bills as a final entry, and in what block or field form locator (FL) does it occur?

____

ASSIGNMENT 17-5 ▸ UB-04 CLAIM FORM QUESTIONS ABOUT EDITING

Performance Objective

Task: Answer questions about editing the blocks on the UB-04 claim form.

Conditions: Use an ink pen.

Standards: Time: ________________ minutes

Accuracy: ________________

(Note: The time element and accuracy criteria may be given by your instructor.)

Directions: You are now ready to learn more about the critical editing process for determining errors and omissions on the UB-04 claim form. This important skill may help you secure a job in the claims processing department. Refer to Figure 17-5 in the *Handbook* and, at the end of the chapter, the procedure for editing a UB-04 paper or electronic claim form, and answer the questions.

1. Where does the editing process begin on the UB-04 claim form? ________________

____

2. What block/field(s) form locator (FL) must be filled in when insurance information on the UB-04 claim form is verified?

____

3. What block/field form locator (FL) should the principal diagnostic code appear in?

____

4. When editing FL 42 through 46, what should you search for besides the room rate and number of inpatient days?

____

____

5. For outpatient claims, what other item/items is/are shown besides the date, description of the service rendered, and fee?

____

6. Where can an insurance editor check when there is doubt about a service shown on a UB-04 claim form?

____

7. Which block/field form locator (FL) should show the estimated amount due from the insurance company?

____

ASSIGNMENT 17-6 ▶ LOCATE ERRORS ON A COMPUTER-GENERATED UB-04 CLAIM FORM

Performance Objective

Task: Locate the blocks on the computer-generated insurance claim form that need completion of missing information or have data that need to be corrected before submission to the insurance company.

Conditions: Use Mary J. Torre's completed insurance claim (Figure 17-1), the checklist for editing a UB-04 claim form, and a red ink pen.

Standards: Time: ______________ minutes

Accuracy: ______________

(Note: The time element and accuracy criteria may be given by your instructor.)

Directions: Refer to Figure 17-5 in the *Handbook* to use the step-by-step approach while editing the computer-generated UB-04 claim form (see Figure 17-1). Use the checklist to help you when reviewing the claim form. Locate the blocks on the claim form that need completion of missing information or that have data to be corrected before submission to the insurance company. Highlight all errors you discover. Insert all corrections and missing information in red. If you cannot locate the necessary information but know it is mandatory, write "NEED" in the corresponding form locator block/field.

In addition, you notice that the second line entry for pharmacy shows a total of $6806. However, you know from reviewing the case that one injection of a drug known as TPA (revenue code 259 and fee $5775), which dissolves clots and opens vessels when a patient has a myocardial infarction, was not broken out of the fee. Handwrite this final entry. On line 2, cross out the total charge $6806 and insert the correct pharmacy-reduced amount.

Checklist for Editing a Uniform Bill (UB-04) Claim Form: Mary J. Torre

Steps	*Form Locator Blocks/Fields*
1	FL 1 ______________ and 5 ______________
2	FL 4: Inpatient ______________ Outpatient ______________
3	FL 8b ______________, 38 ______________, 58 ______________, and 59 ______________
4	FL 10 ______________
5	FL 8b ______________ and 11 ______________
6	FL 50 ______________, 60 ______________, 61 ______________, 62 ______________, and 65 ______________
7	FL 66-67 A-Q ______________ and 69 ______________
8	FL 74 ______________ and 74 a-e ______________
9	FL 76 ______________
10	FL 6 ______________, 12 ______________, and 31 ______________

11 **Inpatient:** FL 42-47: 13 ____________________,

16 ____________________, and 46 ____________________

12 FL 47 ____________________

13 FL 42 ____________________ and 46 ____________________

14 **Outpatient:** FL 43 ____________________, 44 ____________________,

and 45 ____________________

15 Detailed record to be checked

16 FL 42 ____________________, 43 ____________________, and 47 ____________________

17 FL 55 ____________________

1	COLLEGE HOSPITAL 4500 BROAD AVENUE WOODLAND HILLS XY 12345-0001 555-487-6789
2	
3a PAT. CNTL #	10687127
b. MED. REC. #	2018856
4 TYPE OF BILL	0111
5 FED. TAX NO.	95-0731067
6 STATEMENT COVERS PERIOD FROM / THROUGH	071120XX / 071420XX
7	
8 PATIENT NAME	a b TORRE, MARY J.
9 PATIENT ADDRESS	a 452 JEME STREET b WOODLAND HILLS c XY d 12345-0001 e

10 BIRTHDATE	11 SEX	12 ADMISSION DATE	13 HR	14 TYPE	15 SRC	16 DHR	17 STAT	18	19	20	21	22	23	24	25	26	27	28	29 ACDT STATE	30
12031918	F	071120XX	21	2	7	17	01	C5	04											

(18–28: CONDITION CODES)

31 OCCURRENCE CODE	DATE	32 OCCURRENCE CODE	DATE	33 OCCURRENCE CODE	DATE	34 OCCURRENCE CODE	DATE	35 OCCURRENCE SPAN CODE	FROM	THROUGH	36 OCCURRENCE SPAN CODE	FROM	THROUGH	37
11	071120XX													

38
TORRE, MARY J.
452 JEME STREET
WOODLAND HILLS, XY 12345-0001

	39 VALUE CODES CODE	AMOUNT	40 VALUE CODES CODE	AMOUNT	41 VALUE CODES CODE	AMOUNT
a	01	650 00				
b						
c						
d						

	42 REV. CD.	43 DESCRIPTION	44 HCPCS / RATE / HIPPS CODE	45 SERV. DATE	46 SERV. UNITS	47 TOTAL CHARGES	48 NON-COVERED CHARGES	49
1	210	ROOM AND CARE CCU	1600.00		3	4800 00		
2	250	PHARMACY			121	6806 00		
3	270	MED-SUR SUPPLIES			31	700 50		
4	300	LABORATORY			45	1710 50		
5	310	PATHOLOGY LABORATORY			1	99 50		
6	320	RADIOLOGY			3	159 00		
7	450	EMERGENCY ROOM SERVICE			5	196 00		
8	730	ELECTROCARDIOLOGY			7	700 00		
9	001	TOTAL				15171 50		
23		PAGE ___ OF ___	CREATION DATE		TOTALS			

	50 PAYER NAME	51 HEALTH PLAN ID	52 REL. INFO	53 ASG. BEN.	54 PRIOR PAYMENTS	55 EST. AMOUNT DUE	56 NPI 950731067
A	MEDPRIME - HPR		Y	Y			57
B							OTHER
C							PRV ID

	58 INSURED'S NAME	59 P. REL	60 INSURED'S UNIQUE ID	61 GROUP NAME	62 INSURANCE GROUP NO.
A	TORRE, MARY J	01	54626897101		6500-0000
B					
C					

	63 TREATMENT AUTHORIZATION CODES	64 DOCUMENT CONTROL NUMBER	65 EMPLOYER NAME
A			RETIRED 080184
B			
C			

66 DX 9: 41011 | 4589 | 5780 | | | | E9344 | E8497 | 68

69 ADMIT DX 41011 | 70 PATIENT REASON DX | 71 PPS CODE | 72 ECI E9444 | E9424 | E8490 | 73

74 PRINCIPAL PROCEDURE CODE DATE | a. OTHER PROCEDURE CODE DATE | b. OTHER PROCEDURE CODE DATE | 75
c. OTHER PROCEDURE CODE DATE | d. OTHER PROCEDURE CODE DATE | e. OTHER PROCEDURE CODE DATE

76 ATTENDING NPI 642110670 QUAL
LAST CARDI FIRST PERRY
77 OPERATING NPI QUAL
LAST FIRST
78 OTHER NPI QUAL
LAST FIRST
79 OTHER NPI QUAL
LAST FIRST

80 REMARKS | 81CC a b c d

UB-04 CMS-1450 APPROVED OMB NO. THE CERTIFICATIONS ON THE REVERSE APPLY TO THIS BILL AND ARE MADE A PART HEREOF.
NUBC National Uniform Billing Committee LIC9213257

Figure 17-1

ASSIGNMENT 17-7 ▸ LOCATE ERRORS ON A COMPUTER-GENERATED UB-04 CLAIM FORM

Performance Objective

Task: Locate the Form Locator blocks/fields on the computer-generated insurance claim form that need completion of missing information or have data that need to be corrected before submission to the insurance company.

Conditions: Use Henry M. Cosby's completed insurance claim (Figure 17-2), the checklist for editing a UB-04 claim form, and a red ink pen.

Standards: Time: ______________ minutes

Accuracy: ______________

(Note: The time element and accuracy criteria may be given by your instructor.)

Directions: Refer to Figure 17-5 in the *Handbook* to employ the step-by-step approach while editing the computer-generated UB-04 claim form (see Figure 17-2). Use the checklist to help you when reviewing the claim form. Locate the Form Locator blocks/fields on the claim form that need completion of missing information or that have data to be corrected before submission to the insurance company. Highlight all errors you discover. Insert all corrections and missing information in red. If you cannot locate the necessary information but know it is mandatory, write "NEED" in the corresponding Form Locator block/field. State the reason or reasons why the claim may be rejected or delayed or why incorrect payment may be generated because of one or more errors discovered.

Checklist for Editing a Uniform Bill (UB-04) Claim Form: Henry M. Cosby

Steps *Form Locator Blocks/Fields*

1 FL 1 ______________ and 5 ______________

2 FL 4: Inpatient ______________ Outpatient ______________

3 FL 8b ______________, 38 ______________, 58 ______________,

and 59 ______________

4 FL 10 ______________

5 FL 8b ______________ and 11 ______________

6 FL 50 ______________, 60 ______________, 61 ______________,

62 ______________, and 65 ______________

7 FL 66 ______________ and 69 ______________

8 FL 74 ______________ and 74 a-e ______________

9 FL 76 ______________

10 FL 6 ______________, 12 ______________, and 31 ______________

11 **Inpatient:** FL 42-47: 13 ____________________,

16 ____________________, and 46 ____________________

12 FL 47 ____________________

13 FL 42 ____________________ and 46 ____________________

14 **Outpatient:** FL 43 ____________________, 44 ____________________,

and 45 ____________________

15 Detailed record to be checked

16 FL 42 ____________________, 43 ____________________, and 47 ____________________

17 FL 55 ____________________

1 COLLEGE HOSPITAL 4500 BROAD AVENUE WOODLAND HILLS XY 12345-0001 555-487-6789	2	3a PAT. CNTL # 10687127 b. MED. REC. # 2084100 5 FED. TAX NO. 95-0731067	4 TYPE OF BILL 0131 6 STATEMENT COVERS PERIOD FROM 031520XX THROUGH 031520XX 7

8 PATIENT NAME a | b COSBY, HENRY M

9 PATIENT ADDRESS a 1501 PACIFIC WAY | b WOODLAND HILLS | c XY | d 12345-0001 | e

10 BIRTHDATE	11 SEX	12 ADMISSION DATE	13 HR	14 TYPE	15 SRC	16 DHR	17 STAT	18 CONDITION CODES	19	20	21	22	23	24	25	26	27	28	29 ACDT STATE	30
03101956	M	031520XX	13	3	2	99	01	C5												

31 OCCURRENCE CODE	DATE	32 OCCURRENCE CODE	DATE	33 OCCURRENCE CODE	DATE	34 OCCURRENCE CODE	DATE	35 OCCURRENCE SPAN CODE	FROM	THROUGH	36 OCCURRENCE SPAN CODE	FROM	THROUGH	37
05	072120XX													

38
COSBY, HENRY M
1501 PACIFIC WAY
WOODLAND HILLS XY 12345

39 VALUE CODES CODE AMOUNT | 40 VALUE CODES CODE AMOUNT | 41 VALUE CODES CODE AMOUNT (a, b, c, d — blank)

	42 REV. CD.	43 DESCRIPTION	44 HCPCS / RATE / HIPPS CODE	45 SERV. DATE	46 SERV. UNITS	47 TOTAL CHARGES	48 NON-COVERED CHARGES	49
1	110	ROOM-BOARD/SEMI/PVT	650.00		1	650 00		
2	250	PHARMACY			11	207 20		
3	270	MED-SUR SUPPLIES			4	1041 28		
4	360	OPERATING ROOM				865 00		
5	370	ANESTHESIA				64 50		
6	730	ELECTROCARDIOGRAM	93000	031320XX	031320XX	100 00		
7	001	Total				2927 98		
23		PAGE ____ OF ____	CREATION DATE		TOTALS			

50 PAYER NAME	51 HEALTH PLAN ID	52 REL. INFO	53 ASG. BEN.	54 PRIOR PAYMENTS	55 EST. AMOUNT DUE	56 NPI 950731067
A BLUE SHIELD OF CA	Z22C49122	Y	Y			57 OTHER PRV ID

58 INSURED'S NAME	59 P. REL	60 INSURED'S UNIQUE ID	61 GROUP NAME	62 INSURANCE GROUP NO.
A COSBY, HENRY M	01	564729922		PA 0132

63 TREATMENT AUTHORIZATION CODES	64 DOCUMENT CONTROL NUMBER	65 EMPLOYER NAME
		DBA: COSBY AUTO BODY

66 DX 9 | 8408 | 68

69 ADMIT DX | 70 PATIENT REASON DX | 71 PPS CODE | 72 ECI | 73

74 PRINCIPAL PROCEDURE CODE 8301 DATE 031520XX | a. OTHER PROCEDURE CODE DATE | b. OTHER PROCEDURE CODE DATE | 75
c. OTHER PROCEDURE CODE DATE | d. OTHER PROCEDURE CODE DATE | e. OTHER PROCEDURE CODE DATE

76 ATTENDING NPI 126785470 QUAL
LAST SKELETON FIRST RAYMOND
77 OPERATING NPI QUAL
LAST FIRST
78 OTHER NPI QUAL
LAST FIRST
79 OTHER NPI QUAL
LAST FIRST

80 REMARKS
FELL WATERSKIING 7/21/20XX

81CC a b c d

UB-04 CMS-1450 APPROVED OMB NO.

THE CERTIFICATIONS ON THE REVERSE APPLY TO THIS BILL AND ARE MADE A PART HEREOF.

NUBC National Uniform Billing Committee LIC9213257

Figure 17-2

ASSIGNMENT 17-8 ▶ LOCATE ERRORS ON A COMPUTER-GENERATED UB-04 CLAIM FORM

Performance Objective

Task: Locate the blocks on the computer-generated insurance claim form that need completion of missing information or have data that need to be corrected before submission to the insurance company.

Conditions: Use Harold M. McDonald's completed insurance claim (Figure 17-3), the checklist for editing a UB-04 claim form, and a red ink pen.

Standards: Time: ______________ minutes

Accuracy: ______________

(Note: The time element and accuracy criteria may be given by your instructor.)

Directions: Refer to Figure 17-5 in the *Handbook* to use the step-by-step approach while editing the computer-generated UB-04 claim form (see Figure 17-3). Use the checklist to help you when reviewing the claim form. Locate the blocks on the claim form that need completion of missing information or that have data to be corrected before submission to the insurance company. Highlight all errors you discover. Insert all corrections and missing information in red. If you cannot locate the necessary information but know it is mandatory, write "NEED" in the corresponding block.

You notice that the seventh CPT/Healthcare Common Procedure Coding System (HCPCS) code 43450 for operating room is missing. On hospital claims, the entry for operating room is usually blank and must be handwritten in, because this is the code for the surgical procedure.

Checklist for Editing a Uniform Bill (UB-04) Claim Form: Harold M. McDonald

Steps	*Form Locator Blocks/Fields*
1	FL 1 ______________ and 5 ______________
2	FL 4: Inpatient ______________ Outpatient ______________
3	FL 8b ______________, 38 ______________, 58 ______________, and 59 ______________
4	FL 10 ______________
5	FL 8b ______________ and 11 ______________
6	FL 50 ______________, 60 ______________, 61 ______________, 62 ______________, and 65 ______________
7	FL 66-67 A-Q ______________ and 69 ______________
8	FL 74 ______________ and 74 a-e ______________
9	FL 76 ______________
10	FL 6 ______________, 12 ______________, and 31 ______________

11 **Inpatient:** FL 42-47: 13 ____________________, 16 ____________________,

and 46 ____________________

12 FL 47 ____________________

13 FL 42 ____________________ and 46 ____________________

14 **Outpatient:** FL 43 ____________________, 44 ____________________,

and 45 ____________________

15 Detailed record to be checked

16 FL 42 ____________________, 43 ____________________, and 47 ____________________

17 FL 55 ____________________

1	2	3a PAT. CNTL #	10670685	4 TYPE OF BILL
COLLEGE HOSPITAL		b. MED. REC. #	2071307	0131
4500 BROAD AVENUE		5 FED. TAX NO.	6 STATEMENT COVERS PERIOD FROM / THROUGH	7
WOODLAND HILLS XY 12345-0001		95-0731067	070520XX / 070520XX	
555-487-6789				

8 PATIENT NAME	9 PATIENT ADDRESS
a	a 22 BEACON ROAD
b MCDONALD HAROLD M	b WOODLAND HILLS c XY d 12345-0001 e

10 BIRTHDATE	11 SEX	ADMISSION 12 DATE	13 HR	14 TYPE	15 SRC	16 DHR	17 STAT	CONDITION CODES 18	19	20	21	22	23	24	25	26	27	28	29 ACDT STATE	30
04261929	M	070520XX	12	3	1	99	01	C5												

31 OCCURRENCE CODE	DATE	32 OCCURRENCE CODE	DATE	33 OCCURRENCE CODE	DATE	34 OCCURRENCE CODE	DATE	35 OCCURRENCE SPAN CODE	FROM	THROUGH	36 OCCURRENCE SPAN CODE	FROM	THROUGH	37

38

MCDONALD HAROLD M
22 BEACON ROAD
WOODLAND HILLS XY 12345-0001

	39 VALUE CODES CODE	AMOUNT	40 VALUE CODES CODE	AMOUNT	41 VALUE CODES CODE	AMOUNT
a						
b						
c						
d						

	42 REV. CD.	43 DESCRIPTION	44 HCPCS / RATE / HIPPS CODE	45 SERV. DATE	46 SERV. UNITS	47 TOTAL CHARGES	48 NON-COVERED CHARGES	49
1	250	PHARMACY			5	90 90		
2	270	MED - SUR SUPPLIES			16	2519 50		
3	300	DRAWING BLOOD	36415	070520XX	1	8 50		
4	300	13-16 BLOOD/URINE TESTS	80016	070520XX	1	28 00		
5	300	CREATININE CLEARANCE TEST	82575	070520XX	1	20 00		
6	300	CBC	85025 24	070520XX	1	16 50		
7	320	CONTRAST XRAY EXAM, ESOPH	74220	070520XX	1	114 00		
8	320	X-RAY GUIDE, GI DILATION	74360	070520XX	1	750 00		
9	360	OPERATING ROOM				500 00		
10	410	CONT OXIMETER HOURS	82805 22	070520XX	1	8 00		
11	001	Total				4055 40		
12								
13								
14								
15								
16								
17								
18								
19								
20								
21								
22								
23		PAGE ____ OF ____	CREATION DATE		TOTALS			

	50 PAYER NAME	51 HEALTH PLAN ID	52 REL. INFO	53 ASG. BEN.	54 PRIOR PAYMENTS	55 EST. AMOUNT DUE	56 NPI	950731067
A	HEALTH PLAN REDWOOD	278654901	Y	Y			57	
B							OTHER	
C							PRV ID	

	58 INSURED'S NAME	59 P. REL	60 INSURED'S UNIQUE ID	61 GROUP NAME	62 INSURANCE GROUP NO.
A	MCDONALD HAROLD M	01	31424435401		1320-0000 PLAN GO
B					
C					

	63 TREATMENT AUTHORIZATION CODES	64 DOCUMENT CONTROL NUMBER	65 EMPLOYER NAME
A			WC PEDERSON FORD
B			
C			

66 DX 1509 V725 9 — 68

69 ADMIT DX — 70 PATIENT REASON DX — 71 PPS CODE — 72 ECI — 73

74 PRINCIPAL PROCEDURE CODE DATE — a. OTHER PROCEDURE CODE DATE — b. OTHER PROCEDURE CODE DATE — 75

c. OTHER PROCEDURE CODE DATE — d. OTHER PROCEDURE CODE DATE — e. OTHER PROCEDURE CODE DATE

76 ATTENDING NPI 124589770 QUAL
LAST ANTRUM FIRST CONCHA

77 OPERATING NPI QUAL
LAST FIRST

78 OTHER NPI QUAL
LAST FIRST

79 OTHER NPI QUAL
LAST FIRST

80 REMARKS
HPR

81CC a b c d

UB-04 CMS-1450 APPROVED OMB NO. THE CERTIFICATIONS ON THE REVERSE APPLY TO THIS BILL AND ARE MADE A PART HEREOF.

NUBC National Uniform Billing Committee LIC9213257

Figure 17-3

ASSIGNMENT 17-9 ▶ LOCATE ERRORS ON A COMPUTER-GENERATED UB-04 CLAIM FORM

Performance Objective

Task: Locate the blocks on the computer-generated insurance claim form that need completion of missing information or have data that need to be corrected before submission to the insurance company.

Conditions: Use Pedro Martinez's completed insurance claim (Figure 17-4), the checklist for editing a UB-04 claim form, and a red ink pen.

Standards: Time: ____________________ minutes

Accuracy: ____________________

(Note: The time element and accuracy criteria may be given by your instructor.)

Directions: Refer to Figure 17–5 in the *Handbook* to use the step-by-step approach while editing the computer-generated UB-04 claim form (see Figure 17-4). Use the checklist to help you when reviewing the claim form. Locate the blocks on the claim form that need completion of missing information or that have data to be corrected before submission to the insurance company. Highlight all errors you discover. Insert all corrections and missing information in red. If you cannot locate the necessary information but know it is mandatory, write "NEED" in the corresponding block. Then write a list of reasons why the claim may be rejected or delayed or why incorrect payment may be generated because of errors discovered.

Checklist for Editing a Uniform Bill (UB-04) Claim Form: Pedro Martinez

Steps	*Form Locator Blocks/Fields*
1	FL 1 ____________ and 5 ____________
2	FL 4: Inpatient ____________ Outpatient ____________
3	FL 8b ____________, 38 ____________, 58 ____________, and 59 ____________
4	FL 10 ____________
5	FL 8b ____________ and 11 ____________
6	FL 50 ____________, 60 ____________, 61 ____________, 62 ____________, and 65 ____________
7	FL 66-67 A-Q ____________ and 69 ____________
8	FL 74 ____________ and 74 a-e ____________
9	FL 76 ____________
10	FL 6 ____________, 12 ____________, and 32 ____________

11 **Inpatient:** FL 42-47: 13 ________________________, 16 ________________________,

and 46 ________________________

12 FL 47 ________________________

13 FL 42 ________________________ and 46 ________________________

14 **Outpatient:** FL 43 ________________________, 44 ________________________,

and 45 ________________________

15 Detailed record to be checked

16 FL 42 ________________________, 43 ________________________, and 47 ________________________

17 FL 55 ________________________

1	COLLEGE HOSPITAL 4500 BROAD AVENUE WOODLAND HILLS XY 12345-0001 555-487-6789
2	
3a PAT. CNTL #	10630911
b. MED. REC. #	3567811
4 TYPE OF BILL	0111
5 FED. TAX NO.	95-0731067
6 STATEMENT COVERS PERIOD FROM	06120XX
THROUGH	06120XX
7	
8 PATIENT NAME	a / b MARTINEZ PEDRO
9 PATIENT ADDRESS	a 7821 SENSOR AVE b WOODLAND HILLS c XY d 12345-0001 e
10 BIRTHDATE	092218
11 SEX	M
ADMISSION 12 DATE	061120XX
13 HR	20
14 TYPE	1
15 SRC	7
16 DHR	19
17 STAT	03
CONDITION CODES 18	C5
19	04
20–28	
29 ACDT STATE	
30	
31–34 OCCURRENCE CODE / DATE	
35–36 OCCURRENCE SPAN CODE / FROM / THROUGH	
37	
38	MARTINEZ PEDRO 7821 SENSOR AVENUE WOODLAND HILLS XY 12345-0001
39 VALUE CODES CODE / AMOUNT	a 01 650.00
40 VALUE CODES	
41 VALUE CODES	

42 REV. CD.	43 DESCRIPTION	44 HCPCS / RATE / HIPPS CODE	45 SERV. DATE	46 SERV. UNITS	47 TOTAL CHARGES	48 NON-COVERED CHARGES	49
110	ROOM - BOARD/SEMI/PVT	650.00		1	650 00		
120	ROOM AND CARE SEMI	650.00		1	650 00		
210	ROOM AND CARE CCU	1600.00		8	12800 00		
250	PHARMACY			500	7133 90		
270	MED - SUR SUPPLIES			149	3689 50		
300	LABORATORY			97	5399 33		
320	RADIOLOGY			27	1544 00		
350	CT SCAN			1	622 00		
410	RESPIRATORY THERAPY			240	6698 50		
420	PHYSICAL THERAPY			9	470 00		
450	EMERGENCY ROOM SERV			6	197 00		
460	PULMONARY FUNCTION				29 00		
730	ELECTROCARDIOLOGY			1	100 00		
942	EDUCATION			6	82 50		
001	Total				40065 73		
	PAGE ___ OF ___	CREATION DATE		TOTALS			

50 PAYER NAME	51 HEALTH PLAN ID	52 REL. INFO	53 ASG. BEN	54 PRIOR PAYMENTS	55 EST. AMOUNT DUE	56 NPI
A MEDIPRIME-HPR		Y	Y			950731067

57 OTHER PRV ID

58 INSURED'S NAME	59 P. REL	60 INSURED'S UNIQUE ID	61 GROUP NAME	62 INSURANCE GROUP NO.
A MARTINEZ PEDRO	01	55025897001		6500-0000

63 TREATMENT AUTHORIZATION CODES	64 DOCUMENT CONTROL NUMBER	65 EMPLOYER NAME
		RETIRED 1975

66 DX 9: 4169 | 51881 | 49121

68

69 ADMIT DX | 70 PATIENT REASON DX | 71 PPS CODE | 72 ECI | 73

74 PRINCIPAL PROCEDURE CODE DATE | a. OTHER PROCEDURE CODE DATE | b. OTHER PROCEDURE CODE DATE | 75

c. OTHER PROCEDURE CODE DATE | d. OTHER PROCEDURE CODE DATE | e. OTHER PROCEDURE CODE DATE

76 ATTENDING NPI 642110670 QUAL
LAST COCCIDIOIDES FIRST BRADY

77 OPERATING NPI QUAL
LAST FIRST

78 OTHER NPI QUAL
LAST FIRST

79 OTHER NPI QUAL
LAST FIRST

80 REMARKS

81CC a b c d

UB-04 CMS-1450 APPROVED OMB NO. THE CERTIFICATIONS ON THE REVERSE APPLY TO THIS BILL AND ARE MADE A PART HEREOF.

NUBC National Uniform Billing Committee LIC9213257

Figure 17-4

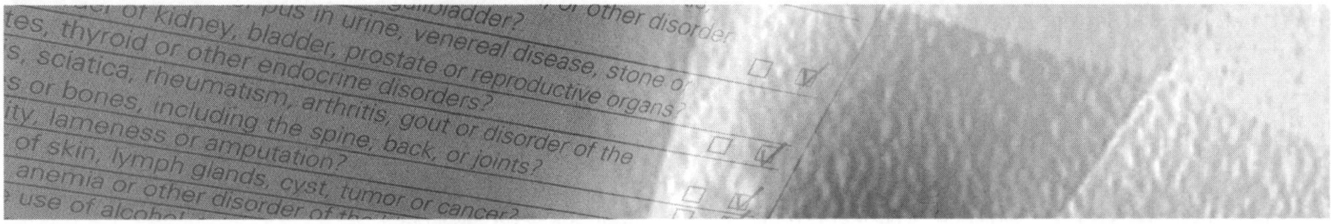

CHAPTER

18

Seeking a Job and Attaining Professional Advancement

KEY TERMS

Your instructor may wish to select some words pertinent to this chapter for a test. For definitions of the terms, further study, and/or reference, the words, phrases, and abbreviations may be found in the glossary at the end of the Handbook. *Key terms for this chapter follow.*

alien
application form
blind mailing
business associate agreement
certification
Certified Coding Specialist
Certified Coding Specialist-Physician
Certified Medical Assistant
Certified Medical Billing Specialist
Certified Professional Coder
chronologic résumé
claims assistance professional
combination résumé
continuing education
cover letter
employment agencies
functional résumé
interview
mentor
National Certified Insurance and Coding Specialist
networking
portfolio
Professional Association of Health Care Office Managers
Registered Medical Assistant
Registered Medical Coder
registration
résumé
self-employment
service contract

KEY ABBREVIATIONS

See how many abbreviations and acronyms you can translate and then use this as a handy reference list. Definitions for the key abbreviations are located near the back of the Handbook *in the glossary.*

AAPC ______________________
AHIMA ______________________
CAP ______________________
CCAP ______________________
CCS ______________________
CCS-P ______________________
CECP ______________________
CMA ______________________
CMBS ______________________
CMRS ______________________
CPC, CPC-A, CPC-H ______________________
ECP ______________________
EEOC ______________________
HRS ______________________
INS ______________________
NCICS ______________________
PAHCOM ______________________
RMA ______________________
RMC ______________________

PERFORMANCE OBJECTIVES

The student will be able to:

- Define and spell the key terms and key abbreviations for this chapter, given the information from the *Handbook* glossary, within a reasonable time period and with enough accuracy to obtain a satisfactory evaluation.
- After reading the chapter, answer the fill-in-the-blank, multiple choice, and true/false review questions with enough accuracy to obtain a satisfactory evaluation.
- Research information in preparation for typing a résumé, given a worksheet to complete, within a reasonable time period and with enough accuracy to obtain a satisfactory evaluation.
- Type an accurate résumé in attractive format, using plain typing paper, within a reasonable time period, to obtain a satisfactory evaluation.
- Compose and type a letter of introduction to go with the résumé and place it in a typed envelope, using one sheet of plain typing paper and a number 10 envelope, within a reasonable time period, to obtain a satisfactory evaluation.
- Complete an application form for a job, given an application for position form, within a reasonable time period and with enough accuracy to obtain a satisfactory evaluation.
- Compose and type a follow-up thank-you letter and place it in a typed envelope, using one sheet of plain typing paper and a number 10 envelope, within a reasonable time period, to obtain a satisfactory evaluation.
- Access the Internet and visit websites to research and/or obtain data, within a reasonable time period and with enough accuracy to obtain a satisfactory evaluation.

STUDY OUTLINE

Employment Opportunities
- Insurance Billing Specialist
- Claims Assistance Professional

Job Search
- Online Job Search
- Job Fairs
- Application
- Letter of Introduction
- Résumé
- Interview
- Follow-up Letter

Self-Employment
- Setting Up an Office
- Finances to Consider
- Marketing, Advertising, Promotion, and Public Relations
- Documentation
- Mentor and Business Incubator Services
- Networking

Procedure: Creating an Electronic Résumé

ASSIGNMENT 18-1 ▶ REVIEW QUESTIONS

Part I Fill in the Blank

Review the objectives, key terms, glossary definitions of key terms, chapter information, and figures before completing the following review questions.

1. You have just completed a 1-year medical insurance billing course at a college. Name some preliminary job search contacts to make on campus.

   a. ____________________

   b. ____________________

   c. ____________________

   d. ____________________

2. Name skills that may be listed on an application form or in a résumé when a person is seeking a position as an insurance billing specialist.

   a. ____________________

   b. ____________________

   c. ____________________

   d. ____________________

   e. ____________________

   f. ____________________

3. A question appears on a job application form about salary. Two ways in which to handle this question are

   a. ____________________

   b. ____________________

4. State the chief purpose of a cover letter when a résumé is sent to a prospective employer.

   ____

5. List the items to be compiled in a portfolio.

   a. ____________________

   b. ____________________

   c. ____________________

   d. ____________________

   e. ____________________

f. ______

g. ______

h. ______

i. ______

6. You are being interviewed for a job and the interviewer asks this question: "What is your religious preference?" How would you respond?

______

______

7. If a short period of time elapses after an interview and the applicant has received no word from the prospective employer, what follow-up steps may be taken?

a. ______

b. ______

8. If an individual creates a billing company and coding services are to be part of the offerings, the coding professional should have what type of professional status?

______

9. Hugh Beason was the owner of XYZ Medical Reimbursement Service. A fire occurred, damaging some of the equipment and part of the office premises and requiring him to stop his work for a month so that repairs could be made. What type/types of insurance would be helpful for this kind of problem?

______

10. Gwendolyn Stevens has an insurance billing company and is attending a professional meeting where she has given business cards to a few attendees. Give two reasons for using this business marketing strategy.

a. ______

b. ______

11. State the difference between *certification* and *registration*.

a. Certification: ______

______

b. Registration: ______

______

12. Name some ways an insurance billing specialist may seek to keep knowledge current.

a. ______________________________

b. ______________________________

c. ______________________________

d. ______________________________

13. Jerry Hahn is pursuing a career as a claims assistance professional. When he markets his business, the target audience should be ______________________________.

14. Jennifer Inouye has been hired as a coding specialist by a hospital and needs to keep documentation when working. This may consist of

a. ______________________________

b. ______________________________

c. ______________________________

15. Give the names of at least two national organizations that certify billers and coders.

a. ______________________________

b. ______________________________

Part II Multiple Choice

Choose the best answer.

16. A résumé format that emphasizes work experience dates is known as

a. functional

b. combination

c. business

d. chronologic

17. When an individual plans to start an insurance billing company, he or she should have enough funds to operate the business for a period of

a. 6 months or more

b. 18 months or more

c. 1 year or more

d. 2 years

18. Under HIPAA regulations, if a physician's insurance billing is outsourced to a person, this individual

    is known as a/an ______________________ because he or she uses and discloses individuals' identifiable health information.

    a. billing specialist

    b. business associate

    c. outside contractor

    d. outside vendor

19. When insurance billing is outsourced to a company, a document should be created, signed, and notarized by both parties known as a

    a. contract agreement

    b. business agreement

    c. service contract

    d. legal contract

20. A guide who offers advice, criticism, and guidance to an inexperienced person to help him or her reach a goal is known as a/an

    a. mentor

    b. counselor

    c. associate

    d. instructor

Part III True/False

Write "T" or "F" in the blank to indicate whether you think the statement is true or false.

_______ 21. A résumé format that stresses job skills is known as functional.

_______ 22. When job applicants have similar skills and education, surveys have shown that hiring by employers has been based on bilingual skills.

_______ 23. Enhancing knowledge and keeping up to date are responsibilities of an insurance billing specialist.

_______ 24. Professional status of an insurance billing specialist may be obtained by passing a national examination for a CMRS.

_______ 25. Professional status of a claims assistance professional may be obtained by passing a national examination as a CCS.

ASSIGNMENT 18-2 ▶ COMPLETE A WORKSHEET AND TYPE A RÉSUMÉ

Performance Objective

Task: Respond to a job advertisement by completing a worksheet and typing a résumé by abstracting data from your worksheet.

Conditions: Use two sheets of plain typing paper, a newspaper advertisement (Figure 18-1), and a computer.

Standards: Time: ______________________ minutes

Accuracy: ______________________

(Note: The time element and accuracy criteria may be given by your instructor.)

Directions: An advertisement appeared in your local newspaper (see Figure 18-1). You decide to apply for the position. Complete a worksheet in preparation for typing your résumé. Some of the information requested on the worksheet should not appear on the résumé but should be available if you are asked to provide it. Ask a classmate to review and comment about the information in your worksheet. Abstract data that you think are relevant from the worksheet, and type a résumé in rough draft. Ask the instructor for suggestions to improve the rough draft. Refer to Chapter 18 and Figure 18-6 in the *Handbook* to help organize your résumé into an attractive format before you type the final copy.

1. Insert title of personal data sheet from worksheet.

2. Insert heading: name, address, telephone number, and so on.

3. Select one of three formats for data.

4. Insert heading and data for education information.

5. Insert heading and data for skill information.

6. Insert heading and data for employment information.

7. Insert reference information.

8. Proofread résumé.

9. Print résumé.

MEDICAL INSURANCE CODING/REIMBURSEMENT SPECIALIST

Mid-Atlantic Clinic, a 20-physician, multi-specialty group practice in Chicago, Illinois, has a need for a coding and reimbursement specialist. Knowledge of medical terminology, CPT and ICD-9-CM coding systems, Medicare regulations, third-party insurance reimbursement and physician billing procedures required. Proficiency in the interpretation and coding of procedural and diagnostic codes is strongly preferred. Successful candidates must have excellent communication and problem-solving skills. This position offers a competitive salary and superior benefits. Please send resume to:

George B. Pason, Personnel Director
Mid-Atlantic Clinic
1230 South Main Street
Chicago, IL 60611

Figure 18-1

ASSIGNMENT 18-3 ▶ COMPLETE A COVER LETTER

Performance Objective

Task: Compose a cover letter to accompany your résumé.

Conditions: Use one sheet of plain typing paper, a number 10 envelope, and a computer, printer, thesaurus, and English dictionary.

Standards: Time: ________________________ minutes

Accuracy: ________________________

(Note: The time element and accuracy criteria may be given by your instructor.)

Directions: Compose a cover letter introducing yourself, and type a rough draft. Consult the instructor for suggestions. Type the cover letter on plain bond paper in a form that can be mailed. Refer to the sample letter in Chapter 18 and Figure 18-5 in the *Handbook* as a guide to help organize your thoughts. Type the name and address of the employer on a number 10 envelope, and insert the letter with the résumé from Assignment 18-2.

ASSIGNMENT 18-4 ▶ COMPLETE A JOB APPLICATION FORM

Performance Objective

Task: Complete a job application form by using data from your résumé.

Conditions: Use application form (see Figure 18-2), your résumé, and a computer.

Standards: Time: ________________________ minutes

Accuracy: ________________________

(Note: The time element and accuracy criteria may be given by your instructor.)

Directions: Assume that the employer asked you to come to his or her place of business to complete an application form and make an appointment for an interview. Using your data and résumé, complete an application form (see Figure 18-2).

APPLICATION FOR POSITION/ Medical or Dental Office
AN EQUAL OPPORTUNITY EMPLOYER

(In answering questions, use extra blank sheet if necessary)

No employee, applicant, or candidate for promotion training or other advantage shall be discriminated against (or given preference) because of race, color, religion, sex, age, physical handicap, veteran status, or national origin.
PLEASE READ CAREFULLY AND WRITE OR PRINT ANSWERS TO ALL QUESTIONS. DO NOT TYPE.

Date of application

A. PERSONAL INFORMATION

Name- Last First Middle	Social Security No.	Area Code/Phone No. ( )
Present Address: -Street (Apt. #) City State Zip		How long at this address?
Previous Address: -Street City State Zip From: To:	Person to notify in case of Emergency or Accident - Name: Address: Telephone:	

B. EMPLOYMENT INFORMATION

For what position are you applying?	☐ Full-time ☐ Part-time ☐ Either	Date available for employment?:	Wage/Salary Expectations:
List hrs./days you prefer to work:	List any hrs./days you are not available: (Except for times required for religious practices or observances)		Can you work overtime, if necessary? ☐ Yes ☐ No
Are you employed now?: ☐ Yes ☐ No	If so, may we inquire of your present employer?: ☐ No ☐ Yes, If yes: Name of employer: Phone number: ( )		
Have you ever been bonded?: ☐ Yes ☐ No	If required for position, are you bondable? ☐ Yes ☐ No ☐ Uncertain	Have you applied for a position with this office before? ☐ No ☐ Yes, If yes, when?:	

Referred by/ or where did you hear of this job?:

Can you, upon employment, submit verification of your legal right to work in the United States? ☐ Yes ☐ No Submit proof that you meet legal age requirement for employment? ☐ Yes ☐ No	Language(s) applicant speaks or writes (if use of a language other than English is relevant to the job for which applicant is applying):

C. EDUCATIONAL HISTORY

Name and address of schools attended (Include current)	Dates From	Thru	Highest grade/level completed	Diploma/degree(s) obtained/areas of study:
High school				
College				Degree/Major
Post graduate				Degree/Major
Other				Course/Diploma/License Certificate

Specific training, education, or experiences which will assist you in the job for which you have applied:

Future educational plans:

D. SPECIAL SKILLS

CHECK BELOW THE KINDS OF WORK YOU HAVE DONE:		☐ MEDICAL INSURANCE FORMS	☐ RECEPTIONIST
☐ BLOOD COUNTS	☐ DENTAL ASSISTANT	☐ MEDICAL TERMINOLOGY	☐ TELEPHONES
☐ BOOKKEEPING	☐ DENTAL HYGIENIST	☐ MEDICAL TRANSCRIPTION	☐ TYPING
☐ COLLECTIONS	☐ FILING	☐ NURSING	☐ STENOGRAPHY
☐ COMPOSING LETTERS	☐ INJECTIONS	☐ PHLEBOTOMY (Draw Blood)	☐ URINALYSIS
☐ COMPUTER INPUT	☐ INSTRUMENT STERILIZATION	☐ POSTING	☐ X-RAY
OFFICE EQUIPMENT USED: ☐ COMPUTER	☐ DICTATING EQUIPMENT	☐ WORD PROCESSOR	☐ OTHER:
Other kinds of tasks performed or skills that may be applicable to position:		Typing speed:	Shorthand speed:

RM NO. 72-110 ©1976 BIBBERO SYSTEMS INC. PETALUMA, CA (MB-CO) # 2-5 (REV. 10/92)
REORDER CALL 800-BIBBERO (800) 242-2376

(PLEASE COMPLETE OTHER SIDE)

Figure 18-2

Continued

E. EMPLOYMENT RECORD

LIST MOST RECENT EMPLOYMENT FIRST — May we contact your previous Employer(s) for a reference? ☐ yes ☐ no

1) Employer | Work performed. Be specific.
Address Street City State Zip code
Phone number ( )
Type of business | Dates From Mo. Yr. To Mo. Yr.
Your position | Hourly rate/Salary Starting Final
Supervisor's name
Reason for leaving

2) Employer | Work performed. Be specific.
Address Street City State Zip code
Phone number ( )
Type of business | Dates From Mo. Yr. To Mo. Yr.
Your position | Hourly rate/Salary Starting Final
Supervisor's name
Reason for leaving

3) Employer | Work performed. Be specific.
Address Street City State Zip code
Phone number ( )
Type of business | Dates From Mo. Yr. To Mo. Yr.
Your position | Hourly rate/Salary Starting Final
Supervisor's name
Reason for leaving

F. REFERENCES: FRIENDS/ACQUAINTANCES NON-RELATED

1) Name Address Telephone Number (☐ Work ☐ Home) Occupation Years acquainted
2) Name Address Telephone Number (☐ Work ☐ Home) Occupation Years acquainted

Please feel free to add any information which you feel will help us consider you for employment.

READ THE FOLLOWING CAREFULLY, THEN SIGN AND DATE THE APPLICATION

I certify that all answers given by me on this application are true, correct and complete to the best of my knowledge. I acknowledge notice that the information contained in this application is subject to check. I agree that, if hired, my continued employment may be contingent upon the accuracy of that information. If employed, I further agree to comply with company/office rules and regulations.

Signature ____________ Date: ____________

RM NO. 72-110 ©1976 BIBBERO SYSTEMS INC. PETALUMA, CA (MB-CO) # 6-7 (REV. 4/92) TO REORDER CALL 800-BIBBERO (800) 242-2376

Figure 18-2, cont'd

ASSIGNMENT 18-5 ▶ PREPARE A FOLLOW-UP THANK-YOU LETTER

Performance Objective

Task: Prepare a follow-up thank-you letter after the interview, sending it to the interviewer.

Conditions: Use one sheet of plain typing paper, a number 10 envelope, and a computer, printer, thesaurus, and English dictionary.

Standards: Time: ______________________ minutes

Accuracy: ______________________

(Note: The time element and accuracy criteria may be given by your instructor.)

Directions: After the interview, you decide to send a follow-up thank-you letter to the person who interviewed you. Type a letter and address a number 10 envelope. Refer to Chapter 18 and Figure 18-11 in the *Handbook* to help organize your thoughts.

ASSIGNMENT 18-6 ▶ VISIT WEBSITES FOR JOB OPPORTUNITIES

Performance Objective

Task: Access the Internet and visit several websites of the World Wide Web.

Conditions: Use a computer with printer and/or a pen or pencil to make notes.

Standards: Time: ______________________ minutes

Accuracy: ______________________

(Note: The time element and accuracy criteria may be given by your instructor.)

Directions: Visit at least five websites by using either a search engine (Yahoo, Excite, AltaVista) or a job search website. Some suggestions are:

http://hotjobs.yahoo.com
www.healthcarejobs.org
www.indeed.com
www.job-search-engine.com
www.flipdog.com
www.topusajobs.com
www.monster.com

Enter a keyword or job title, such as "medical billing specialist" or "medical coder." Enter your city and state to locate listings near you. Click on the search button. If you get some results, print the listings that appeal to you for sharing and discussing in class.

ASSIGNMENT 18-7 ▶ CRITICAL THINKING

Performance Objective

Task: Write a paragraph describing the benefits of becoming certified in this field.

Conditions: Use a computer with printer and/or a pen or pencil.

Standards: Time: ______________________ minutes

Accuracy: ______________________

(Note: The time element and accuracy criteria may be given by your instructor.)

Directions: Write a paragraph or two describing why you would like to become certified in this field, and incorporate a numbered list of benefits. Make sure grammar, punctuation, and spelling are correct.

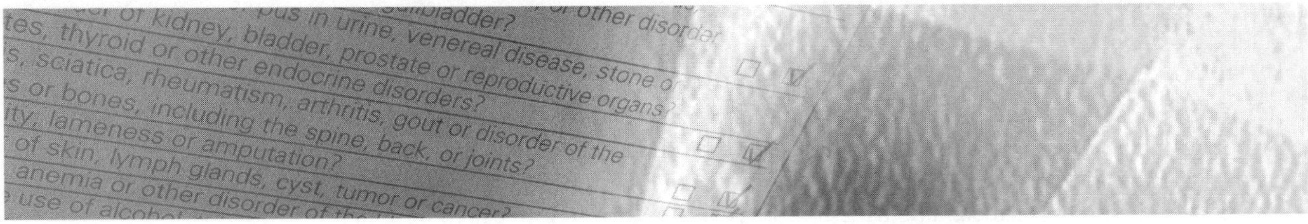

Tests

TEST 1: PROCEDURE (E/M AND MEDICINE SECTIONS) AND DIAGNOSTIC PROCEDURE CODE TEST

Directions: Using a *Current Procedural Terminology* (CPT) code book or Appendix A in this *Workbook*, insert the correct code numbers and modifiers for each service rendered. Give a brief description for each professional service rendered, although this is not needed for completing the CMS-1500 (08-05) claim form. An optional exercise is to abstract the pertinent data from each case, then use the *International Classification of Diseases, Ninth Revision, Clinical Modification* (ICD-9-CM) or ICD-10-CM rough draft code book to insert the diagnosis code.

Insert year of the CPT code book used

____

Insert year of the ICD-9-CM and/or ICD-10-CM code book used

____

1. Dr. Input sees a new patient, Mrs. Post, in the office for acute abdominal distress. The physician spends approximately 1 hour obtaining a comprehensive history and physical examination with high-complexity decision making. Several diagnostic studies are ordered, and Mrs. Post is given an appointment to return in 1 week.

Description

____ CPT # ________

____ ICD-9-CM # ________

____ ICD-10-CM # ________

2. Mr. Nakahara, an established patient, sees Dr. Practon in the office on January 11 for a reevaluation of his type II diabetic condition. Dr. Practon takes a detailed history and performs a detailed examination. Decision making is moderately complex.

Description

____ CPT # ________

____ ICD-9-CM # ________

____ ICD-10-CM # ________

3. Dr. Cardi sees Mrs. Franklin for a follow-up office visit for her hypertension. A problem-focused history and examination of her cardiovascular system are obtained and reveal a blood pressure of 140/100. Decision making is straightforward, with medication being prescribed. The patient is advised to return in 2 weeks to have her blood pressure checked by the nurse. Mrs. Franklin returns 2 weeks later, and the nurse checks her blood pressure.

Description

_______________ CPT # _______

_______________ ICD-9-CM # _______

_______________ ICD-10-CM # _______

_______________ CPT # _______

_______________ ICD-9-CM # _______

_______________ ICD-10-CM # _______

4. Dr. Skeleton receives a call at 7 PM from Mrs. Snyder. Her husband, a patient of Dr. Skeleton's, has been very ill for 2 hours with profuse vomiting. Dr. Skeleton goes to their home to see Mr. Snyder and spends considerable time obtaining a detailed history and examination. The medical decision making is of a highly complex nature. The physician administers an injection of prochlorperazine (Compazine).

Description

_______________ CPT # _______

_______________ CPT # _______

_______________ ICD-9-CM # _______

_______________ ICD-10-CM # _______

5. Dr. Cutis sees an established patient, a registered nurse, for determination of pregnancy. A detailed history and examination are obtained, with moderate-complexity medical decision making. A Papanicolaou smear is taken, a blood sample is drawn, and the specimens are sent to an independent laboratory for a qualitative human chorionic gonadotropin (hCG) test. The patient also complains of something she has discovered under her armpit. On examination, there is a furuncle of the left axilla, which is incised and drained during this visit. The laboratory requires CPT coding on the laboratory requisition. List how these laboratory procedures would appear on the requisition sheet. The Papanicolaou smear is processed according to the Bethesda System and under physician supervision.

Professional Service Rendered by Dr. Cutis

_______________ CPT # _______

_______________ CPT # _______

_______________ CPT # _______

_______________ CPT # _______

_______________ ICD-9-CM # ________

_______________ ICD-10-CM # ________

_______________ ICD-9-CM # ________

_______________ ICD-10-CM # ________

Laboratory Service on Requisition Sheet

_______________ CPT # ________

_______________ CPT # ________

6. Dr. Antrum makes a house call on Betty Mason, an established patient, for a problem-focused history of acute otitis media. A problem-focused examination is performed, with straightforward medical decision making. While there, Dr. Antrum also sees Betty's younger sister, Sandra, whom she has seen previously in the office, for acute tonsillitis. A problem-focused history and examination are performed with low-complexity decision making. In addition to the examinations, Dr. Antrum gives both children injections of penicillin.

Professional Service Rendered to Betty

_______________ CPT # ________

_______________ CPT # ________

_______________ ICD-9-CM # ________

_______________ ICD-10-CM # ________

Professional Service Rendered to Sandra

_______________ CPT # ________

_______________ CPT # ________

_______________ ICD-9-CM # ________

_______________ ICD-10-CM # ________

7. Two weeks later, Dr. Antrum is called to the emergency department at College Hospital at 2 AM on Sunday to see Betty Mason for recurrent chronic otitis media with suppuration. A problem-focused history and examination are performed with straightforward decision making. Dr. Antrum administers a second injection of penicillin.

Description

_______________ CPT # ________

_______________ CPT # ________

_______________ CPT # ________

_______________ ICD-9-CM # ________

_______________ ICD-10-CM # ________

8. While at the hospital, Dr. Antrum is asked to see another patient in the emergency department, who is new to her. A problem-focused history is taken. She performs a problem-focused examination and straightforward decision making for an intermediate 3.5-cm laceration of the scalp. The laceration is sutured, and the patient is advised to come to the office in 4 days for a dressing change. Four days later, the patient comes into the office for a dressing change by the nurse.

Description

____ CPT # ________

____ CPT # ________

____ CPT # ________

____ ICD-9-CM # ________

____ ICD-10-CM # ________

9. Dr. Menter, a psychiatrist, sees the following patients in the hospital. Code each procedure.

Ms. Blake: Consultation, expanded problem-focused history and examination and straightforward decision making; referred by Dr. Practon CPT # ________

Mrs. Clark: Group psychotherapy (50 min) CPT # ________

Mrs. Samson: Group psychotherapy (50 min) CPT # ________

Mr. Shoemaker: Group psychotherapy (50 min) CPT # ________

Miss James: Individual psychotherapy (25 min) CPT # ________

10. Dr. Input, a gastroenterologist, sees Mrs. Chan in the hospital at the request of Dr. Practon for an esophageal ulcer. In addition to the detailed history and examination and the low-complexity decision making, Dr. Input performs an esophageal intubation and washings, and prepares slides for cytology. Two days later, he sees Mrs. Chan in a follow-up hospital visit and obtains a problem-focused interval history and examination with low-complexity decision making. He performs a gastric intubation and collects washings for cytologic evaluation for a gastric ulcer.

Description

____ CPT # ________

____ CPT # ________

____ ICD-9-CM # ________

____ ICD-10-CM # ________

____ CPT # ________

____ CPT # ________

____ ICD-9-CM # ________

____ ICD-10-CM # ________

11. Mrs. Galati, a new patient, goes to Dr. Cardi because of chest pain (moderate to severe), weakness, fatigue, and dizziness. Dr. Cardi takes a comprehensive history and performs a comprehensive examination, followed by a treadmill ECG with interpretation and report. He also performs a vital capacity test and dipstick urinalysis, and draws blood for triiodothyronine (T_3) testing and for analysis by sequential multiple analyzer computer (SMAC) (16 panel tests, including complete blood cell count [CBC]), which are sent to and billed by a laboratory. Medical decision making is of high complexity.

Description

____ CPT # ________

____ CPT # ________

____ CPT # ________

____ CPT # ________

____ CPT # ________

____ CPT # ________

____ ICD-9-CM # ________

____ ICD-10-CM # ________

____ ICD-9-CM # ________

____ ICD-10-CM # ________

____ ICD-9-CM # ________

____ ICD-10-CM # ________

12. Jake Wonderhill has not had his eyes examined by Dr. Lenser for about 5 years. He is seen by Dr. Lenser, who performs the following ophthalmologic procedures in addition to a comprehensive eye examination: fluorescein angioscopy and electroretinography. Mr. Wonderhill receives a diagnosis of retinitis pigmentosa.

Description

____ CPT # ________

____ CPT # ________

____ CPT # ________

____ ICD-9-CM # ________

____ ICD-10-CM # ________

13. Dr. Practon is making rounds at the College Hospital and answers an urgent call on 3rd Floor East. He performs cardiopulmonary resuscitation on Mr. Sanchez for cardiac arrest and orders the patient taken to the critical care unit. Chest radiographs, laboratory work, blood gas measurements, and ECG are performed. The physician is detained 2 hours in constant attendance on the patient.

Description

______________________________ CPT # _______

______________________________ CPT # _______

______________________________ CPT # _______

______________________________ ICD-9-CM # _______

______________________________ ICD-10-CM # _______

14. Mrs. Powers, a new patient, sees Dr. Skeleton for low sciatica. Dr. Skeleton takes a detailed history and performs a detailed examination of the patient's lower back and extremities. Medical decision making is of low complexity. Diathermy (30 minutes) is given. The next day the patient comes in for therapeutic exercises in the Hubbard tank (30 minutes).

Description

______________________________ CPT # _______

______________________________ CPT # _______

______________________________ ICD-9-CM # _______

______________________________ ICD-10-CM # _______

______________________________ CPT # _______

______________________________ ICD-9-CM # _______

______________________________ ICD-10-CM # _______

15. a. Mrs. Garcia, a new patient, is seen by Dr. Caesar for occasional vaginal spotting (detailed history/examination and low-complexity decision making). The doctor determines that the bleeding is coming from the cervix and asks her to return in 3 days for cryocauterization of the cervix. During the initial examination, Mrs. Garcia asks for an evaluation for possible infertility. Dr. Caesar advises her to wait 2 to 3 weeks and make an appointment for two infertility tests.
    b. When the patient returns in 3 days for cryocauterization, the doctor also takes a wet mount for bacteria/fungi, which is sent to and billed by a laboratory.
    c. Three weeks later, an injection procedure for hysterosalpingography and endometrial biopsy are performed.

Description

a. ______________________________ CPT # ________

______________________________ ICD-9-CM # ________

______________________________ ICD-10-CM # ________

b. ______________________________ CPT # ________

______________________________ CPT # ________

______________________________ ICD-9-CM # ________

______________________________ ICD-10-CM # ________

c. ______________________________ CPT # ________

______________________________ CPT # ________

______________________________ ICD-9-CM # ________

______________________________ ICD-10-CM # ________

Multiple Choice

After reading the boxed codes with descriptions, select the answer/answers that is/are best in each case.

59120	surgical treatment of ectopic pregnancy; tubal or ovarian, requiring salpingectomy and/or oophorectomy, abdominal or vaginal approach
59121	tubal or ovarian, without salpingectomy and/or oophorectomy
59130	abdominal pregnancy
59135	interstitial, uterine pregnancy requiring total hysterectomy
59136	interstitial, uterine pregnancy with partial resection of uterus
59140	cervical, with evacuation

16. In regard to this section of CPT codes, which of the following statements is true about codes 59120 through 59140? Mark all that apply.

    a. They refer to abdominal hysterotomy.

    b. They involve laparoscopic treatment of ectopic pregnancy.

    c. They refer to treatment of ectopic pregnancy by surgery.

    d. They involve tubal ligation.

17. In regard to this section of CPT codes, for treatment of a tubal ectopic pregnancy, necessitating oophorectomy, the code to select is

a. 59121

b. 59120

c. 59135

d. 59136

e. 59130

18. In regard to this section of CPT codes, for treatment of an ectopic pregnancy (interstitial, uterine) requiring a total hysterectomy, the code/codes to select is/are

a. 59135

b. 59135 and 59120

c. 59120

d. 59130 and 59120

e. 59121

TEST 2: PROCEDURE CODE WITH MODIFIERS AND DIAGNOSTIC CODE TEST

Match the description given in the right column with the procedure code/modifier combination in the left column. Write the letter in the blank.

Procedure With Modifier		*Description*
1. 99214-25	________	a. Dr. Practon assisted Dr. Caesar with a total abdominal hysterectomy and bilateral salpingo-oophorectomy.
2. 99204-57	________	b. Dr. Skeleton interprets a thoracolumbar x-ray film that was taken at College Hospital.
3. 58150-80	________	c. Mrs. Ulwelling saw Dr. Antrum for an office visit as a new patient, and she recommended that the patient undergo a laryngoscopy, with stripping of vocal cords to be done the following day.
4. 32440-55	________	d. Mrs. Gillenbach walked through a plate glass window and underwent a rhinoplasty, performed by Dr. Graff on February 16, 20xx. On February 26, 20xx, she came to see Dr. Graff for a consultation regarding reconstructive surgery on her right leg.
5. 72080-26	________	e. An established patient, Mrs. Mercado, is seen in follow-up exam for type II diabetes. The patient asks Dr. Langerhans to look at some skin tags. The doctor examines them and says they need to be removed (11200). The evaluation and management service was detailed and of a moderate complexity.
6. 29425-58	________	f. Dr. Cutler performed a bilateral orchiopexy (inguinal approach) on baby Kozak.
7. 54640-50	________	g. Dr. Skeleton applied a short leg walking cast to Mrs. Belchere's right leg 4 weeks after his initial treatment of her fractured tibia.
8. 99253-24	________	h. Dr. Cutler went on vacation, and Dr. Coccidioides took care of Mrs. Ash during the postoperative period after her total pneumonectomy.

Directions: Using a ***Current Procedural Terminology*** (CPT) code book or Appendix A in this Workbook, insert the correct code numbers and modifiers for each service rendered. Give a brief description for each professional service rendered, although this is not needed for completing the CMS-1500 (08-05) claim form.

9. Dr. Input performs a gastrojejunostomy for carcinoma in situ of the duodenum and calls in Dr. Scott to administer the anesthesia and Dr. Cutler to assist. This intraperitoneal surgery takes 2 hours, 30 minutes. The patient is otherwise normal and healthy. List the procedure and diagnostic code numbers with appropriate modifiers for each physician.

Professional Service Rendered by Dr. Input

____________________ CPT # ________

____________________ ICD-9-CM # ________

____________________ ICD-10-CM # ________

Professional Service Rendered by Dr. Scott

____________________ CPT # ________

____________________ ICD-9-CM # ________

____________________ ICD-10-CM # ________

Professional Service Rendered by Dr. Cutler

____________________ CPT # ________

____________________ ICD-9-CM # ________

____________________ ICD-10-CM # ________

10. Dr. Rumsey assists Dr. Cutler with a total colectomy (intraperitoneal procedure) with ileostomy. Dr. Scott is the anesthesiologist. Surgery takes 2 hours, 55 minutes. The patient has a secondary malignant neoplasm of the colon (severe systemic disease). List the procedure code numbers with appropriate modifiers and diagnostic code numbers for each physician.

Professional Service Rendered by Dr. Rumsey

____________________ CPT # ________

____________________ ICD-9-CM # ________

____________________ ICD-10-CM # ________

Professional Service Rendered by Dr. Scott

____________________ CPT # ________

____________________ ICD-9-CM # ________

____________________ ICD-10-CM # ________

Professional Service Rendered by Dr. Cutler

____________________ CPT # ________

____________________ ICD-9-CM # ________

____________________ ICD-10-CM # ________

11. Dr. Cutis removes a malignant tumor from a patient's back (1.5 cm) and does the local anesthesia herself.

Description

____ CPT # ________

____ ICD-9-CM # ________

____ ICD-10-CM # ________

12. Dr. Skeleton sees Mr. Richmond, a new patient worked into the office schedule on an emergency basis after a motor vehicle traffic accident with another car. Mr. Richmond has multiple lacerations of the face, arm, and chest and a fracture of the left tibia. The physician takes a comprehensive history and performs a comprehensive examination. Decision making is moderately complex. Dr. Skeleton orders bilateral radiographs of the tibia and fibula and two views of the chest and left wrist to be taken in his office. Then he closes the following lacerations: 2.6 cm, simple, face; 2.0 cm, intermediate, face; 7.5 cm, intermediate, right arm; 4.5 cm, intermediate, chest. All radiographs are negative except that of the left tibia. Dr. Skeleton performs a manipulative reduction of the left tibial shaft and applies a cast. Code this case as if you were actually listing the codes on the CMS-1500 (08-05) claim form.

Description

____ CPT # ________ and ________

____ CPT # ________

____ CPT # ________

____ CPT # ________

____ CPT # ________

____ CPT # ________

____ CPT # ________

____ CPT # ________

____ CPT # ________

____ CPT # ________

____ ICD-9-CM # ________

____ ICD-10-CM # ________

____ ICD-9-CM # ________

____ ICD-10-CM # ________

____ ICD-9-CM # ________

____ ICD-10-CM # ________

____ ICD-9-CM # ________

______________________________ ICD-10-CM # ________

______________________________ ICD-9-CM # ________

______________________________ ICD-10-CM # ________

Six weeks later, Dr. Skeleton sees the same patient for an office visit and obtains radiographs (two views) of the left tibia and fibula. Treatment involves application of a cast below the patient's left knee to the toes, including a walking heel.

Description

______________________________ CPT # ________

______________________________ CPT # ________

______________________________ CPT # ________

______________________________ ICD-9-CM # ________

______________________________ ICD-10-CM # ________

13. Dr. Cutler performs an incisional biopsy of a patient's breast for a breast lump, which requires 40 minutes of anesthesia. Dr. Scott is the anesthesiologist. The patient is otherwise normal and healthy. List the procedure and diagnostic code numbers for each physician.

Professional Service Rendered by Dr. Cutler

______________________________ CPT # ________

______________________________ ICD-9-CM # ________

______________________________ ICD-10-CM # ________

Professional Service Rendered by Dr. Scott

______________________________ CPT # ________

______________________________ ICD-9-CM # ________

______________________________ ICD-10-CM # ________

14. Mrs. DeBeau is aware that Dr. Input will be out of town for 6 weeks; however, she decides to have him perform the recommended combined anterior-posterior colporrhaphy with enterocele repair for vaginal enterocele. Dr. Practon agrees to perform the follow-up care and assist. Dr. Scott is the anesthesiologist. The anesthesia time is 2 hours, 15 minutes. The patient is normal and healthy. List the procedure and diagnostic code numbers for each physician. Note: Emphasis for this problem should be placed on the choice of CPT modifiers.

Professional Service Rendered by Dr. Input

________________________________ CPT # ________

________________________________ ICD-9-CM # ________

________________________________ ICD-10-CM # ________

Professional Service Rendered by Dr. Practon

________________________________ CPT # ________

________________________________ CPT Modifier ________

________________________________ CPT Modifier ________

________________________________ ICD-9-CM # ________

________________________________ ICD-10-CM # ________

Professional Service Rendered by Dr. Scott

________________________________ CPT # ________

________________________________ ICD-9-CM # ________

________________________________ ICD-10-CM # ________

15. Mr. Wong, a new patient, is seen in the College Hospital and undergoes a comprehensive history and physical examination (H & P) with moderately complex decision making. Dr. Coccidioides performs a bronchoscopy with biopsy. Results of the biopsy confirm the diagnosis: malignant neoplasm of upper left lobe of lung. The following day the physician performs a total pneumonectomy. Dr. Cutler assists on the total pneumonectomy (pulmonary resection), and Dr. Scott is the anesthesiologist. Surgery takes 3 hours, 45 minutes. The patient has mild systemic disease. List the procedure and diagnostic code numbers for each physician.

Professional Service Rendered by Dr. Coccidioides

________________________________ CPT # ________

________________________________ CPT # ________

________________________________ CPT # ________

________________________________ ICD-9-CM # ________

________________________________ ICD-10-CM # ________

Professional Service Rendered by Dr. Cutler

________________________________ CPT # ________

________________________________ ICD-9-CM # ________

________________________________ ICD-10-CM # ________

Professional Service Rendered by Dr. Scott

____ CPT # ________

____ ICD-9-CM # ________

____ ICD-10-CM # ________

When completing the CMS-1500 (08-05) claim form for Dr. Scott, in which block would you list anesthesia minutes? ________________________

TEST 3: PROCEDURE (RADIOLOGY AND PATHOLOGY SECTIONS) AND DIAGNOSTIC CODE TEST

Directions: Using a CPT code book or Appendix A in this ***Workbook***, insert the correct procedure code numbers and modifiers and diagnostic codes for each service rendered. Give a brief description for each professional service rendered, although this is not needed for completing the CMS-1500 (08-05) claim form.

1. Mrs. Cahn sees Dr. Skeleton because of severe pain in her right shoulder. She is a new patient. Dr. Skeleton takes a detailed history and performs a detailed examination. A complete x-ray study of the right shoulder is done. Decision making is of low complexity. A diagnosis of bursitis is made, and an injection into the bursa is administered.

Description

____ CPT # ________

____ CPT # ________

____ CPT # ________

____ ICD-9-CM # ________

____ ICD-10-CM # ________

2. John Murphy comes into the Broxton Radiologic Group, Inc., for an extended radiation therapy consultation for prostatic cancer. The radiologist takes a detailed history and does a detailed examination. Decision making is of low complexity. The physician determines a simple treatment plan involving simple simulation-aided field settings. Basic dosimetry calculations are done, and the patient returns the following day and receives radiation therapy to a single treatment area (6 to 10 MeV).

Description

____ CPT # ________

____ CPT # ________

____ CPT # ________

____ CPT # ________

____ CPT # ________

Diagnosis:

____ ICD-9-CM # ________

____ ICD-10-CM # ________

3. Dr. Input refers Mrs. Horner to the Nuclear Medicine department of the Broxton Radiologic Group, Inc., for a bone marrow imaging of the whole body and imaging of the liver and spleen. List the procedure code numbers after each radiologic procedure to show how the radiology group would bill. Also, list the diagnosis of malignant neoplasm of the bone marrow.

Description

Total body bone marrow, imaging CPT # ________

Radiopharmaceuticals, diagnostic (Iodine I-123) HCPCS #________

Liver and spleen imaging CPT # ________

Radiopharmaceuticals, diagnostic (Iodine I-123) HCPCS # ________

Diagnosis:

____ ICD-9-CM # ________

____ ICD-10-CM # ________

4. Dr. Input also refers Mrs. Horner to XYZ Laboratory for the following tests. List the procedure code numbers to indicate how the laboratory would bill.

Description

CBC, automated and automated differential CPT # ________

Urinalysis, automated with microscopy CPT # ________

Urine culture (quantitative, colony count) CPT # ________

Urine antibiotic sensitivity (microtiter) CPT # ________

5. The general laboratory at College Hospital receives a surgical tissue specimen (ovarian biopsy) for gross and microscopic examination from a patient with Stein-Leventhal syndrome. List the procedure and diagnostic code numbers to indicate what the hospital pathology department would bill.

Description

____ CPT # ________

Diagnosis:

____ ICD-9-CM # ________

____ ICD-10-CM # ________

6. Dr. Langerhans refers Jerry Cramer to XYZ Laboratory for a lipid panel. He has a family history of cardiovascular disease. List the procedure and diagnostic code number or numbers to indicate how the laboratory would bill.

Description

____ CPT # ________

Diagnosis:

____ ICD-9-CM # ________

____ ICD-10-CM # ________

7. Dr. Caesar is an OB/GYN specialist who has her own ultrasound machine. Carmen Cardoza, age 45, is referred to Dr. Caesar for an obstetric consultation and an amniocentesis with ultrasonic guidance. The diagnosis is Rh incompatibility. The doctor performs a detailed history and physical examination, and decision making is of low complexity.

Description

____ CPT # ________

____ CPT # ________

____ ICD-9-CM # ________

____ ICD-10-CM # ________

8. Mr. Marcos's medical record indicates that a retrograde pyelogram followed by a percutaneous nephrostolithotomy, with basket extraction of a 1-cm stone, was performed by Dr. Ulibarri for nephrolithiasis.

Description

____ CPT # ________

____ CPT # ________

Diagnosis:

____ ICD-9-CM # ________

____ ICD-10-CM # ________

9. Broxton Radiologic Group, Inc., performs the following procedures on Mrs. Stephens at the request of Dr. Input. List the procedure code numbers after each radiologic procedure. On the laboratory slip, the following congenital diagnoses are listed: Diverticulum of the stomach and colon; cystic lung. Locate the corresponding diagnostic codes.

Barium enema CPT # ________

Evaluation of upper gastrointestinal tract with small bowel CPT # ________

Complete chest x-ray CPT # ________

Diagnosis:

____ ICD-9-CM # ________

____ ICD-10-CM # ________

Diagnosis:

____ ICD-9-CM # ________

____ ICD-10-CM # ________

Diagnosis:

____ ICD-9-CM # ________

____ ICD-10-CM # ________

10. Two weeks later, Mrs. Stephens is referred again for further radiologic studies for flank pain. List the procedure and diagnostic code numbers after each radiologic procedure.

Intravenous pyelogram (IVP) with drip infusion CPT # ________

Oral cholecystography CPT # ________

Diagnosis:

____ ICD-9-CM # ________

____ ICD-10-CM # ________

TEST 4: COMPLETE A CMS-1500 (08-05) CLAIM FORM

Performance Objective

Task: Complete a CMS-1500 (08-05) claim form for a private case and post transactions to the patient's financial accounting record.

Conditions: Use the patient's record (Figure 1) and financial statement (Figure 2); one health insurance claim form; a computer or pen; procedural and diagnostic code books; and Appendixes A and B in this *Workbook*.

Standards: Claim Productivity Management

Time: ____________________ minutes

Accuracy: ____________________

(Note: The time element and accuracy criteria may be given by your instructor.)

Directions

1. Using OCR guidelines, complete a CMS-1500 (08-05) claim form and direct it to the private carrier. Refer to Jennifer T. Lacey's patient record for information and Appendix A in this *Workbook* to locate the fees to record on the claim, and post them to the financial statement. Date the claim August 15. Dr. Caesar is accepting assignment, and the patient's signatures to release information to the insurance company and to have the payment forwarded directly to the physician are on file.

2. Use your CPT code book or Appendix A in this *Workbook* to determine the correct five-digit code numbers and modifiers for each professional service rendered. Use your HCPCS Level II code book or refer to Appendix B in this *Workbook* for HCPCS procedure codes and modifiers. Use your diagnostic code book to code each active diagnosis. If your instructor tells you to also find the ICD-10-CM codes, a draft version may be downloaded from the following website: http://www.cdc.gov/nchs/icd/icd10cm.htm#10update.

3. Record the proper information on the financial record and claim form, and note the date when you have billed the insurance company.

4. American Commercial Insurance Company sent a check (voucher number 5586) on November 17 in the amount of $880. The patient's responsibility is $220. Post the payment, write off (adjust) the remaining balance, and circle the amount billed to the patient.

PATIENT RECORD NO. T-4

LAST NAME	FIRST NAME	MIDDLE NAME	BIRTH DATE	SEX	HOME PHONE
Lacey	Jennifer	T	11-12-55	F	555-549-0098

ADDRESS	CITY	STATE	ZIP CODE
451 Roberts Street	Woodland Hills	XY	12345

CELL PHONE	PAGER NO.	FAX NO.	E-MAIL ADDRESS
555-443-9899	555-549-0098		lacey@wb.net

PATIENT'S SOC. SEC. NO.	DRIVER'S LICENSE
430-XX-7709	Y0053498

PATIENT'S OCCUPATION	NAME OF COMPANY
legal secretary	Higgins and Higgins Attorneys at Law

ADDRESS OF EMPLOYER	PHONE
430 Second Avenue, Woodland Hills, XY 12345	555-540-6675

SPOUSE OR PARENT	OCCUPATION

EMPLOYER	ADDRESS	PHONE

NAME OF INSURANCE	INSURED OR SUB SCRIBER
American Commercial Insurance Company, 5682 Bendix Blvd., Woodland Hills, XY 12345	

POLICY/CERTIFICATE NO.	GROUP NO.
5789022	444

REFERRED BY: Clarence Cutler, MD

Figure 1

DATE	PROGRESS NOTES No. T-4
8-1-xx	New pt referred by Dr. Cutler, came into office for consultation and additional opinion.
	CC: Full feeling in stomach and low abdominal region.
	Irregular menstruation. Ultrasonic report showed
	leiomyomata uteri and rt ovarian mass; however, visualization of mass poor and type
	cannot be identified. Pap smear Class I. No personal or family hx of CA.
	Comprehensive hx and physical examination performed on healthy appearing white female.
	Wt: 136 lbs. BP 128/60. T 98.6 F. Palpated rt adnexal mass and
	enlarged uterus; vulva and cervix appear normal; LMP 7/16/XX.
	Medical decision making: mod complex
	Tx plan: Adv hospital admit and additional tests to R/O carcinoma.
	Tentatively scheduled abdominal hysterectomy with bilateral salpingo-oophorectomy.
	(M/MDM).
	BC/llf Bertha Caesar, MD
8-2-xx	Adm to College Hosp (C HX/PX M/MDM). Scheduled
	surgery at 7:00 A.M. tomorrow.
	BC/llf Bertha Caesar, MD
8-3-xx	Perf abdominal
	hysterectomy with bilateral salpingo-oophorectomy.
	BC/llf Bertha Caesar, MD
8-4-xx	HV (EPF HX/PX M/MDM) Path report revealed interstitial leiomyomata uteri and corpus
	luteum cyst of rt ovary. Pt C/O PO pain, otherwise doing well.
	BC/llf Bertha Caesar, MD
8-5-xx	HV (EPF HX/PX M/MDM). Pt ambulating well, pain decreased. Dressing changed, wound
	healing well.
	BC/llf Bertha Caesar, MD
8-6-xx	HV (PF HX/PX SF/MDM). Pain minimal. Pt ambulating without assistance.
	Removed staples, no redness or swelling. Pln DC tomorrow.
	BC/llf Bertha Caesar, MD
8-7-xx	Discharge to home; pt doing well. RTO next wk. Disability from 8-1 to 8-23-xx.
	BC/llf Bertha Caesar, MD

Figure 1, cont'd

STATEMENT
COLLEGE CLINIC
4567 Broad Avenue
Woodland Hills, XY 12345-0001
Tel. 555-486-9002
Fax No. 555-487-8976

Acct. No. T-4

Jennifer T. Lacey
451 Roberts Street
Woodland Hills, XY 12345

Phone No. (H) (555) 549-0098 (W) (555) 540-6675 Birthdate 11-12-55

Insurance Co. American Commercial Insurance Company Policy/Group No. 5789022 / 444

DATE	REFERENCE	DESCRIPTION	CHARGES	CREDITS PYMNTS.	CREDITS ADJ.	BALANCE
20XX			**BALANCE FORWARD** →			
8-1-xx		Consult				
8-2-xx		Admit				
8-3-xx		TAH BSO				
8-4-xx		HV				
8-5-xx		HV				
8-6-xx		HV				
8-7-xx		Discharge				

PLEASE PAY LAST AMOUNT IN BALANCE COLUMN

THIS IS A COPY OF YOUR FINANCIAL ACCOUNT AS IT APPEARS ON OUR RECORDS

Figure 2

TEST 5: COMPLETE A CMS-1500 (08-05) CLAIM FORM

Performance Objective

Task: Complete a CMS-1500 (08-05) claim form for a private case and post transactions to the patient's financial accounting record.

Conditions: Use the patient's record (Figure 3) and financial statement (Figure 4); one health insurance claim form; a computer or pen; procedural and diagnostic code books; and Appendixes A and B in this *Workbook*.

Standards: Claim Productivity Management

Time: ____________________ minutes

Accuracy: ____________________

(Note: The time element and accuracy criteria may be given by your instructor.)

Directions

1. Using OCR guidelines, complete a CMS-1500 (08-05) claim form and direct it to the private carrier. Refer to Hortense N. Hope's patient record for information and Appendix A in this *Workbook* to locate the fees to record on the claim, and post them to the financial statement. Date the claim July 31. Dr. Practon is accepting assignment, and the patient's signatures to release information to the insurance company and to have the payment forwarded directly to the physician are on file.

2. Use your CPT code book or Appendix A in this *Workbook* to determine the correct five-digit code numbers and modifiers for each professional service rendered. Use your HCPCS Level II code book or refer to Appendix B in this *Workbook* for HCPCS procedure codes and modifiers. Use your diagnostic code book to code each active diagnosis. If your instructor tells you to also find the ICD-10-CM codes, a draft version may be downloaded from the following website: http://www.cdc.gov/nchs/icd/icd10cm.htm#10update.

3. Record the proper information on the financial record and claim form, and note the date you have billed the insurance company.

PATIENT RECORD NO. T-5

LAST NAME	FIRST NAME	MIDDLE NAME	BIRTH DATE	SEX	HOME PHONE
Hope	Hortense	N	04-12-56	F	555-666-7821

ADDRESS	CITY	STATE	ZIP CODE
247 Lantern Pike	Woodland Hills	XY	12345

CELL PHONE	PAGER NO.	FAX NO.	E-MAIL ADDRESS
	555-323-1687	555-666-7821	hope@wb.net

PATIENT'S SOC. SEC. NO.	DRIVER'S LICENSE
321-XX-8809	N0058921

PATIENT'S OCCUPATION	NAME OF COMPANY
Clerk typist	R and S Manufacturing Company

ADDRESS OF EMPLOYER	PHONE
2271 West 74 Street, Torres, XY 12349	555-466-5890

SPOUSE OR PARENT	OCCUPATION
Harry J. Hope	carpenter

EMPLOYER	ADDRESS	PHONE
Jesse Construction Company,	3861 South Orange Street, Torres, XY 12349	555-765-2318

NAME OF INSURANCE	INSURED OR SUBSCRIBER
Ralston Insurance Company, 2611 Hanley Street, Woodland Hills, XY 12345	Hortense N. Hope

POLICY/CERTIFICATE NO.	GROUP NO.
ATC321458809	T8471811A

REFERRED BY: Harry J. Hope (husband)

DATE	PROGRESS NOTES
7-1-xx	New F pt comes in complaining of lt great toe pain. Incised, drained, and cleaned area
	around nail on lt great toe. Dx: onychia and paronychia. Started on antibiotic and adv to
	retn in 2 days for permanent excision of nail plate (EPF HX/PX SF/MDM).
	GP/llf Gerald Practon, MD
7-3-xx	Pt returns for nail excision. Injected procaine in lt great toe; removed entire toenail.
	Drs applied. PTR in 5 days for PO check.
	GP/llf Gerald Practon, MD
7-7-xx	PO check. Dressing changed, nail bed healing well. Pt to continue on AB until gone.
	Retn PRN (PF HX/PX SF/MDM).
	GP/llf Gerald Practon, MD

Figure 3

Acct No. T-5

STATEMENT
Financial Account
COLLEGE CLINIC
4567 Broad Avenue
Woodland Hills, XY 12345-0001
Tel. 555-486-9002
Fax No. 555-487-8976

Hortense N. Hope
247 Lantern Pike
Woodland Hills, XY 12345

Phone No. (H) 555-666-7821 (W) 555-466-5890 Birthdate 4/12/56

Primary Insurance Co. Ralston Insurance Company Policy/Group No. ATC321458809 / T8471811A

Secondary Insurance Co. None Policy/Group No.

DATE	REFERENCE	DESCRIPTION	CHARGES	CREDITS PYMNTS.	CREDITS ADJ.	BALANCE
20xx		BALANCE FORWARD →				
7-1-xx		NP OV				
7-1-xx		I & D lt great toe				
7-3-xx		Excision lt great toenail				
7-7-xx		PO check				

PLEASE PAY LAST AMOUNT IN BALANCE COLUMN

THIS IS A COPY OF YOUR FINANCIAL ACCOUNT AS IT APPEARS ON OUR RECORDS

Figure 4

TEST 6: COMPLETE A CLAIM FORM FOR A MEDICARE CASE

Performance Objective

Task: Complete a CMS-1500 (08-05) claim form and post transactions to the patient's financial accounting record.

Conditions: Use the patient's record (Figure 5) and financial statement (Figure 6); one health insurance claim form; a computer or pen; procedural and diagnostic code books; and Appendixes A and B in this *Workbook*.

Standards: Claim Productivity Management

Time: ____________________ minutes

Accuracy: ____________________

(Note: The time element and accuracy criteria may be given by your instructor.)

Directions

1. Using OCR guidelines, complete a CMS-1500 (08-05) claim form and direct it to the Medicare fiscal intermediary. To locate your local fiscal intermediary, go to website http://www.cms.hhs.gov/contacts/incardir.asp. Refer to Frances F. Foote's patient record for information and Appendix A in this *Workbook* to locate the fees to record on the claim, and post them to the financial statement. Date the claim October 31. Dr. Practon is a participating provider, and the patient's signatures to release information to the insurance company and to have the payment forwarded directly to the physician are on file.

2. Use your CPT code book or Appendix A in this *Workbook* to determine the correct five-digit code numbers and modifiers for each professional service rendered. Use your HCPCS Level II code book or refer to Appendix B in this *Workbook* for HCPCS procedure codes and modifiers. Use your diagnostic code book to code each active diagnosis. If your instructor tells you to also find the ICD-10-CM codes, a draft version may be downloaded from the following website: http://www.cdc.gov/nchs/icd/icd10cm.htm#10update.

3. Record the proper information on the patient's financial accounting record and claim form, and note the date when you have billed the insurance company.

PATIENT RECORD NO. T-6

LAST NAME	FIRST NAME	MIDDLE NAME	BIRTH DATE	SEX	HOME PHONE
Foote	Frances	F	08-10-32	F	555-678-0943

ADDRESS	CITY	STATE	ZIP CODE
984 North A Street	Woodland Hills	XY	12345

CELL PHONE	PAGER NO.	FAX NO.	E-MAIL ADDRESS
555-443-9908	555-320-7789	555-678-0943	foote@wb.net

PATIENT'S SOC. SEC. NO.	DRIVER'S LICENSE
578-XX-8924	B4309811

PATIENT'S OCCUPATION	NAME OF COMPANY
retired legal secretary	

ADDRESS OF EMPLOYER	PHONE

SPOUSE OR PARENT	OCCUPATION
Harry L. Foote	roofer

EMPLOYER	ADDRESS	PHONE
BDO Construction Company, 340 North 6th Street, Woodland Hills, XY 12345		555-478-9083

NAME OF INSURANCE	INSURED OR SUB SCRIBER
Medicare	self

POLICY/CERTIFICATE NO.	GROUP NO.
578-XX-8924A	

REFERRED BY: G. U. Curette, MD, 4780 Main Street, Ehrlich, XY 12350 Tel: 555-430-8788 NPI #34216600XX

DATE	PROGRESS NOTES
10-11-xx	NP pt referred by Dr. Curette with a CC of foot pain centering around rt great toe and
	sometimes shooting up her leg. PF history taken. PF exam revealed severe overgrowth
	of nail into surrounding tissues. AP and lat right foot x-rays taken & interpreted which
	indicate no fractures or arthritis. Pt has had a N workup for gout by Dr. Curette.
	DX: Severe onychocryptosis both margins of rt hallux. Adv to sched. OP surgery at
	College Hospital for wedge resection of skin of nail fold to repair ingrown nail.
	No disability from work (SF/MDM).
	NP/llf Nick Pedro, MD
10-13-xx	Pt admitted for OP surgery at College Hospital. Complete wedge resection performed for
	repair of rt hallux ingrown nail. Pt will stay off foot over the weekend and retn next wk for
	PO re ch.
	NP/llf Nick Pedro, MD
10-20-xx	PO visit (PF HX/PX SF/MDM). Rt hallux healing well. RTC as necessary.
	NP/llf Nick Pedro, MD

Figure 5

Acct No. T-6

STATEMENT
Financial Account
COLLEGE CLINIC
4567 Broad Avenue
Woodland Hills, XY 12345-0001
Tel. 555-486-9002
Fax No. 555-487-8976

Frances F. Foote
984 North A Street
Woodland Hills, XY 12345

Phone No. (H) 555-678-0943 (W) ______ Birthdate 8/10/32

Primary Insurance Co. Medicare Policy/Group No. 578-XX-8924A

DATE	REFERENCE	DESCRIPTION	CHARGES	CREDITS PYMNTS.	CREDITS ADJ.	BALANCE
20xx		BALANCE FORWARD →				
10-11-xx		NP OV				
10-11-xx		X-rays				
10-13-xx		Wedge excision/skin of nail fold				
10-20-xx		PO				

PLEASE PAY LAST AMOUNT IN BALANCE COLUMN

THIS IS A COPY OF YOUR FINANCIAL ACCOUNT AS IT APPEARS ON OUR RECORDS

Figure 6

TEST 7: COMPLETE A CLAIM FORM FOR A MEDICARE/MEDIGAP CASE

Performance Objective

Task: Complete two CMS-1500 (08-05) claim forms for a Medicare/Medigap case and post transactions to the patient's financial accounting record.

Conditions: Use patient's record (Figure 7) and financial statement (Figure 8); two health insurance claim forms; a computer or pen; procedural and diagnostic code books; and Appendixes A and B in this *Workbook*.

Standards: Claim Productivity Management

Time: ____________________ minutes

Accuracy: ____________________

(Note: The time element and accuracy criteria may be given by your instructor.)

Directions

1. Using OCR guidelines, complete two CMS-1500 (08-05) claim forms and direct them to the Medicare fiscal intermediary. To locate your local fiscal intermediary, go to website http://www.cms.hhs.gov/contacts/incardir.asp. Refer to Charles B. Kamb's patient record for information and Appendix A to locate the fees to record on the claim, and post them to the financial statement. Be sure to include the Medigap information on the claim form so that it will be crossed over (sent to the Medigap insurance carrier) automatically. Date the claim June 30. Dr. Practon is a participating provider with both Medicare and the Medigap program, and the patient's signatures to release information to the insurance companies and to have the payment forwarded directly to the physician are on file.

2. Use your CPT code book or Appendix A in this *Workbook* to determine the correct five-digit code numbers and modifiers for each professional service rendered. Use your HCPCS Level II code book or refer to Appendix B in this *Workbook* for HCPCS procedure codes and modifiers. Use your diagnostic code book to code each active diagnosis. If your instructor tells you to also find the ICD-10-CM codes, a draft version may be downloaded from the following website: http://www.cdc.gov/nchs/icd/icd10cm.htm#10update.

3. Record the proper information on the patient's financial accounting record and claim form, and note the date when you have billed the insurance company.

PATIENT RECORD NO. T-7

LAST NAME	FIRST NAME	MIDDLE NAME	BIRTH DATE	SEX	HOME PHONE
Kamb	Charles	B	01-26-27	M	555-467-2601

ADDRESS	CITY	STATE	ZIP CODE
2600 West Nautilus Street	Woodland Hills	XY	12345

CELL PHONE	PAGER NO.	FAX NO.	E-MAIL ADDRESS

PATIENT'S SOC. SEC. NO.	DRIVER'S LICENSE
454-XX-9569	M3200563

PATIENT'S OCCUPATION	NAME OF COMPANY
Retired TV actor	Amer. Federation of TV & Radio Artists (AFTRA)

ADDRESS OF EMPLOYER	PHONE
30077 Ventura Boulevard, Woodland Hills, XY 12345	555-466-3331

SPOUSE OR PARENT	OCCUPATION
Jane C. Kamb	homemaker

EMPLOYER	ADDRESS	PHONE

NAME OF INSURANCE	INSURED OR SUB SCRIBER	
Medicare (Primary)	self	National Insurance Company (Medigap)

POLICY/CERTIFICATE NO.	GROUP NO.
454-XX-9569A	Medigap Policy No. 5789002

REFERRED BY: Mrs. O. S. Tomy (friend)

National PAYRID NAT234567

DATE	PROGRESS NOTES
6-1-xx	New pt comes into ofc to est new PCP in area; recently moved from Ohio. W obese M c/o
	nasal bleeding for two and a half months c̄ headaches and nasal congestion. Pt states he
	has had HBP for 1 yr. Taking med: Serpasil prescribed by dr in Ohio; does not know dosage.
	Took a C HX and performed a C PX which revealed post nasal hemorrhage. Coagulation
	time (Lee and White) and microhematocrit (spun) done in ofc are WNL. BP 180/100.
	Used nasal cautery and post nasal packs to control hemorrhage. Rx prophylactic antibiotic
	to guard against sinusitis NKA. Adv retn tomorrow, bring hypertensive medication.
	Pt signed authorization to request med records from dr in Ohio. D: Recurrent epistaxis
	due to nonspecific hypertension. No disability from work.
	GP/llf *Gerald Practon, MD*
6-2-xx	Pt retns and nasal hemorrhage is reevaluated (PF HX/PX SF/MDM). Postnasal packs
	removed and replaced. BP 182/98. Pt forgot medication for hypertension but states he is
	taking it 2 X d. Adv retn in 1 day, bring medication.
	GP/llf *Gerald Practon, MD*
6-3-xx	Pt retns and nasal hemorrhage is reevaluated (PF HX/PX SF/MDM). Postnasal packs
	removed. BP 178/100. Verified hypertensive medication. Pt to increase dosage to 4 X d.
	Adv retn in 5 days.
	GP/llf *Gerald Practon, MD*
6-8-xx	Pt retns and nasal hemorrhage is reevaluated (EPF HX/PX L/MDM). Prev medical records
	arrived and reviewed. BP 190/102. Pt referred to Dr. Perry Cardi (int) for future care of
	hypertension.
	GP/llf *Gerald Practon, MD*

Figure 7

Acct No. T-7

STATEMENT
Financial Account

COLLEGE CLINIC
4567 Broad Avenue
Woodland Hills, XY 12345-0001
Tel. 555-486-9002
Fax No. 555-487-8976

Charles B. Kamb
2600 West Nautilus Street
Woodland Hills, XY 12345

Phone No. (H) 555-467-2601 (W) None/retired Birthdate 1-26-27

Primary Insurance Co. Medicare Policy/Group No. 454-XX-9569A

Secondary Insurance Co. National Insurance Company (Medigap) Policy/Group No. 5789002

DATE	REFERENCE	DESCRIPTION	CHARGES	CREDITS PYMNTS.	CREDITS ADJ.	BALANCE
20xx		BALANCE FORWARD →				
6-1-xx		NP OV				
6-1-xx		Coagulation time				
6-1-xx		Microhematocrit				
6-1-xx		Post nasal pack/cautery				
6-2-xx		OV				
6-2-xx		Subsequent nasal pack				
6-3-xx		OV				
6-8-xx		OV				

PLEASE PAY LAST AMOUNT IN BALANCE COLUMN

THIS IS A COPY OF YOUR FINANCIAL ACCOUNT AS IT APPEARS ON OUR RECORDS

Figure 8

TEST 8: COMPLETE A CLAIM FORM FOR A MEDICAID CASE

Performance Objective

Task: Complete a CMS-1500 (08-05) claim form for a Medicaid case and post transactions to the patient's financial accounting record.

Conditions: Use the patient's record (Figure 9) and financial statement (Figure 10); one health insurance claim form; a computer or pen; procedural and diagnostic code books; and Appendixes A and B in this *Workbook*.

Standards: Claim Productivity Management

Time: ____________________ minutes

Accuracy: ____________________

(Note: The time element and accuracy criteria may be given by your instructor.)

Directions

1. Using OCR guidelines, complete a CMS-1500 (08-05) claim form and direct it to the Medicaid fiscal intermediary. Obtain the address of your Medicaid fiscal agent by first going to website http://www.cms.hhs.gov/medicaid/geninfo and then either sending an e-mail message to the Medicaid contact or using the toll-free number to obtain the Medicaid carrier name and address. An option might be to contact your local state medical society. Refer to Louise K. Herman's patient record for information and Appendix A to locate the fees to record on the claim, and post them to the financial statement. Date the claim May 31.

2. Use your CPT code book or Appendix A in this *Workbook* to determine the correct five-digit code numbers and modifiers for each professional service rendered. Use your HCPCS Level II code book or refer to Appendix B in this *Workbook* for HCPCS procedure codes and modifiers. Use your diagnostic code book to code each active diagnosis. If your instructor tells you to also find the ICD-10-CM codes, a draft version may be downloaded from the following website: http://www.cdc.gov/nchs/icd/icd10cm.htm#10update.

3. Record the proper information on the patient's financial accounting record and claim form and note the date when you have billed the insurance company.

4. Post the payment of $350 (voucher number 4300), received from the Medicaid fiscal intermediary 40 days after claim submission, and write off (adjust) the balance of the account.

PATIENT RECORD NO. T-8

LAST NAME	FIRST NAME	MIDDLE NAME	BIRTH DATE	SEX	HOME PHONE
Herman	Louise	K	11-04-60	F	555-266-9085

ADDRESS	CITY	STATE	ZIP CODE
13453 Burbank Boulevard	Woodland Hills	XY	12345

CELL PHONE	PAGER NO.	FAX NO.	E-MAIL ADDRESS
555-466-7003		555-266-9085	herman@wb.net

PATIENT'S SOC. SEC. NO.	DRIVER'S LICENSE
519-XX-0018	T0943995

PATIENT'S OCCUPATION	NAME OF COMPANY
unemployed budget analyst	

ADDRESS OF EMPLOYER	PHONE

SPOUSE OR PARENT	OCCUPATION
Harold D. Herman	retired salesman

EMPLOYER	ADDRESS	PHONE

NAME OF INSURANCE	INSURED OR SUBSCRIBER
Medicaid	self

MEDICAID NO.	GROUP NO.
0051936001X	

REFERRED BY: Raymond Skeleton, MD

DATE	PROGRESS NOTES
5-6-xx	NP pt referred by Dr. Skeleton. CC: Rectal bleeding. Took a comprehensive history and
	performed a comprehensive physical examination. Diagnostic anoscopy revealed
	bleeding int and ext hemorrhoids and 2 infected rectal polyps. Rx antibiotics. Retn in
	2 days for removal of hemorrhoids and polyps (M/MDM)
	RR/llf Rex Rumsey, MD
5-8-xx	Pt returned to office for simple internal/external hemorrhoidectomy. Rigid
	proctosigmoidoscopy also perf for removal of polyps using snare technique. Adv. sitz
	baths daily. Continue on AB until gone. Retn in 1 wk.
	RR/llf Rex Rumsey, MD
5-15-xx	DNS Telephoned pt and rescheduled.
	Mary Bright, CMA
5-17-xx	PO OV (EPF HX/PX LC/MDM). Pt progressing well. No pain, discomfort or bleeding.
	Discharged from care, retn PRN.
	RR/llf Rex Rumsey, MD

Figure 9

Acct No. T-8

STATEMENT
Financial Account
COLLEGE CLINIC
4567 Broad Avenue
Woodland Hills, XY 12345-0001
Tel. 555-486-9002
Fax No. 555-487-8976

Louise K. Herman
13453 Burbank Boulevard
Woodland Hills, XY 12345

Phone No. (H) 555-266-9085 (W) ______ Birthdate 11/4/60

Primary Insurance Co. Medicaid Policy/Group No. 0051936001X

Secondary Insurance Co. ______ Policy/Group No. ______

DATE	REFERENCE	DESCRIPTION	CHARGES	CREDITS PYMNTS.	CREDITS ADJ.	BALANCE
20xx		BALANCE FORWARD →				
5-6-xx		NP OV				
5-6-xx		Dx anoscopy				
5-8-xx		Int/Ext Hemorrhoidectomy				
5-8-xx		Proctosigmoidoscopy with removal of polyps				
5-17-xx		PO OV				

PLEASE PAY LAST AMOUNT IN BALANCE COLUMN

THIS IS A COPY OF YOUR FINANCIAL ACCOUNT AS IT APPEARS ON OUR RECORDS

Figure 10

TEST 9: COMPLETE A CLAIM FORM FOR A TRICARE CASE

Performance Objective

Task: Complete a CMS-1500 (08-05) claim form for a TRICARE case and post transactions to the patient's financial accounting record.

Conditions: Use the patient's record (Figure 11) and financial statement (Figure 12); one health insurance claim form; a computer or pen; procedural and diagnostic code books; and Appendixes A and B in this *Workbook*.

Standards: Claim Productivity Management

Time: ____________________ minutes

Accuracy: ____________________

(Note: The time element and accuracy criteria may be given by your instructor.)

Directions

1. Using OCR guidelines, complete a CMS-1500 (08-05) claim form and direct it to the TRICARE carrier. To locate your local fiscal intermediary, go to website http://www.tricare.osd.mil. Click on the area of the map you are residing in and then choose a state to access claims information for that state. Refer to Darlene M. Cash's patient record for information and Appendix A to locate the fees to record on the claim, and post them to the financial statement. Date the claim February 27. Dr. Cutler is accepting assignment, and the patient's signatures to release information to the insurance company and to have the payment forwarded directly to the physician are on file.

2. Use your CPT code book or Appendix A in this *Workbook* to determine the correct five-digit code numbers and fees for each professional service rendered. Use your HCPCS Level II code book or refer to Appendix B in this *Workbook* for HCPCS procedure codes and modifiers. Use your diagnostic code book to code each active diagnosis. If your instructor tells you to also find the ICD-10-CM codes, a draft version may be downloaded from the following website: http://www.cdc.gov/nchs/icd/icd10cm.htm#10update.

3. Record the proper information on the patient's financial accounting record and claim form, and note the date when you have billed the insurance company.

PATIENT RECORD NO. T-9

Cash	Darlene	M	3-15-70	F	555-666-8901
LAST NAME	FIRST NAME	MIDDLE NAME	BIRTH DATE	SEX	HOME PHONE

5729 Redwood Avenue — Woodland Hills — XY — 12344
ADDRESS — CITY — STATE — ZIP CODE

555-290-5400 — — 555-666-8901 — cash@wb.net
CELL PHONE — PAGER NO. — FAX NO. — E-MAIL ADDRESS

298-XX-6754 — J3457789
PATIENT'S SOC. SEC. NO. — DRIVER'S LICENSE

Teacher — City Unified School District
PATIENT'S OCCUPATION — NAME OF COMPANY

Century High School, 2031 West Olympic Boulevard, Dorland, XY 12345 — 555-678-1076
ADDRESS OF EMPLOYER — PHONE

David F. Cash — Navy Petty Officer—Grade 8 (active status)
SPOUSE OR PARENT — OCCUPATION

United States Navy — HHC, 2nd Batt, 26th Infantry, APO New York, NY, 10030
EMPLOYER — ADDRESS — PHONE

TRICARE Standard — David Cash (DOB 4-22-70)
NAME OF INSURANCE — INSURED OR SUBSCRIBER

767-XX-9080
POLICY/CERTIFICATE NO. — GROUP NO.

REFERRED BY: Hugh R. Foot, MD, 2010 Main St., Woodland Hills, XY 12345 — NPI #61 25099XX

DATE	PROGRESS NOTES
1-4-xx	New pt, referred by Dr. Foot comes in complaining of head pain which began yesterday. Performed an EPF history and physical exam. Lt parietal area of skull slightly tender, some redness of scalp. Pain localized and not consistent with HA syndromes. Rest of exam N. Imp: head pain, undetermined nature, possible cyst. Apply hot compresses and observe. Take Ibuprofen for pain prn (200 mg up to 2 q. 4 h). Retn in 1 wk, no disability from work (SF/MDM).
	CC/llf Clarence Cutler, MD
1-11-xx	Pt retns and states that the hot compresses have helped but is concerned with some swelling in area. On exam noticed slt elevation of skin in lt parietal area of scalp, no warmth over area. Slt pain on palpation. Exam otherwise neg. Imp: Subcutaneous nodule. Continue with same tx plan: Hot compresses daily and Ibuprofen prn. Retn in 2 to 3 wks if not resolved (PF HX/PX SF/MDM).
	CC/llf Clarence Cutler, MD
2-3-xx	Pt retns for reexamination of parietal skull. Elevation of skin still persisting. It has now come to a head, is warm to the touch, and consistent with an inflammatory cystic lesion. A decision is made to excise the benign lesion. Scalp cyst, 1.5 cm removed under procaine block with knife dissection; closed wound with six #000 black silk sutures. Adv to retn 1 wk for removal of sutures (EPF HX/PX LC/MDM).
	CC/llf Clarence Cutler, MD
2-10-xx	Pt presents for suture removal. Sutures removed and slight oozing occurs in midsection of wound. Wound dressed and pt advised to apply antibacterial cream daily. Retn in 4 to 5 days for final check (PF HX/PX SF/MDM).
	CC/llf Clarence Cutler, MD
2-15-xx	Pt presents for PO check of head wound. Parietal area healed well. RTO prn (PF HX/PX SF/MDM).
	CC/llf Clarence Cutler, MD

Figure 11

Acct No. T-9

STATEMENT
Financial Account
COLLEGE CLINIC
4567 Broad Avenue
Woodland Hills, XY 12345-0001
Tel. 555-486-9002
Fax No. 555-487-8976

Darlene M. Cash
5729 Redwood Avenue
Woodland Hills, XY 12345

Phone No. (H) 555-666-8901 (W) 555-678-1076 Birthdate 3/15/70

Primary Insurance Co. TRICARE Standard Policy/Group No. 767-XX-9080

Secondary Insurance Co. Policy/Group No.

DATE	REFERENCE	DESCRIPTION	CHARGES	CREDITS PYMNTS.	CREDITS ADJ.	BALANCE
20xx		BALANCE FORWARD →				
1-4-xx		NP OV				
1-11-xx		OV				
2-3-xx		OV				
2-3-xx		Excision inflammatory cystic scalp lesion				
2-10-xx		OV				
2-15-xx		OV				

PLEASE PAY LAST AMOUNT IN BALANCE COLUMN

THIS IS A COPY OF YOUR FINANCIAL ACCOUNT AS IT APPEARS ON OUR RECORDS

Figure 12

TEST 10: COMPLETE TWO CLAIM FORMS FOR A PRIVATE PLAN

Performance Objective

Task: Complete two CMS-1500 (08-05) claim forms for a private case and post transactions to the patient's financial accounting record.

Conditions: Use the patient's record (Figure 13) and financial statement (Figure 14); two health insurance claim forms; a computer or pen; procedural and diagnostic code books; and Appendixes A and B in this *Workbook*.

Standards: Claim Productivity Management

Time: ____________________ minutes

Accuracy: ____________________

(Note: The time element and accuracy criteria may be given by your instructor.)

Directions

1. Using OCR guidelines, complete two CMS-1500 (08-05) claim forms and direct them to the private carrier. Refer to Gertrude C. Hamilton's patient record for information and Appendix A in this *Workbook* to locate the fees to record on the claim, and post them to the financial statement. Date the first claim August 15 and the second one October 15. Dr. Cardi is accepting assignment, and the patient's signatures to release information to the insurance company and to have the payment forwarded directly to the physician are on file.

2. Use your CPT code book or Appendix A in this *Workbook* to determine the correct five-digit code numbers and modifiers for each professional service rendered. Use your HCPCS Level II code book or refer to Appendix B in this *Workbook* for HCPCS procedure codes and modifiers. Use your diagnostic code books to code each active diagnosis. Frequently, surgeons wait to receive the pathology report before entering a final diagnosis on the claim form. In this case, the claim was submitted before the pathology report was received. If your instructor tells you to also find the ICD-10-CM codes, a draft version may be downloaded from the following website: http://www.cdc.gov/nchs/icd/icd10cm.htm#10update.

3. Record the proper information on the financial record and claim form, and note the date when you have billed the insurance company.

4. Mrs. Hamilton makes a payment of $200, check number 5362, on her account on October 26. Post the proper entry for this transaction.

PATIENT RECORD NO. T-10

LAST NAME	FIRST NAME	MIDDLE NAME	BIRTH DATE	SEX	HOME PHONE
Hamilton	Gertrude	C	03-06-57	F	555-798-3321

ADDRESS	CITY	STATE	ZIP CODE
5320 Phillips Street	Woodland Hills	XY	12345

CELL PHONE	PAGER NO.	FAX NO.	E-MAIL ADDRESS
555-399-4990	555-312-6677	555-798-3321	hamilton@wb.net

PATIENT'S SOC. SEC. NO.	DRIVER'S LICENSE
540-XX-7677	D9043557

PATIENT'S OCCUPATION	NAME OF COMPANY
retired secretary	

ADDRESS OF EMPLOYER	PHONE

SPOUSE OR PARENT	OCCUPATION
deceased	

EMPLOYER	ADDRESS	PHONE

NAME OF INSURANCE	INSURED OR SUBSCRIBER
Colonial Health Insurance, 1011 Main Street, Woodland Hills, XY 12345	self

POLICY/CERTIFICATE NO.	GROUP NO.
540XX7677	4566 (through previous employment)

REFERRED BY: Gerald Practon, MD, 4567 Broad Avenue, Woodland Hills, XY 12345

Figure 13

DATE	PROGRESS NOTES No. T-10
7-29-xx	Dr. Practon asked me to consult on this 57-year-old pt adm to College Hosp today.
	Duplex carotid ultrasonography indicates bilateral carotid stenosis. C/HX: Suffered CVA lt
	hemisphere 1 yr prior to adm. Marked rt arm & leg weakness c̄ weakness of rt face and
	slurring of speech. C/PE revealed lt carotid bruit, II/IV, & right carotid bruit, II/IV.
	Performed hand-held Doppler vascular study on bilateral carotids which indicated
	decreased blood flow. Adv brain scan and lt carotid thromboendarterectomy; rt carotid
	thromboendarterectomy at a later date H/MDM.
	PC/llf Perry Cardi, MD
7-30-xx	HV (EPF HX/PX MC/MDM). Dr. Practon asked me to take over pt's care. Pt had brain scan
	done today, ECG, and lab work.
	PC/llf Perry Cardi, MD
7-31-xx	HV (EPF HX/PX MC/MDM). Brain scan indicates prior CVA; no new findings. ECG, normal
	sinus rhythm with occasional premature ventricular contractions. Lab work WNL.
	Discussed test results with Mrs. Hamilton.
	PC/llf Perry Cardi, MD
8-1-xx	HV (PF HX/PX LC/MDM). Decision made for surgery, to be scheduled tomorrow.
	PC/llf Perry Cardi, MD
8-2-xx	Pt taken to the operative suite. Performed lt carotid thromboendarterectomy by neck
	incision (see op report). Surgery went as planned, pt in recovery.
	PC/llf Perry Cardi, MD
8-3-xx	HV (PF HX/PX SF/MDM). Operative site appears normal. Pt resting comfortably.
	PC/llf Perry Cardi, MD
8-4-xx	DC from hosp. Pt to be seen in ofc in 1 week.
	PC/llf Perry Cardi, MD
8-12-xx	PO OV (D HX/PX M/MDM). Discussed outcome of surgery. Pt making satisfactory
	progress. Adv rt carotid thromboendarterectomy. Pt would like it done as soon as possible;
	next month if there is an operative time. Scheduled surgery for September 16, 20XX at
	College Hospital.
	PC/llf Perry Cardi, MD
9-16-xx	Adm to College Hospital. Performed a D history, D physical examination, and SF medical
	decision making. Rt. carotid thromboendarterectomy performed by neck incision.
	DX: Rt carotid stenosis.
	PC/llf Perry Cardi, MD
9-17-xx	HV (PF HX/PX SF/MDM). Pt stable and doing well. Operative site looks good. Plan for
	discharge tomorrow.
	PC/llf Perry Cardi, MD
9-18-xx	DC from hosp to home. RTC 1 wk.
	PC/llf Perry Cardi, MD
9-25-xx	PO visit (PF HX/PX SF/MDM). Pt making satisfactory recovery. Her neighbor will monitor
	BP daily. Retn 1 month.
	PC/llf Perry Cardi, MD

Figure 13, cont'd

Acct. No . T-10

STATEMENT

COLLEGE CLINIC
4567 Broad Avenue
Woodland Hills, XY 12345-0001
Tel. 555-486-9002
Fax No. 555-487-8976

Gertrude C. Hamilton
5320 Phillips Street
Woodland Hills, XY 12345

Phone No. (H) (555) 798-3321 (W) ______ Birthdate 03-06-57

Insurance Co Colonial Health Insurance Policy/Group No. 540Xx7677 / 4566

	REFERENCE	DESCRIPTION	CHARGES	CREDITS PYMNTS.	CREDITS ADJ.	BALANCE
20xx		BALANCE FORWARD →				
7-29-xx		Inpatient consult				
7-30-xx		HV				
7-31-xx		HV				
8-1-xx		HV				
8-2-xx		L carotid thromboendarterectmy				
8-3-xx		HV				
8-4-xx		Discharge				
8-12-xx		PO OV				
9-16-xx		Admit				
9-16-xx		R carotid thromboendarterectomy				
9-17-xx		HV				
9-18-xx		Discharge				
9-25-xx		PO OV				

PLEASE PAY LAST AMOUNT IN BALANCE COLUMN

THIS IS A COPY OF YOUR FINANCIAL ACCOUNT AS IT APPEARS ON OUR RECORDS

Figure 14

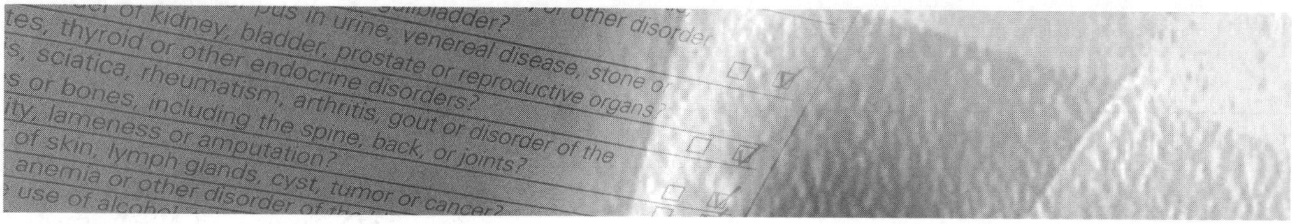

APPENDIX

A

College Clinic Office Policies and Mock Fee Schedule

College Clinic

In this simulation, you are employed as an insurance billing specialist for a group of medical doctors, other allied health specialists, and podiatrists. Each clinic is configured in its own unique way. The College Clinic has staff physicians that are employed, receive monthly pay checks, and are given Wage and Tax Statements (Forms W-2) at the end of the tax year. These doctors are on the staff of a nearby hospital, College Hospital.

Medical practices can have different configurations. For example, individuals or groups can be incorporated. Physicians can be independent contractors, running their own practices outside of the clinic, receive payment by the job and not a salary, and receive a Form 1099 at the end of the tax year.

Reference information to complete insurance claim forms for each assignment follows. Claim forms are to be submitted for the group unless a case involves a physician working as an independent contractor.

Office address:
College Clinic
4567 Broad Avenue
Woodland Hills, XY 12345-0001
Telephone: 555–486–9002
FAX: 555–487–8976
Clinic e-mail: cclinic@cmail.net
Staff e-mail: insert physician's last name followed by a period (.) then cclinic@cmail.net
(example: Pedro Atrics, MD, would have an e-mail address of atrics.cclinic@cmail.net)
Group practice, national provider identifier (NPI): 3664021CC
Medicare Durable Medical Equipment (DME) supplier number: 3400760001
Group tax ID #: XX12210XX

Hospital address:
College Hospital
4500 Broad Avenue
Woodland Hills, XY 12345-0001
Telephone: 555–487–6789
FAX: 555–486–8900
Hospital (NPI) national provider identifier: X950731067.

College Clinic Staff

Patient records in this *Workbook* include the doctors' names, specialties, subspecialties, and physicians' identification numbers of the College Clinic staff. They begin on the next page.

Table 1. College Clinic Staff

Name	Specialty (abbreviation)	Social Security No.*	State License No.	EIN No. or Federal Tax Identification No.	Medicare CMS-Assigned National Provider Identifier (NPI)†
Concha Antrum, MD	Otolaryngologist (OTO) or Ear, Nose, and Throat Specialist (ENT)	082–XX–1707	C 01602X	74–10640XX	12458977XX
Pedro Atrics, MD	Pediatrician (PD)	134–XX–7600	D 06012X	71–32061XX	37640017XX
Bertha Caesar, MD	Obstetrician and Gynecologist (OBG)	230–XX–6700	A 01817X	72–57130XX	43056757XX
Perry Cardi, MD	Internist (I) Subspecialty: Cardiovascular Disease (CD)	557–XX–9980	C 02140X	70–64217XX	67805027XX
Brady Coccidioides, MD	Internist (I) Subspecialty: Pulmonary Disease (PUD)	670–XX–0874	C 04821X	75–67321XX	64211067XX
Vera Cutis, MD	Dermatologist (D)	409–XX–8620	C 06002X	71–80561XX	70568717XX
Clarence Cutler, MD	General Surgeon (GS)	410–XX–5630	B 07600X	71–57372XX	43050047XX
Max Glutens, RPT	Physical Therapist (PT)	507–XX–4300	87610X	79–36500XX	65132277XX
Cosmo Graff, MD	Plastic Surgeon (PS)	452–XX–9899	C 08104X	74–60789XX	50307117XX
Malvern Grumose, MD	Pathologist (Path)	470–XX–2301	A 01602X	72–73651XX	72315621XX
Gaston Input, MD	Internist (I) Subspecialty: Gastroenterologist (GE)	211–XX–6734	C 08001X	75–67210XX	32783127XX
Adam Langerhans, MD	Endocrinologist	447–XX–6720	C 06051X	60–57831XX	47680657XX
Cornell Lenser, MD	Ophthalmologist (OPH)	322–XX–8963	C 06046X	61–78941XX	54037217XX
Michael Menter, MD	Psychiatrist (P)	210–XX–5302	C 07140X	73–66577XX	67301237XX
Astro Parkinson, MD	Neurosurgeon (NS)	210–XX–8533	C 02600X	75–44530XX	46789377XX
Nick Pedro, DPM	Podiatrist	233–XX–4300	E 08340X	62–74109XX	54022287XX
Gerald Practon, MD	General Practitioner (GP) or Family Practitioner (FP)	123–XX–6789	C 01402X	70–34597XX	46278897XX
Walter Radon, MD	Radiologist (R)	344–XX–6540	C 05001X	95–46137XX	40037227XX
Rex Rumsey, MD	Proctologist (Proct)	337–XX–9743	C 03042X	95–32601XX	01999047XX
Sensitive E. Scott, MD	Anesthesiologist (Anes)	220–XX–5655	C 02041X	72–54203XX	99999267XX
Raymond Skeleton, MD	Orthopedist (ORS, Orthop)	432–XX–4589	C 04561X	74–65412XX	12678547XX
Gene Ulibarri, MD	Urologist (U)	990–XX–3245	C 06430X	77–86531XX	25678831XX

*Social Security numbers are shown in the table because each individual is issued one and this is a realistic picture since they would be on file.
†Providers began using the NPI on May 23, 2007, except for small health plans, whose compliance date was May 23, 2008.

Abbreviations and Symbols

Abbreviations and symbols may appear on patient records, prescriptions, hospital charts, and patient ledger cards. Abbreviation styles differ, but the current trend is to omit periods in capital letter abbreviations except for doctors' academic degrees. For information on official American Hospital Association policy, refer to p. 108 in the *Handbook*. Following is a list of abbreviations and symbols used in this *Workbook* and their meanings.

Abbreviations

A	allergy
AB	antibiotics
Abdom	abdomen
abt	about
a.c.	before meals
Adj*	adjustment
adm	admit; admission; admitted
adv	advise(d)
aet	at the age of
agit	shake or stir
$AgNO_3$	silver nitrate
ALL	allergy
AM, a.m.	ante meridian (time—before noon)
ant	anterior
ante	before
AP	anterior-posterior; anteroposterior
approx	approximate
appt	appointment
apt	apartment
ASA	acetylsalicylic acid (aspirin)
ASAP	as soon as possible
ASCVD	arteriosclerotic cardiovascular disease
ASHD	arteriosclerotic heart disease
asst	assistant
auto	automated, automobile
AV	atrioventricular
Ba	barium (enema)
Bal/fwd*	balance forward
BE	barium enema
B/F*	balance forward; brought forward
b.i.d.	two times daily
BM	bowel movement
BMR	basal metabolic rate
BP	blood pressure
Brev	Brevital sodium
BX, bx	biopsy
C	cervical (vertebrae); comprehensive (history/examination)
Ca, CA	cancer, carcinoma
c/a*	cash on account
CABG	coronary artery bypass graft
CAT	computed axial tomography
cau	Caucasian
CBC	complete blood count
CBS	chronic brain syndrome
cc	cubic centimeter
CC	chief complaint
chr	chronic
ck*	check
cm	centimeter
CO, c/o	complains of; care of
compl, comp	complete; comprehensive
Con, CON, Cons	consultation
Cont	continue
CPX	complete physical examination
C&R	compromise and release
Cr*	credit
C&S	culture and sensitivity
cs, CS*	cash on account
C-section	cesarean section
CT	computed or computerized tomography
CVA	cardiovascular accident; cerebrovascular accident
CXR	chest radiograph
cysto	cystoscopy
D, d	diagnosis; detailed (history/examination); day(s)
D & C	dilatation and curettage
dc	discontinue
DC	discharge
DDS	Doctor of Dental Surgery
def*	charge deferred
Del	delivery; obstetrics and gynecology
Dg	diagnosis
dia	diameter
diag	diagnosis; diagnostic
dil	dilate (stretch, expand)
Disch	discharge
DM	diabetes mellitus
DNA	does not apply
DNS	did not show
DPM	Doctor of Podiatric Medicine
DPT	diphtheria, pertussis, and tetanus
Dr	Doctor
Dr*	debit
DRG	diagnosis-related group
Drs	dressing
DUB	dysfunctional uterine bleeding
Dx	diagnosis
E	emergency
EC*	error corrected
ECG, EKG	electrocardiogram; electrocardiograph
echo	echocardiogram; echocardiography
ED	emergency department
EDC	estimated date of confinement
EEG	electroencephalograph
EENT	eye, ear, nose, and throat
EGD	esophagogastroduodenoscopy
EKG, ECG	electrocardiogram; electrocardiograph
E/M	Evaluation and Management (*Current Procedural Terminology* code)
EMG	electromyogram
EPF	expanded problem-focused (history/examination)
epith	epithelial
ER	emergency room
Er, ER*	error corrected
ESR	erythrocyte sedimentation rate
est	established (patient); estimated

*Bookkeeping abbreviation.

Ex, exam	examination
exc	excision
Ex MO*	express money order
ext	external
24F, 28F	French (size of catheter)
F	female
FBS	fasting blood sugar
FH	family history
ft	foot, feet
FU	follow-up (examination)
fwd*	forward
Fx	fracture
gb, GB	gallbladder
GGE	generalized glandular enlargement
GI	gastrointestinal
Grav, grav	gravida, a pregnant woman; used with Roman numerals (I, II, III) to indicate the number of pregnancies
GU	genitourinary
H	hospital call
HA	headache
HBP	high blood pressure
HC	hospital call or consultation; high-complexity (decision-making)
HCD	house call (day)
HCN	house call (night)
Hct	hematocrit
HCVD	hypertensive cardiovascular disease
Hgb	hemoglobin
hist	history
hosp	hospital
H & P	history and physical (examination)
hr, hrs	hour, hours
h.s.	before bedtime
HS	hospital surgery
Ht	height
HV	hospital visit
HX, hx	history
HX PX	history and physical examination
I	injection
IC	initial consultation
I & D	incision and drainage
I/f*	in full
IM	intramuscular (injection)
imp, imp.	impression (diagnosis)
incl.	include; including
inflam	inflammation
init	initial (office visit)
inj, INJ	injection
ins, INS*	insurance
int	internal
intermed	intermediate (office visit)
interpret	interpretation
IUD	intrauterine device
IV	intravenous (injection)
IVP	intravenous pyelogram
K 35	Kolman (instrument used in urology)
KUB	kidneys, ureters, and bladder
L	left; laboratory

*Bookkeeping abbreviation.

lab, LAB	laboratory
lat	lateral; pertaining to the side
lbs	pounds
LC	low complexity (decision-making)
LMP	last menstrual period
LS	lumbosacral
lt	left
ltd	limited (office visit)
L & W	living and well
M	medication; married
MC	moderate-complexity (decision-making)
MDM	medical decision making
med	medicine
mg	milligram(s)
mg/dL	milligrams per deciliter
MI	myocardial infarction
micro	microscopy
mL, ml	milliliter
mo	month(s)
MO*	money order
N	negative
NA	not applicable
NAD	no appreciable disease
NC, N/C*	no charge
NEC	not elsewhere classifiable
neg	negative
NKA	no known allergies
NOS	not otherwise specified
NP	new patient
NYD	not yet diagnosed
OB, Ob-Gyn	obstetrics and gynecology
OC	office call
occ	occasional
OD	right eye
ofc	office
OP	outpatient
Op, op	operation
OR	operating room
orig	original
OS	office surgery; left eye
OV	office visit
oz	ounce
PA	posterior-anterior; posteroanterior
Pap	Papanicolaou (smear, stain, test)
Para I	woman having borne one child
PC	present complaint
p.c.	after meals
PCP	primary care physician
PD	permanent disability
Pd, PD*	professional discount
PE	physical examination
perf	performed
PF	problem-focused (history/examination)
PFT	pulmonary function test
PH	past history
Ph ex	physical examination
phys	physical
PID	pelvic inflammatory disease
PM, p.m.	post meridian (time—after noon)

PND	postnasal drip
PO, P Op	postoperative
p.o.	by mouth (per os)
post	posterior
postop	postoperative
PPD	purified protein derivative (such as in tuberculin test)
preop	preoperative
prep	prepared
PRN, p.r.n.	as necessary (pro re nata)
Proc	procedure
Prog	prognosis
P & S	permanent and stationary
PSA	prostate-specific antigen (blood test to determine cancer in prostate gland)
Pt, pt	patient
PT	physical therapy
PTR	patient to return
PVC	premature ventricular contraction
PVT ck*	private check received
PX	physical examination
q	every
qd	one time daily, every day
qh	every hour
q.i.d.	four times daily
QNS	quantity not sufficient
qod	every other day
R	right; residence call; report
RBC, rbc	red blood cell (count)
rec	recommend
rec'd	received
re ch	recheck
re-exam	reexamination
Reg	regular
ret, retn, rtn	return
rev	review
RHD	rheumatic heart disease
RN	registered nurse
R/O	rule out
ROA*	received on account
RPT	registered physical therapist
rt	right
RTC	return to clinic
RTO	return to office
RTW	return to work
RX, Rx, R_x	prescribe; prescription; any medication or treatment ordered
S	surgery
SC	subcutaneous
sched.	scheduled
SD	state disability
SE	special examination
SF	straightforward (decision-making)
Sig	directions on prescription
SLR	straight leg raising
slt	slight
Smr	smear
SOB	shortness of breath
Sp gr	specific gravity
SQ	subcutaneous (injection)
STAT	immediately
strep	Streptococcus
surg	surgery
Sx	symptom(s)
T	temperature
T & A	tonsillectomy and adenoidectomy
Tb, tb	tuberculosis
TD	temporary disability
tech	technician
temp	temperature
tet. tox.	tetanus toxoid
t.i.d.	three times daily
TPR	temperature, pulse, and respiration
Tr, trt	treatment
TURB	transurethral resection of bladder
TURP	transurethral resection of prostate
TX	treatment
u	units
UA, ua	urinalysis
UCHD	usual childhood diseases
UCR	usual, customary, and reasonable (fees)
UGI	upper gastrointestinal
UPJ	ureteropelvic junction or joint
UR	urinalysis
URI	upper respiratory infection
Urn	urinalysis
UTI	urinary tract infection
W	work; white
WBC, wbc	white blood cell (count); well baby care
WC	workers' compensation
wk	week; work
wks	weeks
WNL	within normal limits
Wr	Wassermann reaction (test for syphilis)
Wt, wt	weight
X	-xray, x-ray(s) times (e.g., 3X means three times)
XR	xray, x-ray(s)
yr(s)	year(s)

Symbols

+	positive
#	pound(s)
c̄, /c	with
s̄, /s	without
c̄c, c̄/c	with correction (eye glasses)
s̄c, s̄/c	without correction (eye glasses)
-	negative
ō	negative
⊕, +	positive
(L)	left
(R)	right
♂	male
♀	female
–*	charge already made
θ*	no balance due
√*	posted
($0.00)*	credit

*Bookkeeping abbreviation.

Laboratory Abbreviations

Abbreviation	*Definition*
ABG	arterial blood gas(es)
AcG	factor V (AcG or proaccelerin); a factor in coagulation that converts prothrombin to thrombin
ACTH	adrenocorticotropic hormone
AFB	acid-fast bacilli
A/C ratio	albumin-coagulin ratio
AHB	alpha-hydroxybutyric (dehydrogenase)
AHG	antihemophilic globulin; antihemolytic globulin (factor)
ALA	aminolevulinic acid
ALT	alanine aminotransferase (*see* SGPT)
AMP	adenosine monophosphate
APT test	aluminum-precipitated toxoid test
AST	aspartate aminotransferase (*see* SGOT)
ATP	adenosine triphosphate
BSP	bromsulfophthalein (Bromsulphalein; sodium sulfobromophthalein) (test)
BUN	blood urea nitrogen
CBC	complete blood count
CNS	central nervous system
CO	carbon monoxide
CPB	competitive protein binding: plasma
CPK	creatine phosphokinase
CSF	cerebrospinal fluid
D hemoglobin	hemoglobin fractionation by electrophoresis for hemoglobin D
DAP	direct agglutination pregnancy (Gravindex and DAP)
DEAE	diethylaminoethanol
DHT	dihydrotestosterone
diff	differential
DNA	deoxyribonucleic acid
DRT	test for syphilis
EACA	epsilon-aminocaproic acid (a fibrinolysin)
EMIT	enzyme-multiplied immunoassay technique (for drugs)
ENA	extractable nuclear antigen
esr, ESR	erythrocyte sedimentation (sed) rate
FDP	fibrin degradation products
FIGLU	formiminoglutamic acid
FRAT	free radical assay technique (for drugs)
FSH	follicle-stimulating hormone
FSP	fibrinogen split products
FTA	fluorescent-absorbed treponema antibodies
Gc, Gm, Inv	immunoglobulin typing
GG, gamma G, A, D, G, M	gamma-globulin (immunoglobulin fractionation by electrophoresis)
GG, gamma G E, RIA	immunization E fractionation by radioimmunoassay
GGT	gamma-glutamyl transpeptidase
GLC	gas liquid chromatography
GMP	guanosine monophosphate
GTT	glucose tolerance test
G6PD	glucose-6-phosphate dehydrogenase
HAA	hepatitis-associated agent (antigen)
HBD, HBDH	hydroxybutyrate dehydrogenase
HCT	hematocrit
hemoglobin, electrophoresis	letters of the alphabet used for different types or factors of hemoglobins (includes A_2, S, C, etc.)
Hgb	hemoglobin, qualitative
HGH	human growth hormone
HI	hemagglutination inhibition
HIA	hemagglutination inhibition antibody
HIAA	hydroxyindoleacetic acid (urine), 24-hour specimen
HIV	human immunodeficiency virus
HLA	human leukocyte antigen (tissue typing)

HPL	human placental lactogen
HTLV-III	antibody detection; confirmatory test
HVA	homovanillic acid
ICSH	interstitial cell–stimulating hormone
IFA	intrinsic factor, antibody (fluorescent screen)
IgA, IgE, IgG, IgM	immunoglobulins: quantitative by gel diffusion
INH	isonicotinic hydrazide, isoniazid
LAP	leucine aminopeptidase
LATS	long-acting thyroid-stimulating (hormone)
LDH	lactic dehydrogenase
LE Prep	lupus erythematosus cell preparation
L.E. factor	antinuclear antibody
LH	luteinizing hormone
LSD	lysergic acid diethylamide
L/S ratio	lecithin-sphingomyelin ratio
MC *(Streptococcus)*	antibody titer
MIC	minimum inhibitory concentration
NBT	nitro-blue tetrazolium (test)
OCT	ornithine carbamyl transferase
PAH	para-aminohippuric acid
PBI	protein-bound iodine
pco_2	arterial carbon dioxide pressure (or tension)
PCP	phencyclidine piperidine
pcv	packed cell volume
pH	symbol for expression of concentration of hydrogen ions (degree of acidity)
PHA	phenylalanine
PIT	prothrombin inhibition test
PKU	phenylketonuria—a metabolic disease affecting mental development
PO_2	oxygen pressure
P & P	prothrombin-proconvertin
PSP	phenolsulfonphthalein
PT	prothrombin time
PTA	plasma thromboplastin antecedent
PTC	plasma thromboplastin component; phenylthiocarbamide
PTT	prothrombin time; partial thromboplastin time (plasma or whole blood)
RBC, rbc	red blood cells (count)
RIA	radioimmunoassay
RISA	radioiodinated human serum albumin
RIST	radioimmunosorbent test
RPR	rapid plasma reagin (test)
RT_3U	resin triiodothyronine uptake
S-D	strength-duration (curve)
SGOT	serum glutamic oxaloacetic transaminase (*see* AST)
SGPT	serum glutamic pyruvic transaminase (*see* ALT)
STS	serologic test for syphilis
T_3	triiodothyronine (uptake)
TB	tubercle bacillus, tuberculosis
TBG	thyroxine-binding globulin
T & B differentiation, lymphocytes	thymus-dependent lymphs and bursa-dependent lymphs
THC	tetrahydrocannabinol (marijuana)
TIBC	total iron-binding capacity, chemical
TLC screen	thin-layer chromatography screen
TRP	tubular reabsorption of phosphates
UA	urinalysis
VDRL	Venereal Disease Research Laboratory (agglutination test for syphilis)
VMA	vanillylmandelic acid
WBC, wbc	white blood cells (count)

Mock Fee Schedule

Refer to the mock fee schedule (Table 2) to complete the financial accounting statements (ledgers) and claim forms in this *Workbook*. The fees listed are hypothetical and are intended only for use in completing the questions. For the cases that are private, Medicaid, TRICARE, and workers' compensation, use the amounts in the column labeled Mock Fees. For Medicare cases, refer to the three columns pertaining to Medicare and use the amounts in the column labeled Limiting Charge. Follow these instructions unless your instructor wishes you to round out the amounts on the fee schedule to the next dollar.

In a real medical practice, some offices round out the amounts to the next dollar unless the physician is nonparticipating with Medicare and then by Medicare regulations the provider can only bill the exact limiting amount on nonassigned claims. Other offices may have two fee schedules. Schedule B is for Medicare participating physicians and amounts are listed in dollars and cents. Schedule A is used for other plans and the amounts are rounded to the next dollar. However, if a fee schedule is sent by the insurance plan, then the medical practice may use the dollars and cents provided.

When completing the insurance claim forms, use the latest edition of *Current Procedural Terminology* (CPT), the professional code book published by the American Medical Association, to find the correct code numbers and modifiers for the services rendered. If you do not have access to the latest edition of CPT, you may use the code numbers provided in the mock fee schedule; however, do so with the understanding that the code numbers and descriptions provided in this schedule are not comprehensive. They are based on the information found in CPT; however, students are cautioned not to use it as a substitute for CPT. Because the code numbers are subject to change, every medical office must have on hand the most recent edition of CPT.

The mock fee schedule (Tables 2 and 3) is arranged in the same sequence as the six CPT code book sections (i.e., Evaluation and Management; Anesthesia; Surgery; Radiology, Nuclear Medicine, and Diagnostic Ultrasound; Pathology and Laboratory; and Medicine), with a comprehensive list of modifiers placed at the beginning. An index at the end of the mock fee schedule can assist you in locating code numbers. Mock fees for the modifiers are not listed, because these can vary from one claim to another, depending on the circumstances.

Remember that fees can vary with the region of the United States (West, Midwest, South, East), the specialty of the practitioner, the type of community (urban, suburban, or rural), the type of practice (incorporated or unincorporated, solo, partners, or shareholders), the overhead, and a number of other factors.

Table 2. College Clinic Mock Fee Schedule

Modifier Code Number	Description	Mock Fee ($)
-22	*Unusual Services:* When the service(s) provided is substantially greater than that usually required for the listed procedure, it may be identified by adding modifier -22 to the usual procedure code number. Documentation must support the substantial work and the reason for the additional work. This modifier cannot be appended to an E/M service.	Increase fee
-23	*Unusual Anesthesia:* Occasionally a procedure that usually requires either no anesthesia or local anesthesia must be done under general anesthesia because of unusual circumstances. These circumstances may be reported by adding the modifier -23 to the procedure code number of the basic service.	Increase fee
-24	*Unrelated Evaluation and Management Service by the Same Physician During a Postoperative Period:* The physician may need to indicate that an evaluation and management service was performed during a postoperative period for a reason(s) unrelated to the original procedure. This circumstance may be reported by adding the modifier -24 to the appropriate level of E/M service.	Variable per E/M fee
-25	*Significant, Separately Identifiable Evaluation and Management Service by the Same Physician on the Same Day of a Procedure or Other Service:* The physician may need to indicate that on the day a procedure or service identified by a CPT code was performed, the patient's condition required a significant, separately identifiable E/M service above and beyond the other service provided or beyond the usual preoperative and postoperative care associated with the procedure that was performed. The E/M service may be prompted by the symptom or condition for which the procedure and/or service was provided. As such, different diagnoses are not required for reporting of the E/M services on the same date. This circumstance may be reported by adding the modifier -25 to the appropriate level of E/M service. NOTE: This modifier is not used to report an E/M service that resulted in a decision to perform surgery. See modifier -57.	Variable per E/M fee

Table 2. College Clinic Mock Fee Schedule—cont'd

Modifier Code Number	Description	Mock Fee ($)
-26	*Professional Component:* Certain procedures are a combination of a physician component and a technical component. When the physician component is reported separately, the service may be identified by adding the modifier -26 to the usual procedure code number.	Decrease fee
-32	*Mandated Services:* Services related to mandated consultation and/or related services (e.g., PRO, third-party payer) may be identified by adding the modifier -32 to the basic procedure.	Use standard fee
-47	*Anesthesia by Surgeon:* Regional or general anesthesia provided by the surgeon may be reported by adding the modifier -47 to the basic service (this does not include local anesthesia). **Note:** Modifier -47 would not be used as a modifier for the anesthesia procedures 00100 through 01999.	Increase fee
-50	*Bilateral Procedure:* Unless otherwise identified in the listings, bilateral procedures that are performed at the same operative session should be identified by the appropriate five-digit code number describing the first procedure. The second (bilateral) procedure is identified by adding modifier -50 to the procedure code number.	Paid at 50% of standard fee
-51	*Multiple Procedures:* When multiple procedures other than E/M services are performed at the same session by the same provider, the primary procedure or service may be reported as listed. The additional procedure(s) or service(s) may be identified by adding the modifier -51 to the additional procedure or service code(s). **Note:** This modifier should not be appended to designated "add-on" codes.	Second procedure usually paid at 50% of fee. Third procedure usually paid at 25% of fee. Fourth and subsequent procedures usually paid at 10% of fee.
-52	*Reduced Services:* Under certain circumstances a service or procedure is partially reduced or eliminated at the physician's discretion. Under these circumstances, the service provided can be identified by its usual procedure number and the addition of the modifier -52, signifying that the service is reduced. This provides a means of reporting reduced services without disturbing the identification of the basic service. **Note:** For hospital outpatient reporting of a previously scheduled procedure/service that is partially reduced or canceled as a result of extenuating circumstances or those that threaten the well-being of the patient before or after administration of anesthesia, see modifiers -73 and -74.	Decrease fee
-53	*Discontinued Procedure:* Under certain circumstances, the physician may elect to terminate a surgical or diagnostic procedure. Due to extenuating circumstances or those that threaten the well-being of the patient, it may be necessary to indicate that a surgical or diagnostic procedure was started but discontinued. This circumstance may be reported by adding modifier -53 to the code reported by the physician for the discontinued procedure. **Note:** This modifier is not used to report the elective cancellation of a procedure before the patient's anesthesia induction and/or surgical preparation in the operating suite. For outpatient hospital/ambulatory surgery center (ASC) reporting of a previously scheduled procedure/service that is partially reduced or canceled as a result of extenuating circumstances or those that threaten the well-being of the patient before or after administration of anesthesia, see modifiers -73 and -74 (see modifiers approved for ASC hospital outpatient use).	Decrease fee
-54	*Surgical Care Only:* When one physician performs a surgical procedure and another provides preoperative and/or postoperative management, surgical services may be identified by adding the modifier -54 to the usual procedure number.	Decrease fee

Continued

Table 2. College Clinic Mock Fee Schedule—cont'd

Modifier Code Number	Description	Mock Fee ($)
-55	*Postoperative Management Only:* When one physician performs the postoperative management and another physician performs the surgical procedure, the postoperative component may be identified by adding modifier -55 to the usual procedure number.	Decrease fee
-56	*Preoperative Management Only:* When one physician performs the preoperative care and evaluation and another physician performs the surgical procedure, the preoperative component may be identified by adding the modifier -56 to the usual procedure number.	Decrease fee
-57	*Decision for Surgery:* An evaluation and management service that resulted in the initial decision to perform the surgery may be identified by adding the modifier -57 to the appropriate level of E/M service.	Use standard fee
-58	*Staged or Related Procedure or Service by the Same Physician During the Postoperative Period:* The physician may need to indicate that the performance of a procedure or service during the postoperative period was: (a) planned prospectively at the time of the original procedure (staged); (b) more extensive than the original procedure; or (c) for therapy following a diagnostic surgical procedure. This circumstance may be reported by adding the modifier -58 to the staged or related procedure. NOTE: This modifier is not used to report the treatment of a problem that requires a return to the operating room. See modifier -78.	Variable
-59	*Distinct Procedural Service:* Under certain circumstances, the physician may need to indicate that a procedure or service was distinct or independent from other services performed on the same day. Modifier -59 is used to identify procedures/services that are not normally reported together, but are appropriate under the circumstances. This may represent a different session or patient encounter, different procedure or surgery, different site or organ system, separate incision/excision, separate lesion, or separate injury (or area of injury in extensive injuries) not ordinarily encountered or performed on the same day by the same physician. However, when another already established modifier is appropriate it should be used rather than modifier -59. Only if no more descriptive modifier is available, and the use of modifier -59 best explains the circumstances, should modifier -59 be used.	Variable
-62	*Two Surgeons:* Under certain circumstances the skills of two surgeons (usually with different skills) may be required in the management of a specific surgical procedure. Under such circumstances the separate services may be identified by adding the modifier -62 to the procedure number used by each surgeon for reporting his or her services. NOTE: If a co-surgeon acts as an assistant in the performance of additional procedure(s) during the same surgical session, those services may be reported using separate procedure code(s) with the modifier -80 or modifier -81 added, as appropriate.	Use standard fee
-63	*Procedure Performed on Infants less than 4 kg:* Procedures performed on neonates and infants up to a present body weight of 4 kg may involve significantly increased complexity and physician work commonly associated with these patients. This circumstance may be reported by adding the modifier -63 to the procedure number (20000 through 69990).	
-66	*Surgical Team:* Under some circumstances, highly complex procedures (requiring the concomitant services of several physicians, often of different specialties, plus other highly skilled, specially trained personnel and various types of complex equipment) are carried out under the "surgical team" concept. Such circumstances may be identified by each participating physician with the addition of the modifier -66 to the basic procedure code number used for reporting services.	Variable

Table 2. College Clinic Mock Fee Schedule—cont'd

Modifier Code Number	Description	Mock Fee ($)
–76	*Repeat Procedure by Same Physician:* The physician may need to indicate that a procedure or service was repeated subsequent to the original procedure or service. This circumstance may be reported by adding modifier –76 to the repeated service/procedure.	Decrease fee
–77	*Repeat Procedure by Another Physician:* The physician may need to indicate that a basic procedure or service performed by another physician had to be repeated. This situation may be reported by adding modifier –77 to the repeated procedure/service.	Decrease fee
–78	*Unplanned Return to the Operating Room for a Related Procedure During the Postoperative Period by the Same Physician:* The physician may need to indicate that another procedure was performed during the postoperative period of the initial procedure. When this subsequent procedure is related to the first and requires the use of the operating room, it may be reported by adding the modifier –78 to the related procedure. (For repeat procedures on the same day, see –76.)	Decrease fee
–79	*Unrelated Procedure or Service by the Same Physician During the Postoperative Period:* The physician may need to indicate that the performance of a procedure or service during the postoperative period was unrelated to the original procedure. This circumstance may be reported by using the modifier –79. (For repeat procedures on the same day, see –76.)	Use standard fee
–80	*Assistant Surgeon:* Surgical assistant services may be identified by adding the modifier –80 to the usual procedure number(s).	Billed and/or paid at approximately 20% of surgeon's fee
–81	*Minimum Assistant Surgeon:* Minimum surgical assistant services are identified by adding the modifier –81 to the usual procedure number.	Billed and/or paid at approximately 10% of surgeon's fee
–82	*Assistant Surgeon When Qualified Resident Surgeon Not Available:* The unavailability of a qualified resident surgeon is a prerequisite for use of modifier –82 appended to the usual procedure code number(s).	Decrease fee
–90	*Reference (Outside) Laboratory:* When laboratory procedures are performed by a party other than the treating or reporting physician and billed by the treating physician, the procedure may be identified by adding the modifier –90 to the usual procedure number.	Fee according to contract
–91	*Repeat Clinical Diagnostic Laboratory Test:* In the course of treatment of the patient, it may be necessary to repeat the same laboratory test on the same day to obtain subsequent (multiple) test results. Under these circumstances, the laboratory test performed can be identified by its usual procedure number and the addition of modifier –91. **Note:** This modifier may not be used when tests are rerun to confirm initial results; due to testing problems with specimens or equipment; or for any other reason when a normal, one-time, reportable result is all that is required. This modifier may not be used when other code(s) describe a series of test results (e.g., glucose tolerance tests, evocative/suppression testing). This modifier may only be used for laboratory test(s) performed more than once on the same day on the same patient.	Decrease fee
–92	*Alternative Laboratory Platform Testing:* When laboratory testing is performed using a kit or transportable instrument that wholly or in part consists of a single use, disposable analytical chamber, the service may be identified by adding modifier –92 to the usual laboratory procedure code (HIV testing 86701–86703). The test does not require permanent dedicated space; hence by its design, it may be hand carried or transported to the vicinity of the patient for immediate testing at the site, although location of the testing is not in itself determinative of the use of the modifier.	Use standard fee
–99	*Multiple Modifiers:* Under certain circumstances two or more modifiers may be necessary to completely delineate a service. In such situations modifier –99 should be added to the basic procedure, and other applicable modifiers may be listed as part of the description of the service.	Variable

Table 3. Mock Fee Schedule

			Medicare*		
Code Number	**Description**	**Mock Fees**	**Participating**	**Nonparticipating**	**Limiting Charge**
EVALUATION AND MANAGEMENT†					
Office					
New Patient					
99201	Level 1 Problem Focused	33.25	30.43	28.91	33.25
99202	Level 2 Expanded Prob Foc	51.91	47.52	45.14	51.91
99203	Level 3 Detailed	70.92	64.92	61.67	70.92
99204	Level 4 Comprehensive	106.11	97.13	92.27	106.11
99205	Level 5 Comprehensive	132.28	121.08	115.03	132.28
Established Patient					
99211	Level 1 Nurse Visit	16.07	14.70	13.97	16.07
99212	Level 2 Problem Focused	28.55	26.14	24.83	28.55
99213	Level 3 Expanded Prob Foc	40.20	36.80	34.96	40.20
99214	Level 4 Comprehensive	61.51	56.31	53.79	61.51
99215	Level 5 Comprehensive	96.97	88.76	84.32	96.97
Hospital					
Observation Services (new or established patient)					
99217	Observation Care Dischg	66.88	61.22	58.16	66.88
99218	Dhx/exam SF/LC MDM	74.22	67.94	64.54	74.22
99219	Chx/exam MC MDM	117.75	107.78	102.39	117.75
99220	Chx/exam HC MDM	147.48	134.99	128.24	147.48
Inpatient Services (new or established patient)					
99221	30 min Dhx, Dpx, SF or low MDM	73.00	66.84	63.48	73.00
99222	50 min Comp/Comp/Moderate	120.80	110.57	105.04	120.80
99223	70 min Comp/Comp/High MDM	152.98	140.03	133.03	152.98
Subsequent Hospital Care					
99231	15 min PF, PF, SF MDM	37.74	34.55	32.82	37.74
99232	25 min EPF, EPF, Moderate	50.85	48.31	55.56	
99233	35 min D, D, HC MDM	76.97	70.45	66.93	76.97
99238	Discharge <30 min	65.26	59.74	56.75	65.26
99239	Discharge >30 min				
Consultations					
Office (new or established patient)					
99241	Level 1 PF, PF, SF	51.93	47.54	45.16	51.93
99242	Level 2 EPF, EPF, SF	80.24	73.44	69.77	80.24
99243	Level 3 D, D, LC MDM	103.51	94.75	90.01	103.51
99244	Level 4 C, C, Moderate MDM	145.05	132.77	126.13	145.05
99245	Level 5 C, C, HC MDM	195.45	178.93	169.98	195.45
Inpatient (new or established patient)					
99251	Level 1 PF, PF, SF	53.29	48.78	46.34	53.29
99252	Level 2 EPF, EPF, SF	80.56	73.74	70.05	80.56
99253	Level 3 D, D, LC MDM	106.10	97.12	92.26	106.10
99254	Level 4 C, C, Moderate MDM	145.26	132.96	126.31	145.26
99255	Level 5 C, C, HC MDM	196.55	179.91	170.91	196.55
Emergency Department (new/established patient)					
99281	PF hx/exam SF MDM	24.32	22.26	21.15	24.32
99282	EPF hx/exam LC MDM	37.02	33.88	32.19	37.02
99283	EPF hx/exam MC MDM	66.23	60.62	57.59	66.23
99284	D hx/exam MC MDM	100.71	92.18	87.57	100.71
99285	C hx/exam HC MDM	158.86	145.41	138.14	158.86

*Some services and procedures may not be considered a benefit under the Medicare program and when listed on a claim form, no reimbursement may be received. However, it is important to include these codes when billing because Medicare policies may change without an individual knowing of a new benefit. For this reason, some of the services shown in this mock fee schedule do not have any amounts listed under the three Medicare columns.

†See Tables 6–3 and 6–4 in the *Handbook* for more descriptions of E/M codes 99201 through 99255.

Table 3. Mock Fee Schedule—cont'd

Code Number	Description	Mock Fees	Medicare* Participating	Medicare* Nonparticipating	Medicare* Limiting Charge
Critical Care Services					
99291	First hour	208.91	191.22	181.66	208.91
99292	Each addl. 30 min	102.02	92.46	87.84	102.02
Neonatal Intensive Care					
99468	Initial	892.74	817.16	776.30	892.74
99469	Subsequent unstable case	418.73	383.27	364.11	418.73
Initial Nursing Facility					
99304	25 min (Low Severity)	64.11	58.68	55.75	64.11
99305	35 min (Moderate Severity)	90.55	82.88	78.74	90.55
99306	45 min (High Severity)	136.76	125.18	118.92	136.76
Subsequent NF Care					
99307	PF hx/exam SF DM	37.95	34.74	33.00	37.95
99308	15 min EPF hx/exam LC DM	55.11	50.44	47.92	55.11
99309	25 min D hx/exam MC DM	69.61	63.72	60.53	69.61
99310	35 min C hx/exam HC DM	84.73	77.00	73.14	84.73
Domiciliary, Rest Home, Custodial Care					
New Patient					
99324	PF hx/exam SF DM	46.10	42.20	40.09	46.10
99325	EPF hx/exam LC DM	65.02	59.53	56.54	65.02
99326	D hx/exam MC DM	86.18	78.88	74.94	86.18
99327	C hx/exam MC DM	107.34	98.23	93.34	107.34
99328	C hx/exam HC DM	128.50	117.58	111.74	128.50
Established Patient					
99334	PF hx/exam SF MDM	37.31	34.15	32.44	37.31
99335	EPF hx/exam LC MDM	49.22	45.05	42.80	49.22
99336	D hx/exam Moderate MDM	60.61	55.47	52.70	60.61
99337	C hx/exam M-H DM	72.00	65.89	62.60	72.00
Home Services					
New Patient					
99341	PF hx/exam SF DM	70.32	64.37	61.15	70.32
99342	EPF hx/exam LC DM	91.85	84.07	79.87	91.85
99343	D hx/exam MC DM	120.24	110.06	104.56	120.24
99344	C hx/exam MC DM	148.63	136.05	129.25	148.63
99345	C hx/exam HC DM	177.02	162.04	153.50	177.02
Established Patient					
99347	PF hx/exam SF DM	54.83	50.19	47.68	54.83
99348	EPF hx/exam LC DM	70.06	64.13	60.92	70.06
99349	D hx/exam MC DM	88.33	80.85	76.81	88.33
99350	C hx/exam M-H DM	106.60	97.57	92.70	106.60
Prolonged Services With Direct (Face-to-Face) Patient Contact (Report in Addition to the Designated E/M Service at Any Level)					
Outpatient					
99354	First hour	96.97	88.76	84.32	96.97
99355	Each addl. 30 min	96.97	88.76	84.32	96.97
Inpatient					
99356	First hour	96.42	88.25	83.84	96.42
99357	Each addl. 30 min	96.42	88.25	83.84	96.42

*Some services and procedures may not be considered a benefit under the Medicare program and when listed on a claim form, no reimbursement may be received. However, it is important to include these codes when billing because Medicare policies may change without an individual knowing of a new benefit. For this reason, some of the services shown in this mock fee schedule do not have any amounts listed under the three Medicare columns.

Continued

Table 3. Mock Fee Schedule—cont'd

Code Number	Description	Mock Fees	Medicare*		
			Participating	Nonparticipating	Limiting Charge
Prolonged Services Without Direct Contact					
99358	First hour	90.00			
99359	Each addl. 30 min	90.00			
Physician Standby Service					
99360	Each 30 min	95.00			
Case Management Services					
Team Conferences					
99366		85.00			
99367-99368		105.00			
Telephone Calls					
99441	5-10 min	30.00			
99442	11-20 min	40.00			
99443	21-30 min	60.00			
Care Plan Oversight Services					
99375	30 min or more/month	93.40	85.49	81.22	93.40
Preventive Medicine					
New Patient					
99381	Infant younger than 1 year	50.00			
99382	1-4 years	50.00			
99383	5-11 years	45.00			
99384	12-17 years	45.00			
99385	18-39 years	50.00			
99386	40-64 years	50.00			
99387	65 years and older	55.00			
Established Patient					
99391	Infant younger than year	35.00			
99392	1-4 years	35.00			
99393	5-11 years	30.00			
99394	12-17 years	30.00			
99395	18-39 years	35.00			
99396	40-64 years	35.00			
99397	65 years and older	40.00			
Counseling (new/est pt)					
Individual					
99401	15 min	35.00			
99402	30 min	50.00			
99403	45 min	65.00			
99404	60 min	80.00			
Group					
99411	30 min	30.00			
99412	60 min	50.00			
Other Preventive Medicine Services					
99420	Health hazard appraisal	50.00			
99429	Unlisted preventive med service	variable			
Newborn Care					
99460	Birthing room delivery	102.50	93.50	88.83	102.15
99461	Other than birthing room	110.16	100.83	95.79	110.16
99462	Subsequent hospital care	54.02	49.44	46.97	54.02
99465	Newborn resuscitation	255.98	234.30	222.59	255.98

*Some services and procedures may not be considered a benefit under the Medicare program and when listed on a claim form, no reimbursement may be received. However, it is important to include these codes when billing because Medicare policies may change without an individual knowing of a new benefit. For this reason, some of the services shown in this mock fee schedule do not have any amounts listed under the three Medicare columns.

Table 3. Mock Fee Schedule—cont'd

Code Number	Description	Mock Fees	Medicare* Participating	Medicare* Nonparticipating	Medicare* Limiting Charge
Anesthesiology					
Anesthesiology fees are presented here for CPT codes. However, each case would require a fee for time, e.g., every 15 minutes would be worth $55. This fee is determined according to the relative value system, calculated, and added into the anesthesia (CPT) fee. Some anesthetists may list a surgical code using an anesthesia modifier on a subsequent line for carriers that do not acknowledge anesthesia codes.					
99100	Anes for pt younger than 1 yr or older than 70 years	55.00			
99116	Anes complicated use total hypothermia	275.00			
99135	Anes complicated use hypotension	275.00			
99140	Anes complicated emer cond	110.00			
Physician Status Modifier Codes					
P-1	Normal healthy patient	00.00			
P-2	Patient with mild systemic disease	00.00			
P-3	Patient with severe systemic disease	55.00			
P-4	Patient with severe systemic disease that is a constant threat to life	110.00			
P-5	Moribund pt not expected to survive without operation	165.00			
P-6	Declared brain-dead pt, organs being removed for donor	00.00			
Head					
00160	Anes nose/sinus (NEC)	275.00			
00172	Anes repair cleft palate	165.00			
Thorax					
00400	Anes for proc ant integumentary system of chest, incl SC tissue	165.00			
00402	Anes breast reconstruction	275.00			
00546	Anes pulmonary resection with thoracoplasty	275.00			
00600	Anes cervical spine and cord	550.00			
Lower Abdomen					
00800	Anes for proc lower ant abdominal wall	165.00			
00840	Anes intraperitoneal proc lower abdomen: NOS	330.00			
00842	Amniocentesis	220.00			
00914	Anes TURP	275.00			
00942	Anes colporrhaphy, colpotomy, colpectomy	220.00			
Upper Leg					
01210	Anes open proc hip joint; NOS	330.00			
01214	Total hip replacement	440.00			
Upper Arm and Elbow					
01740	Anes open proc humerus/elbow; NOS	220.00			
01758	Exc cyst/tumor humerus	275.00			

*Some services and procedures may not be considered a benefit under the Medicare program and when listed on a claim form, no reimbursement may be received. However, it is important to include these codes when billing because Medicare policies may change without an individual knowing of a new benefit. For this reason, some of the services shown in this mock fee schedule do not have any amounts listed under the three Medicare columns.

Continued

Table 3. Mock Fee Schedule—cont'd

Code Number	Description	Mock Fees	Medicare* Participating	Medicare* Nonparticipating	Medicare* Limiting Charge
Radiologic Procedures					
01922	Anes CAT scan	385.00			
Miscellaneous Procedure(s)					
01999	Unlisted anes proc	variable			
Neurology					
95812	Electroencephalogram	129.32	118.37	112.45	129.32
95819	Electroencephalogram—awake	126.81	116.07	110.27	126.81
95860	Electromyography, 1 extremity	88.83	81.31	77.24	88.83
95864	Electromyography, 4 extremities	239.99	219.67	208.69	239.99
96101	Psychological testing (per hour)	80.95	74.10	70.39	80.95
Physical Medicine					
97024	Diathermy	14.27	13.06	12.41	14.27
97036	Hubbard tank, each 15 min	24.77	22.67	21.54	24.77
97110	Therapeutic proc, one or more areas, each 15 min	23.89	21.86	20.77	23.89
97140	Manual therapy (manipulation, traction), one or more regions, each 15 min	16.93	15.49	14.72	16.93
Special Services and Reports					
99000	Handling of specimen (transfer from Dr.'s office to lab)	5.00			
99024	Postoperative visit (bundled)	No Charge			
99050	Services provided, in the office at times other than regularly scheduled office hours or days when office is normally closed (e.g., holidays, Saturday or Sunday) in addition to basic service	25.00			
99053	Services between 10:00 PM and 8:00 AM in addition to basic service (24 hr fac)	35.00			
99056	Services normally provided in office requested by pt in location other than office in addition to basic service	20.00			
99058	Office services provided on an emergency basis which causes disruption of other sched svcs.				
99070	Supplies and materials (itemize drugs and materials provided)	10.00			
99080	Special reports: insurance forms				
	Review of data to clarify pt's status	20.00			
	WC reports	50.00			
	WC extensive review report	250.00			

*Some services and procedures may not be considered a benefit under the Medicare program and when listed on a claim form, no reimbursement may be received. However, it is important to include these codes when billing because Medicare policies may change without an individual knowing of a new benefit. For this reason, some of the services shown in this mock fee schedule do not have any amounts listed under the three Medicare columns.

Table 3. Mock Fee Schedule—cont'd

			Medicare			
Code Number	Description	Mock Fees	Participating	Non-participating	Limiting Charge	Follow-Up Days*
10060	I & D furuncle, onychia, paronychia; single	75.92	69.49	66.02	75.92	10
11040	Débridement; skin, partial thickness	79.32	75.60	68.97	79.32	10
11044	Débridement; skin, subcu. muscle, bone	269.28	246.48	234.16	269.28	10
11100	Biopsy of skin, SC tissue &/or mucous membrane; 1 lesion	65.43	59.89	56.90	65.43	10
11200	Exc, skin tags; up to 15	55.68	50.97	45.42	55.68	10
11401	Exc, benign lesion, 0.6-1.0 cm trunk, arms, legs	95.62	87.53	83.15	96.62	10
11402	1.1-2.0 cm	121.52	111.23	105.67	121.52	10
11403	2.1-3.0 cm	151.82	138.97	132.02	151.82	10
11420	Exc, benign lesion, 0.5 cm or less scalp, neck, hands, feet, genitalia	75.44	69.05	65.60	75.44	10
11422	Exc, benign lesion scalp, neck, hands, feet, or genitalia; 1.1-2.0 cm	131.35	120.23	114.22	131.35	10
11441	Exc, benign lesion face, ears, eyelids, nose, lips, or mucous membrane	119.08	109.00	103.55	119.08	10
11602	Exc, malignant lesion, trunk, arms, or legs; 1.1-2.0 cm dia	195.06	178.55	169.62	195.06	10
11719	Trimming of nondystrophic nails, any number	30.58	27.82	26.33	30.58	0
11720	Débridement of nails, any method, 1-5	32.58	29.82	28.33	32.58	0
11721	6 or more	32.58	29.82	28.33	32.58	0
11730	Avulsion nail plate, partial or complete, simple repair; single	76.91	70.40	66.88	76.91	0
11750	Exc, nail or nail matrix, partial or complete	193.45	177.07	168.22	193.45	10
11765	Wedge excision of nail fold	57.95	53.04	50.39	57.95	10
12001	Simple repair (scalp, neck, axillae, ext genitalia, trunk, or extremities incl hands & feet); 2.5 cm or less	91.17	83.45	79.28	91.17	10
12011	Simple repair (face, ears, eyelids, nose, lips, or mucous membranes); 2.5 cm or less	101.44	92.85	88.21	101.44	10
12013	2.6–5.0 cm	123.98	113.48	107.81	123.98	10
12032	Repair, scalp, axillae, trunk (intermediate)	169.73	155.36	147.59	169.73	10

*Data for the surgical follow-up days from St. Anthony's *CPT '96 Companion: A Guide to Medicare Billing.*

Continued

Table 3. Mock Fee Schedule—cont'd

Code Number	Description	Mock Fees	Medicare: Participating	Medicare: Non-participating	Medicare: Limiting Charge	Medicare: Follow-Up Days*
12034	Repair, intermediate, wounds (scalp, axillae, trunk, or extremities) excl hands or feet; 7.6-12.5 cm	214.20	196.06	186.26	214.20	10
12051	Repair, intermediate, layer closure of wounds (face, ears, eyelids, nose, lips, or mucous membranes); 2.5 cm or less	167.60	153.41	145.74	167.60	10
17000	Cauterization, 1 lesion	52.56	48.11	45.70	52.56	10
17003	Second through 14 lesions, each	15.21	17.77	16.88	15.21	
17004	Destruction (laser surgery), 15 or more lesions	52.56	48.11	45.70	52.56	10
19020	Mastotomy, drainage/ exploration deep abscess	237.36	217.26	206.40	237.36	90
19100	Biopsy, breast, needle	96.17	88.03	83.63	96.17	0
19101	Biopsy, breast, incisional	281.51	257.67	244.79	281.51	10
20610	Arthrocentesis, aspiration or injection major joint (shoulder, hip, knee, or bursa)	52.33	47.89	45.50	52.33	0
21330	Nasal fracture, open treatment complicated	599.46	548.71	521.27	599.46	90
24066	Biopsy, deep, soft tissue, upper arm, elbow	383.34	350.88	333.34	383.34	90
27455	Osteotomy, proximal tibia	1248.03	1142.36	1085.24	1248.03	90
27500	Treatment closed femoral shaft fracture without manipulation	554.90	507.92	482.52	554.90	90
27530	Treatment closed tibial fracture, proximal, without manipulation	344.24	315.09	299.34	344.24	90
27750	Treatment closed tibial shaft fracture, without manipulation	400.94	366.99	348.64	400.94	90
27752	With manipulation	531.63	486.62	462.29	531.63	90
29280	Strapping of hand or finger	35.13	31.36	29.79	35.13	0
29345	Appl long leg cast (thigh to toes)	123.23	112.80	107.16	123.23	0
29355	Walker or ambulatory type	133.75	122.42	116.30	133.75	0
29425	Appl short leg walking cast	102.10	93.45	88.78	102.10	0
30110	Excision, simple nasal polyp	145.21	132.92	126.27	145.21	10
30520	Septoplasty	660.88	604.93	574.68	660.88	90
30903	Control nasal hemorrhage; unilateral	118.17	108.17	102.76	118.17	0

*Data for the surgical follow-up days from St. Anthony's *CPT '96 Companion: A Guide to Medicare Billing.*

Table 3. Mock Fee Schedule—cont'd

Code Number	Description	Mock Fees	Medicare Participating	Medicare Non-participating	Medicare Limiting Charge	Medicare Follow-Up Days*
30905	Control nasal hemorrhage, posterior with posterior nasal packs and/or cautery; initial	190.57	174.43	165.71	190.57	0
30906	Subsequent	173.01	158.36	150.44	173.01	0
31540	Laryngoscopy with excision of tumor and/or stripping of vocal cords	488.95	447.55	425.17	488.95	0
31541	With operating microscope	428.33	392.06	372.46	428.33	0
31575	Laryngoscopy, flexible fiberoptic; diagnostic	138.48	126.76	120.42	138.48	0
31625	Bronchoscopy with biopsy	312.87	286.38	272.06	312.87	0
32310	Pleurectomy	1234.79	1130.24	1073.73	1234.79	90
32440	Pneumonectomy, total	1972.10	1805.13	1714.87	1972.10	90
33020	Pericardiotomy	1289.25	1180.09	1121.09	1289.25	90
33206	Insertion of pacemaker; atrial	728.42	666.75	633.41	728.42	90
33208	Atrial and ventricular	751.57	687.89	653.50	751.57	90
35301	Thromboendarterectomy, with or without patch graft; carotid, vertebral, subclavian, by neck incision	1585.02	1450.82	1378.28	1585.02	90
36005	Intravenous injection for contrast venography	59.18	54.17	51.46	59.18	0
36248	Catheter placement (selective) arterial system, 2nd, 3rd order and beyond	68.54	62.74	59.60	68.54	0
36415	Routine venipuncture for collection of specimen(s)	10.00	—	—	—	XXX
38101	Splenectomy, partial	994.44	910.24	864.73	994.44	90
38220	Bone marrow; aspiration only	73.52	67.29	63.93	73.52	NA
38221	Biopsy, needle or trocar	90.65	82.98	78.83	90.65	NA
38510	Biopsy/excision deep cervical node/s	327.42	299.69	284.71	327.42	10
39520	Hernia repair	1436.50	1314.87	1249.13	1436.50	90
42820	T & A under age 12 years	341.63	312.71	297.07	341.63	90
42821	T & A over age 12 years	410.73	375.96	357.16	410.73	90
43234	Upper GI endoscopy, simple primary exam	201.86	184.77	175.53	201.86	0
43235	Upper GI endoscopy incl esophagus, stomach, duodenum, or jejunum; complex	238.92	218.69	207.76	238.92	0
43255	With control of bleeding, any method	281.51	257.67	244.79	281.51	0
43456	Dilation esophagus	254.52	232.97	221.32	254.52	0
43820	Gastrojejunostomy	971.86	889.58	845.10	971.86	90
44150	Colectomy, total, abdominal	1757.81	108.98	1528.53	1757.81	90
44320	Colostomy or skin level cecostomy	966.25	884.44	840.22	966.25	90

*Data for the surgical follow-up days from St. Anthony's *CPT'96 Companion: A Guide to Medicare Billing.*
NA = Not Applicable

Continued

Table 3. Mock Fee Schedule—cont'd

			Medicare			
Code Number	Description	Mock Fees	Participating	Non-participating	Limiting Charge	Follow-Up Days*
44950	Appendectomy	568.36	520.24	494.23	568.36	90
45308	Proctosigmoidoscopy; removal of polyp	135.34	123.88	117.69	135.34	0
45315	Multiple polyps	185.12	169.44	160.97	185.12	0
45330	Sigmoidoscopy (flexible), diagnostic (with or without biopsy or collection of specimen by brushing or washing)	95.92	87.80	83.41	95.92	0
45333	Sigmoidoscopy (flexible) with removal of polyps	183.99	168.41	159.99	183.99	0
45380	Colonoscopy with biopsy	382.35	349.98	332.48	382.35	0
46255	Hemorrhoidectomy int & ext, simple	503.57	460.94	437.89	503.57	90
46258	Hemorrhoidectomy with fistulectomy	636.02	582.17	553.06	636.02	90
46600	Anoscopy; diagnostic	32.86	30.07	28.57	32.86	0
46614	With control of hemorrhage	182.10	166.68	158.35	182.10	0
46700	Anoplasty, for stricture, adult	657.39	601.73	571.64	657.39	90
47562	Cholecystectomy; laparoscopic	714.99	654.45	621.73	714.99	90
47600	Cholecystectomy; abdominal excision	937.74	858.35	815.43	937.74	90
49505	Inguinal hernia repair, age 5 or over	551.07	504.41	479.19	551.07	90
49520	Repair, inguinal hernia, any age; reducible	671.89	615.00	584.25	671.89	90
50080	Nephrostolithotomy, percutaneous	1323.93	1211.83	1151.24	1323.93	90
50780	Ureteroneocystostomy	1561.23	1429.84	1357.59	1561.23	90
51900	Closure of vesicovaginal fistula, abdominal approach	1196.82	1095.48	1040.71	1196.82	90
52000	Cystourethroscopy	167.05	152.90	145.26	167.05	0
52601	Transurethral resection of prostate	1193.53	1092.47	1037.85	1193.53	90
53040	Drainage of deep periurethral abscess	379.48	347.35	329.98	379.48	90
53060	Drainage of Skene's gland	147.45	134.97	128.22	147.45	10
53230	Excision, female diverticulum (urethral)	859.69	786.91	747.56	859.69	90
53240	Marsupialization of urethral diverticulum, M or F	520.11	476.07	452.27	520.11	90
53270	Excision of Skene's gland(s)	184.39	168.78	160.34	184.39	10
53620	Dilation, urethra, male	100.73	92.20	87.59	100.73	0
53660	Dilation urethra, female	48.32	44.23	42.02	48.32	0
54150	Circumcision	111.78	102.32	97.20	111.78	10
54520	Orchiectomy, simple	523.92	479.56	455.58	523.92	90
55700	Biopsy of prostate, needle or punch	156.22	142.99	135.84	156.22	0

*Data for the surgical follow-up days from St. Anthony's *CPT'96 Companion: A Guide to Medicare Billing*.

Table 3. Mock Fee Schedule—cont'd

Code Number	Description	Mock Fees	Medicare			
			Participating	Non-participating	Limiting Charge	Follow-Up Days*
55801	Prostatectomy, perineal subtotal	1466.56	1342.39	1275.27	1466.56	90
57265	Colporrhaphy AP with enterocele repair	902.24	825.85	784.56	902.24	90
57452	Colposcopy	84.18	77.05	73.20	84.18	0
57510	Cauterization of cervix, electro or thermal	115.15	105.40	100.13	115.15	10
57520	Conization of cervix with or without D & C, with or without repair	387.08	354.30	336.59	387.08	90
58100	Endometrial biopsy	71.88	65.79	62.50	71.88	0
58120	D & C, diagnostic and/or therapeutic (non-OB)	272.83	249.73	237.24	272.83	10
58150	TAH w/without salpingo-oophorectomy	1167.72	1068.85	1015.41	1167.72	90
58200	Total hysterectomy, extended, corpus	1707.24	1562.69	1484.56	1707.24	90
58210	Radical abdominal hysterectomy with bilateral total pelvic lymphadenectomy	2160.78	1977.83	1878.94	2160.78	90
58300	Insertion of intrauterine device	100.00	93.45	88.78	100.00	0
58340	Hysterosalpingography, inj proc for	73.06	66.87	63.53	73.06	0
58720	Salpingo-oophorectomy, complete or partial, unilateral or bilateral surgical treatment of ectopic pregnancy	732.40	670.39	636.87	732.40	90
59120	Ectopic pregnancy requiring salpingectomy and/or oophorectomy	789.26	722.43	686.31	789.26	90
59121	Without salpingectomy and/or oophorectomy	638.84	584.75	555.51	638.84	90
59130	Abdominal pregnancy	699.12	639.93	607.93	699.12	90
59135	Total hysterectomy, interstitial, uterine pregnancy	1154.16	1056.44	1003.62	1154.16	90
59136	Partial uterine resection, interstitial uterine pregnancy	1154.16	1056.44	1003.62	1154.16	90
59140	Cervical, with evacuation	489.68	448.22	425.81	489.68	90
59160	Curettage postpartum hemorrhage (separate proc)	293.46	268.61	255.18	293.46	10
59400	OB care—routine, inc. antepartum/postpartum care	1864.30	1706.45	1621.13	1864.30	N/A
59510	C-section including antepartum and postpartum care	2102.33	1924.33	1828.11	2102.33	N/A
59515	C-section, postpartum care only	1469.80	1345.36	1278.09	1469.80	N/A

*Data for the surgical follow-up days from St. Anthony's *CPT'96 Companion: A Guide to Medicare Billing.*

Continued

Table 3. Mock Fee Schedule—cont'd

			Medicare			
Code Number	Description	Mock Fees	Participating	Non-participating	Limiting Charge	Follow-Up Days*
59812	Treatment of incompl abortion, any trimester;	357.39	327.13	310.77	357.39	90
	completed surgically	357.39	327.13	310.77	357.39	90
61314	Craniotomy infratentorial	2548.09	2332.35	2215.73	2548.09	90
62270	Spinal puncture, lumbar; diagnostic	77.52	70.96	67.41	77.52	0
65091	Evisceration of eye, without implant	708.22	648.25	615.84	708.22	90
65205	Removal of foreign body, ext eye	56.02	51.27	48.71	56.02	0
65222	Removal of foreign body, corneal, with slit lamp	73.81	67.56	64.18	73.81	0
69420	Myringotomy	97.76	89.48	85.01	97.76	10

*Data for the surgical follow-up days from St. Anthony's *CPT'96 Companion: A Guide to Medicare Billing.*

Table 3. Mock Fee Schedule—cont'd

Code Number	Description	Mock Fees	Medicare* Participating	Medicare* Nonparticipating	Medicare* Limiting Charge
RADIOLOGY, NUCLEAR MEDICINE, AND DIAGNOSTIC ULTRASOUND					
70120	X-ray mastoids, less than 3 views per side	38.96	35.66	33.88	38.96
70130	Complete, min., 3 views per side	56.07	51.33	48.76	56.07
71010	Chest x-ray, 1 view	31.95	29.24	27.78	31.95
71020	Chest x-ray, 2 views	40.97	37.50	35.63	40.97
71030	Chest x-ray, compl, 4 views	54.02	49.44	46.97	54.02
71060	Bronchogram, bilateral	143.75	131.58	125.00	143.75
72100	X-ray spine, LS; 2 or 3 views	43.23	39.57	37.59	43.23
72114	Complete, incl. bending views	74.97	68.62	65.19	74.97
73100	X-ray wrist, 2 views	31.61	28.94	27.49	31.61
73500	X-ray hip, 1 view, 1 side	31.56	28.88	27.44	31.56
73540	X-ray pelvis & hips, infant or child, minimum 2 views	37.94	34.73	32.99	37.94
73590	X-ray tibia & fibula, 2 views	33.35	30.53	29.00	33.35
73620	Radiologic exam, foot; 2 views	31.61	28.94	27.49	31.61
73650	X-ray calcaneus, 2 views	30.71	28.11	26.70	30.71
74241	Radiologic exam, upper gastrointestinal tract; with/without delayed films with KUB	108.93	99.71	94.72	108.93
74245	With small bowel, serial films	161.70	148.01	140.61	161.70
74270	Barium enema	118.47	108.44	103.02	118.47
74290	Cholecystography, oral contrast	52.59	48.14	45.73	52.59
74400	Urography (pyelography), intravenous, with or without KUB	104.78	95.90	91.11	104.78
74410	Urography, infusion	116.76	106.87	101.53	116.76
74420	Urography, retrograde	138.89	127.13	120.77	138.89
75982	Percutaneous placement of drainage catheter	359.08	328.67	312.24	359.08
76805	Ultrasound, pregnant uterus, or real time; complete, first gestation	154.18	141.13	134.07	154.18
76810	Ultrasound, pregnant uterus, complete: each additional gestation, after first trimester	306.54	280.59	266.56	306.54
76946	Ultrasonic guidance for amniocentesis	91.22	83.49	79.32	91.22
77055	Mammography, unilateral	62.57	57.27	54.41	62.57
77056	Mammography, bilateral	82.83	75.82	72.03	82.83
77300	Radiation dosimetry	97.58	89.32	84.85	97.58
77315	Teletherapy, isodose plan, complex	213.59	195.51	185.73	213.59
78104	Bone marrow imaging, whole body	230.56	211.04	200.49	230.56
78215	Liver and spleen imaging	160.44	146.85	139.51	160.44
78800	Tumor localization, limited area	191.53	175.32	166.55	191.53

*Some services and procedures may not be considered a benefit under the Medicare program and when listed on a claim form, no reimbursement may be received. However, it is important to include these codes when billing because Medicare policies may change without an individual knowing of a new benefit. For this reason, some of the services shown in this mock fee schedule do not have any amounts listed under the three Medicare columns.

PATHOLOGY AND LABORATORY[1]

Laboratory tests done as groups or combination "profiles" performed on multichannel equipment should be billed using the appropriate code number (80048 through 80076). Following is a list of the tests. The subsequent listing illustrates how to find the correct code.

Alanine aminotransferase (ALT, SGPT)
Albumin
Aspartate aminotransferase (AST, SGOT)
Bilirubin, direct
Bilirubin, total
Calcium
Carbon dioxide content
Chloride
Cholesterol
Creatinine
Glucose (sugar)
Lactate dehydrogenase (LD)
Phosphatase, alkaline
Phosphorus (inorganic phosphate)
Potassium
Protein, total
Sodium
Urea nitrogen (BUN)
Uric acid

[1]Mock fees for laboratory tests presented in this schedule may not be representative of fees in your region due to the variety of capitation and managed care contracts, as well as discount policies made by laboratories. At the time of this edition, Medicare guidelines may or may not pay for automatic multichannel tests where a large number of tests are performed per panel. Some cases require documentation and a related diagnostic code for each test performed. Provider must have the CLIA level of licensure to bill for tests, and test results must be documented.

Table 3. Mock Fee Schedule—cont'd

Code Number	Description	Mock Fees	Medicare* Participating	Medicare* Nonparticipating	Medicare* Limiting Charge
ORGAN OR DISEASE-ORIENTED PANELS					
80048	Basic metabolic panel	15.00	14.60	13.87	16.64
80050	General health panel	20.00	19.20	15.99	21.87
80051	Electrolyte panel	20.00	19.20	15.99	21.87
80053	Comprehensive metabolic panel	25.00	20.99	19.94	23.93
80055	Obstetric panel	25.00	20.99	19.94	23.93
80061	Lipid panel	30.00	28.60	25.97	32.16
80074	Acute hepatitis panel	27.00	25.00	20.88	24.88
80076	Hepatic function panel	27.00	25.00	20.88	24.98
81000	Urinalysis, non-automated, with microscopy	8.00	7.44	5.98	8.84
81001	Urinalysis, automated, with microscopy	8.00	7.44	5.98	8.84
81002	Urinalysis, non-automated without microscopy	8.00	7.44	5.98	8.84
81015	Urinalysis, microscopy only	8.00	7.44	5.98	8.84
82270	Blood, occult; feces screening 1-3	4.05	3.56	3.31	4.05
82565	Creatinine; blood	10.00	9.80	8.88	12.03
82947	Glucose; quantitative	15.00			
82951	Glucose tol test, 3 spec	40.00	41.00	36.8	45.16
82952	Each add spec beyond 3	30.00	28.60	25.97	32.16
83020	Hemoglobin, electrophoresis	25.00	20.00	19.94	23.93
83700	Lipoprotein, blood; electrophoretic separation	25.00	20.00	19.94	23.93
84478	Triglycerides, blood	20.00	19.20	15.999	21.87
84480	Triiodothyronine (T–3)	20.00	19.20	15.99	21.87
84520	Urea nitrogen, blood (BUN); quantitative	25.00	20.99	19.94	23.93
84550	Uric acid, blood chemical	20.00	19.20	15.99	21.87
84702	Gonadotropin, chorionic; quantitative	20.00	19.20	15.99	21.87
84703	Gonadotropin, chorionic; qualitative	20.00	19.20	15.99	21.87
85013	Microhematocrit (spun)	20.00	19.20	15.99	21.87
85025	Complete blood count (hemogram), platelet count, automated, differential WBC count	25.00	20.00	19.94	23.93
85032	Manual cell count (erythrocyte, leukocyte, or platelet) each	20.00	19.20	15.99	21.87
85345	Coagulation time; Lee & White	20.00	19.20	15.99	21.87
86038	Antinuclear antibodies	25.00	20.00	19.94	23.93
86580	Skin test; TB, intradermal	11.34	10.38	9.86	11.34
87081	Culture, bacterial, screening for single organisms	25.00	20.00	19.94	23.93
87181	Sensitivity studies, antibiotic; per antibiotic	20.00	19.20	15.99	21.87
87184	Disk method, per plate (12 disks or less)	20.00	19.20	15.99	21.87
87210	Smear, primary source, wet mount with simple stain, for bacteria, fungi, ova, and/or parasites	35.00	48.35	45.93	55.12
88150	Papanicolaou, cytopath	35.00	48.35	45.93	55.12
88302	Surgical pathology, gross & micro exam (skin, fingers, nerve, testis)	24.14	22.09	20.99	24.14
88305	Bone marrow, interpret	77.69	71.12	67.56	77.69

*Some services and procedures may not be considered a benefit under the Medicare program and when listed on a claim form, no reimbursement may be received. However, it is important to include these codes when billing because Medicare policies may change without an individual knowing of a new benefit. For this reason, some of the services shown in this mock fee schedule do not have any amounts listed under the three Medicare columns.

Table 3. Mock Fee Schedule—cont'd

Code Number	Description	Mock Fees	Medicare* Participating	Medicare* Nonparticipating	Medicare* Limiting Charge
MEDICINE PROCEDURES					
Immunization Injections					
90701	Diphtheria, tetanus, pertussis	34.00			
90703	Tetanus toxoid	28.00			
90712	Poliovirus vaccine, oral	28.00			
Therapeutic Injections					
96372	Therapeutic prophylactic or Dx injection; IM or SC	5.22	4.37	4.15	5.22
96374	Intravenous push, single or initial substance/drug	21.33	19.53	18.55	21.33
96379	Intravenous therapeutic, prophylactic, or diagnostic	21.33	19.53	18.55	21.33
Psychiatry					
90816	Individual psychotherapy 20-30 min	60.25	55.15	52.39	60.25
90853	Group therapy	29.22	26.75	25.41	29.22
Hemodialysis					
90935	Single phys evaluation	117.23	107.31	101.94	117.23
90937	Repeat evaluation	206.24	188.78	179.34	206.24
Gastroenterology					
91000	Esophageal incubation	69.82	63.91	60.71	69.82
91055	Gastric incubation	87.41	80.01	76.01	87.41
Ophthalmologic Services					
92004	Comprehensive eye exam	90.86	83.17	79.01	90.86
92100	Tonometry	47.31	43.31	41.14	47.31
92230	Fluorescein angioscopy	55.49	50.79	48.25	55.49
92275	Electroretinography	81.17	74.29	70.58	81.17
92531	Spontaneous nystagmus	26.00			
Audiologic Function Tests					
92557	Comprehensive audiometry	54.33	49.73	47.24	54.33
92596	Ear measurements	26.81	24.54	23.31	26.81
Cardiovascular Therapeutic Services					
93000	Electrocardiogram (ECG)	34.26	31.36	29.79	34.26
93015	Treadmill ECG	140.71	128.80	122.36	140.71
93040	Rhythm ECG, 1-3 leads	18.47	16.90	16.06	18.47
93306	Doppler echocardiography	250.73	229.50	218.03	250.73
93307	Echocardiography without Doppler	114.60	104.90	99.65	114.60
Pulmonary					
94010	Spirometry	38.57	35.31	33.54	38.57
94060	Spirometry before and after bronchodilator	71.67	65.60	62.32	71.67
94150	Vital capacity, total	13.82	12.65	12.02	13.82
Allergy and Clinical Immunology					
95024	Intradermal tests; immediate reaction	6.58	6.02	5.72	6.85
95028	Intradermal tests; delayed reaction	9.32	8.85	10.18	9.32
95044	Patch tests	8.83	8.08	7.68	8.83
95115	Treatment for allergy, single inj.	17.20	15.75	14.96	17.20
95117	2 or more inj.	22.17	20.29	19.28	22.17
95165	Allergen immunotherapy, single or multiple antigens, multiple-dose vials (professional svcs for preparation supervision)	7.11	6.50	6.18	7.11

*Some services and procedures may not be considered a benefit under the Medicare program and when listed on a claim form, no reimbursement may be received. However, it is important to include these codes when billing because Medicare policies may change without an individual knowing of a new benefit. For this reason, some of the services shown in this mock fee schedule do not have any amounts listed under the three Medicare columns.

Continued

Table 3. Mock Fee Schedule—cont'd

Code Number	Description	Mock Fees	Medicare*		
			Participating	Nonparticipating	Limiting Charge
Neurology					
95812	Electroencephalogram, 41-60 min	129.32	118.37	112.45	129.32
95819	Electroencephalogram—awake and	126.81	116.07	110.27	126.81
95860	Electromyography, 1 extremity	88.83	81.31	77.24	88.83
96101	Psychological testing (per hour)	80.95	74.10	70.39	80.95
Physical Medicine					
97024	Diathermy	14.27	13.06	12.41	14.27
97036	Hubbard tank, each 15 min	24.77	22.67	21.54	24.77
97110	Physical therapy, initial 30 min	23.89	21.86	20.77	23.89
97140	Manual therapy (manipulation, traction), one or more regions, each 15 min	16.93	15.49	14.72	16.93
Special Services and Reports					
99000	Handling of specimen (transfer from Dr.'s office to lab)	5.00			
99050	Services provided after office hours, or on Sundays and holidays in addition to basic service in the office	25.00			
99053	Services between 10 pm and 8 am in addition to basic service	35.00			
99056	Services normally provided in office requested by pt in location other than office	20.00			
99058	Office services provided on an emergency basis	65.00			
99070	Supplies and materials (itemize drugs and materials provided)	25.00			
99080	Special reports:				
	Insurance forms	10.00			
	Review of data to clarify pt's status	20.00			
	WC reports	50.00			
	WC extensive review report	250.00			

*Some services and procedures may not be considered a benefit under the Medicare program and when listed on a claim form, no reimbursement may be received. However, it is important to include these codes when billing because Medicare policies may change without an individual knowing of a new benefit. For this reason, some of the services shown in this mock fee schedule do not have any amounts listed under the three Medicare columns.

INDEX

A

Abortion 59100, 59812-9852
Abscess, periurethral 53040
Allergy and clinical immunology 95004-95199
Allergy testing 95004-95199
Amniocentesis, ultrasonic guidance 76946
Anesthesia procedures 00100-01999, 99100-99140
Anoplasty 46700-46705
Anoscopy 46600-46614
Antinuclear antibodies 86038-86039
Appendix surgery 44900-44960
Arm, excision, malignant lesion 11600-11606
Arthrocentesis 20600-20610
Aspiration
  bone marrow 85095
  joint or bursa 20600-20610
Audiometry 92551-92596
Avulsion, nail plate 11730-11732
Axillae
  layer closure, wounds 12031-12037
  repair, simple 12001-12007

B

Barium enema 74270-74280
Biopsy
  breast 19100-19101
  cervical nodes 38510-38520
  cervix 57454, 57500
  endometrium 58100
  prostate 55700-55705
  skin 11100, 11101
  soft tissue (arm) 24065-24066
Blood urea nitrogen, BUN 84520-84525
Bone marrow
  aspiration 85095-85097
  interpretation 88305
  needle biopsy 85102
Bronchography 71040-71060
Bronchoscopy 31622-31656

C

Calcaneus, radiologic exam 73650
Care Plan Oversight Services 99374-99380
Case management 99366-99368
Casts and strapping 29000-29799
Catheter, drainage 75982
Cauterization benign lesion—see destruction
Cauterization, cervix 57510-57513
Cesarean section 59510-59525
  standby 99360
Chest, radiographs 71010-71270
Cholecystectomy 47562-47620
Cholecystography 74290, 74291
Circumcision 54150-54161
Coagulation time 85345-85348

Colectomy	44140-44160
Colonoscopy, fiberoptic	45355-45385
Colostomy, separate procedure	44320
Colporrhaphy	57240-57265, 57289
Colposcopy	57452-57460
Complete blood count	85022-85031
Conization, cervix	57520-57522
Consultation	
during surgery (pathology)	88329-88332
initial	99251-99255
office	99241-99245
telephone calls	99371-99373
with examination and evaluation	99241-99255
Counseling—Preventative Medicine	
group	99411, 99412
individual	99401-99404
Craniotomy	61314
Creatinine	82540, 82565-82570
Critical care	
first 30-74 minutes	99291
each additional 30 minutes	99292
neonatal	99295-99297
Culture, bacterial	87040-87088
Custodial care medical services	
established patient	99334-99337
new patient	99324-99328
Cystourethroscopy	52000-52340

D

Débridement	
nails	11720-11721
skin	11040-11044
Destruction benign lesion, any method	
face	17000-17010
other than face	17100-17105
Dentition, prolonged physician attendance	99354-99360
Dilation	
dilatation and curettage	57820, 58120, 59160, 59840, 59851
esophagus	43450-43460
urethra, female	53660-53661
urethra, male	53620-53621
Diathermy	97024
Domiciliary visits	
established patient	99334-99337
new patient	99324-99328
Dosimetry	77300, 77331

E

Ear	
excision, benign lesion, external	11440-11446
layer closure, wounds	12051-12057
simple repair, wounds	12011-12018
Echocardiography	93307
Echography, pregnant uterus	76805-76816
Electrocardiogram	93000-93042
Electroencephalogram	95819-95827
Electromyography	95858, 95860-95869
Electroretinography	92275

Emergency department services	99281-99288
Endoscopy, gastrointestinal, upper	43234-43264
Esophageal intubation	91000
Excision—see organ, region, or structure involved	
Eye	
excision	65091
removal foreign body	65205-65222
Eyelid	
excision, benign lesion	11440-11446
layer closure, wounds	12051-12057
repair, simple	12011-12018

F

Face	
excision, benign lesion	11440-11446
layer closure, wounds (intermediate)	12051-12057
simple repair, wounds	12011-12018
Feces screening; blood occult	82270
Feet—see foot	
Fluorescein angioscopy, ophthalmoscopy	92230
Foot	
excision, benign lesion, skin	11420-11426
radiologic exam	73620-73630
simple repair, wounds	12001-12007
Fracture	
femur shaft	27500-27508
nasal	21300-21339
tibia proximal, plateau	27530-27537
tibia shaft	27750-27758

G

Gastric intubation	91055
Gastrointestinal tract, radiologic examination	74210-74340
Gastrojejunostomy	43632, 43820-43825, 43860-43865
Genitalia	
excision, benign lesion	11420-11426
repair, simple	12001-12007
Glucose, quantitative	82947
Glucose tolerance test	82951, 82952
Gonadotropin, chorionic	84702, 84703

H

Handling of specimen	99000
Hands	
excision, benign lesion	11420-11426
simple repair, wounds	12001-12007
Hemodialysis	90935-90937
insertion of cannula	36800-36815
placement, venous catheter	36245-36248
Hemoglobin electrophoresis	83020
Hemorrhage, nasal	30901-30906
Hemorrhoidectomy	46221-46262
Hernia, inguinal	49495-49525
Hip, radiologic examination	73500-73540
Home visits	
established patient	99347-99350
new patient	99341-99345

Hospital visits
  discharge day 99238-99239
  first day 99221-99223
  newborn, initial care 99460
  prolonged service 99356, 99357
  subsequent care 99231-99233
  newborn, subsequent day 99462
Hubbard tank 97036, 97113
Hysterectomy 58150-58285
  ectopic pregnancy 59135-59140
  supracervical 58180
  total 58150-58152, 58200-58240
  vaginal 58260-58285
Hysterosalpingography 74740
  injection procedure for 58340

I

Imaging
  bone marrow 78102-78104
  liver 78201-78220
Immunotherapy 95120-95199
Incision and drainage, furuncle 10060
Incision, breast 19000-19030
Injection
  allergies, steroids 95115-95117
  antibiotic 96372
  arthrocentesis, small joint or bursa 20600-20610
  catheter placement 36245-36248
  immunization 90700-90749
  intravenous 96365
IV for contrast venography 36005
  medication, intravenous 96365
  medication, subcutaneous or intramuscular 96372
  therapeutic 96372-96379
Intrauterine device (IUD)
  insertion 58300
  removal 58301

J

Joint fluid, cell count 89050, 89051

K

KUB 74400-74405, 74420

L

Laryngoscopy 31540-31575
Leg, excision, malignant lesion 11600-11606
Lip
  excision, benign lesion 11440-11446
  layer closure, wounds 12051-12057
  repair, superficial wound 12011-12018
Lipoprotein 83700-83701

M

Mammography 76090, 76091
Manipulation, spine 22505, 97260

Manipulation (physical therapy)	97260, 97261
Marsupialization, urethral diverticulum	53240
Mastoids, radiologic exam	70120, 70130
Mucous membrane, cutaneous	
excision, benign lesion	11440-11446
layer closure, wounds	12051-12057
simple repair, wounds	12011-12018
Myringotomy	69420

N

Nail	
excision	11750
trim	11719
wedge excision	11765
Nasal polyp, excision	30110
Neck	
excision, benign lesion	11420-11426
simple repair, wounds	12001-12007
Neonatal critical care	99295-99297
Nephrostolithotomy	50080
Newborn care	99460-99480
Nose	
excision, benign lesion	11440-11446
layer closure	12051-12057
simple repair	12011-12018
Nursing facility care	
initial (new or established)	99304-99306
subsequent care	99307-99310
Nystagmus	
optokinetic	92534
optokinetic test	92544
positional	92532
spontaneous	92531
spontaneous test	92541

O

Obstetric care	59400-59410
Office medical service	
after hours	99050-99053
emergency care	99058
Office visit	
established patient	99211-99215
new patient	99201-99205
service at another location	99056
Ophthalmologic examination	92002-92019
Orchiectomy	54520-54535
Organ- or disease-oriented laboratory panels	80049-80091
Osteotomy, tibia	27455, 27457, 27705, 27709
Outpatient visit	
established patient	99211-99215
new patient	99201-99205

P

Pacemaker, insertion	33200-33217, 71090
Papanicolaou cytopathology	88150-88155
Patch skin test	95044-95052
Pathology, surgical gross and microscopic	88302-88309

Pericardiotomy	33020
Physical medicine services	97010-97150
Platelet count	85590
Pleurectomy	32310
Pneumonectomy	32440-32450
Preventive medicine	
established patient	99391-99397
health hazard appraisal	99420
new patient	99381-99387
unlisted	99429
Proctosigmoidoscopy	45300-45321
Prolonged services	
inpatient or outpatient setting	99354-99359
Prostatectomy, perineal, subtotal	55801
Psychiatric evaluation of records, reports, and/or tests	90825
Psychological testing	96101
Psychotherapy	
pharmacologic management	90862
family (conjoint)	90847
group medical	90853
individual	90816
multiple-family	90849
Puncture, lumbar spine	62270, 62272

Q

Quadriceps repair	27430

R

Radiology	
dosimetry	77300, 77331
teletherapy	77305-77315, 77321
therapeutic	77261-77799
treatment delivery	77401-77417
Repair—see procedure, organ, structure, or region involved	
Reports, special	99080
Resection, prostate, transurethral	52601-54640

S

Salpingo-oophorectomy	58720
Salpingectomy and/or oophorectomy	59120-59140
excision, benign lesion	11420-11422
layer closure, wounds	12031-12037
simple repair, wounds	12001-12007
Sensitivity studies, antibiotic	87181-87192
Septum, nasal septoplasty	30520
Sigmoidoscopy	45330-45333
Skene's gland	53060-53270
Skin excision, skin tags	11200, 11201
Splenectomy	38100-38115
Smear, primary source	87205-87211
Spine, radiologic exam	72010-72120
Spirometry	94010-94070
Standby services	99360
Supplies and materials	99070, 99071

T

TB skin test	86580
Teletherapy	77305-77321
Telephone calls	99441-99443
Thromboendarterectomy	35301-35381
Tibia, radiologic exam	73590
Tonometry	92100
Tonsillectomy	42820-42826
TURP	52601-52648
Treadmill exercise	93015-93018
Triglycerides	84478
Triiodothyronine	84479-84482
Trunk	
excision, malignant lesion	11600-11606
layer closure—intermediate	12031-12037
simple repair	12001-12007
Tumor localization	78800-78803

U

Ureteroneocystostomy	50780-50800
Urethral diverticulum, excision	53230-53235
Uric acid	84550-84560
Urinalysis	81000-81099
Urography	74400-74425

V

Venipuncture	36400-36425
Vesicovaginal fistula, closure	51900, 57320, 57330
Vital capacity (pulmonary function)	94010, 94150, 94160

W

Wrist, radiologic examination	73100, 73110

X

Xenograft	15400

Y

Y-plasty, bladder	51800

Z

Z-plasty	14000, 26121, 41520

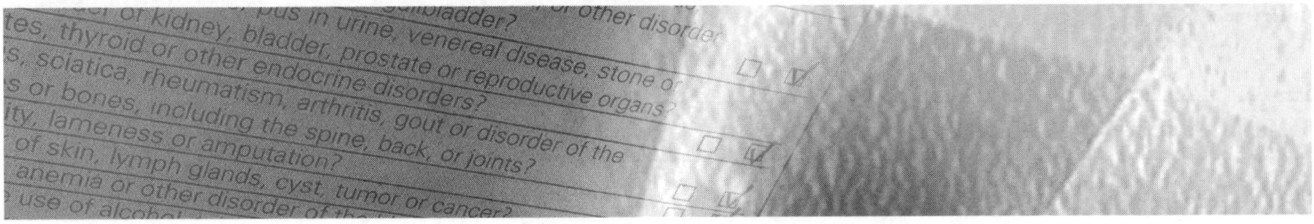

APPENDIX

B

Medicare Level II HCPCS Codes

The following pages provide a partial alphanumeric list of the Centers for Medicare and Medicaid Services (CMS), referred to as Healthcare Common Procedure Coding System (HCPCS) (pronounced "hick-picks"). These Level II codes and modifiers were adopted by the Medicare program in 1984; additional codes and modifiers are added and deleted every year. This system was developed to code procedures not listed in the American Medical Association's Current Procedural Terminology (CPT) code book. This second level is a national standard used by all regional Medicare carriers.

Partial List of the Medicare Healthcare Common Procedure Coding System (HCPCS)

In certain circumstances, a code may need a modifier to show that the procedure has been changed by a specific situation. Remember that CPT and national modifiers apply to both CPT and HCPCS code systems. When applicable, indicate the appropriate modifier on the insurance claim form (Tables 1 and 2). Sometimes a special report may be needed to clarify the use of the modifier to the insurance company.

Table 1. Medicare HCPCS Modifiers

Modifier	Short Description
A1	Dressing for one wound
A2	Dressing for two wounds
A3	Dressing for three wounds
A4	Dressing for four wounds
A5	Dressing for five wounds
A6	Dressing for six wounds
A7	Dressing for seven wounds
A8	Dressing for eight wounds
A9	Dressing for nine or more wounds
AA	Anesthesia performed personally by anesthesiologist
AD	Physician supervision; more than four concurrent anesthesia procedures
AE	Registered dietitian
AF	Specialty physician
AG	Primary physician
AH	Clinical psychologist
AJ	Clinical social worker
AK	Nonparticipating physician
AM	Physician, team member service
AP	No determination of refractive state
AR	Physician scarcity area
AS	Non-NPP assistant-at-surgery service
AT	Acute treatment
AU	Uro, ostomy, or trach item
AV	Item with prosthetic/orthotic
AW	Item with a surgical dressing
AX	Item with dialysis services
AY	Item or service furnished to an end-stage renal disease patient that is not for the treatment of ESRD
AZ	Physician providing service in dental health professional–shortage area for electronic health record incentive pmt
BA	Item with pen services
BO	Nutrition oral admin no tube
BP	Beneficiary elected to purchase item
BR	Beneficiary elected to rent item
BU	Beneficiary undecided on purch/rent
CA	Procedure payable inpatient
CB	ESRD beneficiary Part A SNF-sep pay
CC	Procedure code change

Table 1. Medicare HCPCS Modifiers—cont'd

Modifier	Short Description
CD	AMCC test for ESRD or MCP physician
CE	Med necessity AMCC test sep reimbursement
CF	AMCC test not composite rate
DA	Oral health assessment by licensed health professional other than dentist
E1	Upper left eyelid
E2	Lower left eyelid
E3	Upper right eyelid
E4	Lower right eyelid
EJ	Subsequent claim
EM	Emergency reserve supply (ESRD)
EP	Medicaid EPSDT program SVC
ET	Emergency treatment
EY	No physician/healthcare provider order for item/service
FA	Left hand, thumb
FP	Service provided as part of family planning program
F1	Left hand, second digit
F2	Left hand, third digit
F3	Left hand, fourth digit
F4	Left hand, fifth digit
F5	Right hand, thumb
F6	Right hand, second digit
F7	Right hand, third digit
F8	Right hand, fourth digit
F9	Right hand, fifth digit
G1	URR reading of less than 60
G2	URR reading of 60 to 64.9
G3	URR reading of 65 to 69.9
G4	URR reading of 70 to 74.9
G5	URR reading of 75 or greater
G6	ERSD patient less than 6 dialysis/mth
G7	Pregnancy as result of rape, incest or pregnancy certified by physician as life threatening
G8	Monitored anesthesia care
G9	MAC for at risk patient
GA	Waiver of liability statement issued, as required by payer policy (for covered charges)
GB	Claim resubmitted
GC	Resident/teaching phys serv
GE	Resident primary care exception
GF	Nonphysician serv C A hosp
GG	Payment screen mam diag mam, same pt, same day
GH	Diag mammo to screening mamo
GJ	Opt out physician or practitioner of ER serv
GK	Reasonable and necessary service associated with modifier GA or GZ
GL	Upgraded item, no charge
GM	Multiple transports per ambulance
GN	OP speech language service
GO	OP occupational therapy serv
GP	OP PT services
GQ	Telehealth store and forward
GT	Interactive telecommunication
GU	Waiver of liability statement issued as required by payer policy, routine notice
GV	Attending phys not hospice
GW	Service unrelated to terminal condition of hospice pt
GX	Notice of liability issued, voluntary under payer policy (services excluded from coverage) for noncovered charges
GY	Statutorily excluded
GZ	Not reasonable and necessary
H9	Court ordered
HA	Child/adolescent program
HB	Adult program nongeriatric
HC	Adult program geriatric
HD	Pregnant/parenting women's program
HE	Mental health program
HF	Substance abuse program
HG	Opioid addiction tx program
HH	Mental hlth/substance abs pr
HI	M health/m retrdtn/dev dis pro
HJ	Employee assistance program
HK	Spec high risk mntl hlth pop p
HL	Intern
HM	Less than bachelor degree level
HN	Bachelors degree level
HO	Masters degree level
HP	Doctoral level
HQ	Group setting
HR	Family/couple W client present
HS	Family/couple W/O client present
HT	Multi-disciplinary team
HU	Child welfare agency funded
HV	Funded state addiction agency
HW	State mntl hlth agency funded
HX	County/local agency funded
HY	Funded by juvenile justice agency
HZ	Criminal justice agency fund
JW	Discarded drug not administered
K0	LWR EXT PROST FUNCTNL LVL 0
K1	LWR EXT PROST FUNCTNL LVL 1
K2	LWR EXT PROST FUNCTNL LVL 2
K3	LWR EXT PROST FUNCTNL LVL 3
K4	LWR EXT PROST FUNCTNL LVL 4
KA	Wheelchair add-on option/acc
KB	More than 4 modifiers on claim, based on beneficiary request for ABN upgrade
KC	Replace special power wheelchair interface
KD	Drug/biological dme infused
KF	FDA class III device
KH	DME POS INI CLM, PUR/1 MO RNT
KI	DME POS 2nd or 3rd mo rental

Table 1. Medicare HCPCS Modifiers—cont'd

Modifier	Short Description	Modifier	Short Description
KJ	DME POS PEN PMP or 4-15 mo rent	QS	Monitored anesthesia care
KM	RPLC facial prosth new imp	QT	Recording/storage tape analog recorder
KN	RPLC facial prosth old mod	QU	Physician providing service urban HPSA
K0	Single drug unit dose form	QW	CLIA waived test
KP	First drug of multidrug UD	QX	CRNA service with physician med direction
KQ	2nd/subsqnt drg multi DRG UD	QY	Medically directed CRNA
KR	Rental item partial month	QZ	CRNA service: without medical direction by physician
KS	Glucose monitor supply		
KX	Documentation on file	RC	Right coronary artery
KZ	New cov not implement by MC	RD	Drug admin not incident-to
LC	Left circumflex coronary artery	RR	Rental (DME)
LD	Left anterior descending coronary artery	RT	Right side
LL	Lease/rental (Appld to pur)	SA	Nurse practitioner with physician
LR	Laboratory round trip	SB	Nurse midwife
LS	FDA-monitored intraocular lens implant	SC	Medically necessary serv/sup
LT	Left side	SD	Service by home infusion RN
MS	6 mo maint/svc fee parts/lbr if services not covered under warranty	SE	State/Fed funded program/ser
		SF	2nd opinion ordered by PRO
NB	Nebulizer system, any type, FDA cleared for use with specific drug	SG	Ambulatory surgical center facility service
		SH	2nd concurrent infusion therapy
NR	New when rented	SJ	3rd concurrent infusion therapy
NU	New equipment	SK	High-risk population
PL	Progressive addition lenses	SL	State supplied vaccine
PT	Colorectal cancer screening test; converted to diagnostic test or other procedure	SM	Second opinion
		SN	Third opinion
Q0	Investigational clinical service provided in a clinical research study that is in an approved clinical research study	SQ	Item ordered by home health
		ST	Related to trauma or injury
		SU	Performed in phys office
Q1	Routine clinical service provided in a clinical research study that is in an approved clinical research study	SV	Drugs delivered not used
		SW	Serv by cert diab educator
		SY	Contact w/high-risk pop
Q2	HCFA/ord demo procedure/svc	Tl	Left foot, second digit
Q3	Live donor surgery/services	T2	Left foot, third digit
Q4	Service exempt ordering/referring physician	T3	Left foot, fourth digit
Q5	Substitute physician service, recip bill arrangement	T4	Left foot, fifth digit
		T5	Right foot, great toe
Q6	Locum tenens physician service	T6	Right foot, second digit
Q7	One Class A finding	T7	Right foot, third digit
Q8	Two Class B findings	T8	Right foot, fourth digit
Q9	One Class B and two Class C findings	T9	Right foot, fifth digit
QB	Physician providing SVC in rural HPSA	TA	Left foot, great toe
QC	Single-channel monitoring	TC	Technical component
QD	Recording/storage in solid-state memory	TD	RN
QE	Prescribed oxygen <1 LPM	TE	LPN/LVN
QF	Prescribed oxygen >4 LPM & port	TF	Intermediate level of care
QG	Prescribed oxygen >4 LPM	TG	Complex/high tech level care
QH	Oxygen-conserving device with delivery system	TH	OB tx/servcs prenatl/postpart
		TJ	Child/adolescent program GP
QJ	Patient in state/local custody	TK	Extra patient or passenger
QK	Med dir 2-4 concurrent anes proc	TL	Early intervention IFSP
QL	Patient died after Amb call	TM	Individualized ED prrm (EP)
QM	Ambulance arrangement by hospital	TN	Rural/out of service area
QN	Ambulance furnished by provider	TP	Med transprt unloaded vehicle
QP	Individually ordered lab test	TQ	Bls by volunteer amb provider
QQ	SOI submitted with claim	TR	School-based IEP out of district

Continued

Table 1. Medicare HCPCS Modifiers—cont'd

Modifier	Short Description	Modifier	Short Description
TS	Follow-up service	UB	Medicaid care Level 11 state def
TT	Additional patient	UC	Medicaid care Level 12 state def
TU	Overtime payment rate	UD	Medicaid care Level 13 state def
TV	Holiday/weekend payment rate	UE	Used durable medical equipment
TW	Back-up equipment	UF	Services provided, morning
U1	Medicaid care Level 1 state def	UG	Services provided afternoon
U2	Medicaid care Level 2 state def	UH	Services provided, evening
U3	Medicaid care Level 3 state def	UJ	Services provided, night
U4	Medicaid care Level 4 state def	UK	Service on behalf client-collateral
U5	Medicaid care Level 5 state def	UN	Two patients served
U6	Medicaid care Level 6 state def	UP	Three patients served
U7	Medicaid care Level 7 state def	UQ	Four patients served
U8	Medicaid care Level 8 state def	UR	Five patients served
U9	Medicaid care Level 9 state def	US	Six or more patients served
UA	Medicaid care Level 10 state def	VP	Aphakic patient

Table 2. HCPCS Alphanumeric Index

Description	Code
A	
above-elbow endoskeletal prostheses	L6500
above-elbow prostheses	L6250
acetazolamide sodium (Diamox), injection	J1120
actinomycin D, injection	J9120
adjustable arms, wheelchair	E0973
adjustable chair, dialysis	E1570
adrenaline, injection	J0170
ambulance oxygen and oxygen supplies	A0422
air bubble detector, dialysis	E1530
air travel and nonemergency transport	A0140
alarm, pressure dialysis	E1540
alcohol	A4244
alcohol wipes	A4245
alternating pressure pad, powered pressure	E0181
aminophylline, injection	J0280
amitriptyline HCl (Elavil), injection	J1320
ammonia test paper	A4774
amobarbital sodium (Amytal sodium), injection	J0300
ampicillin, injection	J0290
ampicillin sodium (Omnipen-N), injection	J2430
amputee adapter, wheelchair	E0959
amputee wheelchair, detachable elevating leg rests	E1170
amputee wheelchair, detachable foot rests	E1200
amygdalin, injection	J3570
anesthetics, topical, for dialysis	A4736
ankle prostheses, Symes, metal frame	L5060
ankle prostheses, Symes, molded socket	L5050
antineoplastic drugs, not otherwise classified (NOC)	J9999
antitipping device, wheelchair	E0971
appliance, pneumatic	E0655
arm rest, wheelchair	E0994
arms, adjustable, wheelchair	E0973
asparaginase (Elspar), injection	J9020

Table 2. HCPCS Alphanumeric Index—cont'd

Description	Code
atropine sulfate, injection	J0460
aurothioglucose (Solganal), injection	J2910
axillary crutch extension	L0978
B	
bath conductivity meter, dialysis	E1550
BCNU (carmustine, bis-chloroethyl-nitrosourea), injection	J9050
bed accessories: boards, tables	E0315
bed pan	E0276
below-elbow endoskeletal prostheses	L6400
belt, extremity	E0945
belt, ostomy	A4367
belt, pelvic	E0944
bench, bathtub	E0245
benztropine, injection	J0515
bethanechol chloride, injection	J0520
bethanechol chloride (Myotonachol), injection	J0520
bethanechol chloride (Urecholine), injection	J0520
bicarbonate concentrate for hemodialysis per gallon	A4706
bilirubin (phototherapy) light	E0202
biperiden HCl (Akineton), injection	J0190
bis-chloroethyl-nitrosourea, injection	J9050
bleomycin sulfate, injection	J9040
blood, mucoprotein	P2038
blood (split unit), specify amount	P9011
blood (whole), for transfusion, per unit	P9010
blood leak detector, dialysis	El560
blood pressure monitor	A4670
blood pump, dialysis	El620
blood strips	A4253
blood testing supplies	A4770
bond or cement, ostomy skin	A4364
brompheniramine maleate (Dehist), injection	J0945
C	
calcitonin (salmon) (Calcimar), injection	J0630
calcium disodium edetate (Versenate), injection	J0600
calcium gluconate, injection	J0610
calcium glycerophosphate and calcium lactate (Calphosan), injection	J0620
calcium leucovorin, injection	J0640
calf rest, wheelchair	E0995
calibrator solution	A4256
canes	E0100
carbon filters	A4680
carmustine, injection	J9050
cast supplies	
long leg, adult (11 years), cylinder, fiberglass	Q4034
long leg, adult (11 years), cylinder, plaster	Q4033
long leg, adult (11 years), fiberglass	Q4030
catheter caps, disposable (dialysis)	A4860
catheter insertion tray	A4354
catheter irrigation set	A4355
cefazolin sodium, injection	J0690
ceftriaxone sodium (Rocepin), 250-mg injection	J0696
cellular therapy	M0075

Continued

Table 2. HCPCS Alphanumeric Index—cont'd

Description	Code
cement, ostomy	A4364
centrifuge	A4650
cephalin flocculation, blood	P2028
cephalothin sodium (Keflin), injection	J1890
cephapirin sodium, injection	J0710
cervical head harness/halter	E0942
chair, adjustable, dialysis	E1570
chelation therapy, intravenous (chemical endarterectomy)	M0300
chin cup, cervical	L0150
chloramphenicol (Chloromycetin Sodium Succinate), injection	J0720
chlordiazepoxide HCl (Librium), injection	J1990
chloroprocaine HCl (Nesacaine), injection	J2400
chloroquine HCl (Aralen HCl), injection	J0390
chlorothiazide sodium (Diuril), injection	J1205
chlorpromazine (Thorazine), injection	J3230
chorionic gonadotropin, injection	J0725
clamps, dialysis, venous pressure	A4918
clotting time tube	A4771
codeine phosphate, injection	J0745
colistimethate sodium (Coly-Mycin M), injection	J0770
commode seat, wheelchair	E0968
compressor	E0565
compressor, pneumatic	E0650
conductive paste or gel	A4558
Congo red blood	P2029
contracts, repair and maintenance, ESRD	A4890
corticotropin, injection	J0800
crutches	E0110
cryoprecipitate, each unit	P9012
culture sensitivity study	P7001
Cycler, hemodialysis	E1590
Cycler dialysis machine	E1594
cyclophosphamide, injection	J9070
D	
dactinomycin (Cosmegen) or actinomycin, injection	J9120
daunorubicin HCl, injection	J9150
decubitus care pad	E0185
deionizer, water purification system	El615
detector, blood leak, dialysis	El560
dexamethasone sodium phosphate, injection	J1100
dextrose/normal saline, solution	J7042
Dextrostix	A4772
dialysate concentrate additives	A4765
dialysate testing solution	A4760
dialysis, bath conductivity, meter	E1550
dialysis supplies, miscellaneous	A4913
dialyzers	A4690
diazepam (Valium), injection	J3360
diazoxide (Hyperstat), injection	J1730
dicyclomine HCl (Bentyl), injection	J0500
digoxin, injection	J1160
dihydroergotamine mesylate (D.H.E. 45), injection	J1110
dimenhydrinate (Dramamine), injection	J1240
dimercaprol in peanut oil (BAL in Oil), injection	J0470

Table 2. HCPCS Alphanumeric Index—cont'd

Description	Code
dimethyl imidazole carboxamide (DIC) (dacarbazine, DTIC-DOME), 100-mg vial	J9130
dimethyl sulfoxide (DMSO) (Rimso-50), injection	J1212
diphenhydramine HCl (Benadryl), injection	J1200
disarticulation, elbow, prostheses	L6200
doxorubicin (Adriamycin), injection	J9000
drainage bag	A4358
drainage board	E0606
droperidol (Inapsine), injection	J1790
droperidol and fentanyl citrate (Innovar), injection	J1810
drugs, nonprescription	A9150
dyphylline (Dilor), injection	J1180
E	
elbow protector	E0191
electrical work or plumbing, home, dialysis equipment	A4870
electrocardiogram, routine ECG with 12 leads, with interpret and report	G0403
electrocardiogram, routine ECG with 12 leads, without interpret and report	G0404
electrocardiogram, routine ECG with 12 leads, interpret and report only	G0405
electrodes	A4556
elevating leg rest, wheelchair	E0990
endarterectomy, chemical	M0300
epinephrine, injection	J0170
ergonovine maleate (Ergotrate Maleate), injection	J1330
estradiol cypionate (Depo-Estradiol Cypionate), injection	J1000
estradiol valerate (Delestrogen), injection	J0970
estradiol valerate, up to 20 mg (Estraval-2X), injection	J1390
estradiol valerate, up to 10 mg (Estraval P.A.), injection	J1380
estrone, injection	J1435
etoposide, 50 mg, injection	J9181
examination, initial preventive physical	G0402
external ambulatory infusion pump with administration equipment	E0781
extremity belt-harness	E0945
F	
faceplate, ostomy	A4361
fentanyl citrate (Sublimaze), injection	J3010
fistula cannulation set	A4730
flotation mattress	E0184
flotation pad gel pressure	E0185
floxuridine, 500 mg, injection	J9200
fluid barriers, dialysis	E1575
fluorouracil, injection	J9190
fluphenazine decanoate (Prolixin Decanoate), injection	J2680
foot rest, for use with commode chair	E0175
footplates, wheelchair	E0970
forearm crutches	E0110
furosemide (Lasix), injection	J1940
G	
gamma globulin, 1 ml, injection	J1460
gel, conductive	A4558
gel flotation pad	E0185
gentamicin, injection	J1580
gentamicin sulfate (Garamycin), injection	J1580
gloves, dialysis	A4927

Continued

Table 2. HCPCS Alphanumeric Index—cont'd

Description	Code
glucose test strips	A4772
gold sodium thiosulfate, injection	J1600
Grade-Aid, wheelchair	E0974
gravity traction device	E0941
Gravlee Jet Washer	A4470
H	
hair analysis	P2031
hallux-valgus dynamic splint	L3100
haloperidol (Haldol), injection	J1630
halter, cervical head	E0942
hand rims, wheelchair	E0967
harness, extremity	E0945
harness, pelvic	E0944
harness/halter, cervical head	E0942
head rest extension, wheelchair	E0966
heater for nebulizer	E1372
heel or elbow protector	E0191
heel stabilizer	L3170
hemipelvectomy prostheses	L5280
hemodialysis, monthly capitation	E0945
hemodialysis unit	E1590
Hemostix	A4773
heparin infusion pump, dialysis	E1520
hexachlorophene (pHisoHex) solution	A4246
Hexcelite, cast material—see Q codes under “cast supplies” for specific casts	A4590
HN2 (nitrogen mustard)	J9230
hot water bottle	E0220
hyaluronidase (Wydase), injection	J3470
hydralazine HCl (Apresoline), injection	J0360
hydrocortisone, injection	J1720
hydrocortisone acetate, up to 25 mg, injection	J1700
hydrocortisone phosphate, injection	J1710
hydrocortisone sodium succinate (Solu-Cortef), injection	J1720
hydromorphone (Dilaudid), injection	J1170
hydroxyzine HCl (Vistaril), injection	J3410
hyoscyamine sulfate (Levsin), injection	J1980
hypertonic saline solution	J7130
I	
ice cap or collar	E0230
incontinence clamp	A4356
infusion pump, external ambulatory with administration equipment	E0781
infusion pump, heparin, dialysis	E1520
infusion pump, implantable	E0782
installation and/or delivery charges for ESRD equipment	E1600
insulin, injection	J1815
intercapsular thoracic endoskeletal prostheses	L6570
interferon, injection	J9213
intermittent peritoneal dialysis (IPD) system, automatic	E1592
intermittent positive-pressure breathing (IPPB) machine	E0500
intraocular lenses, anterior chamber	V2630
intraocular lenses, iris supported	V2631
intraocular lenses, posterior chamber	V2632
iodine I-123 sod. iodide capsule(s) diag.	A9516

Table 2. HCPCS Alphanumeric Index—cont'd

Description	Code
iodine swabs/wipes	A4247
irrigation kits, ostomy	A4400
irrigation set, catheter	A4355
IV pole	E0776
K	
kanamycin sulfate, injection	J1840
kanamycin sulfate (Kantrex), up to 75 mg, pediatric, injection	J1850
Kartop patient lift, toilet or bathroom	E0625
L	
laetrile, amygdalin (vitamin B17), injection	J3570
lancets	A4259
lead wires	A4557
leg rest, wheelchair, elevating	E0990
leukocyte-poor blood, each unit	P9016
levorphanol tartrate (Levo-Dromoran), injection	J1960
lightweight wheelchair	E1087
lincomycin, injection	J2010
liquid barrier, ostomy	A4363
lubricant, ostomy	A4402
M	
mannitol, injection	J2150
mechlorethamine HCl (Mustargen), injection	J9230
meperidine, injection	J2175
meperidine HCl and promethazine HCl (Mepergan), injection	J2180
metaraminol bitartrate (Aramine), injection	J0380
meter, bath conductivity, dialysis	E1550
methadone HCl, injection	J1230
methocarbamol (Robaxin), injection	J2800
methyldopate HCl (Aldomet Ester HCl)	J0210
methylergonovine maleate (Methergine), injection	J2210
methylprednisolone acetate (Depo-Medrol), injection	J1020
methylprednisolone sodium succinate (Solu Medrol), injection	
up to 40 mg	J2920
up to 125 mg	J2930
metoclopramide HCl (Reglan)	J2765
microbiology tests	P7001
mini-bus, nonemergency transportation	A0120
miscellaneous dialysis supplies	A4913
mithramycin, injection	J9270
mitomycin (Mutamycin), injection	J9280
monitor, blood pressure	A4670
morphine, injection	J2270
mucoprotein, blood	P2038
N	
nandrolone decanoate, up to 50 mg, injection	J2320
nandrolone decanoate, up to 200 mg, injection	J2322
narrowing device, wheelchair	E0969
nasal vaccine inhalation	J3530
nebulizer, with compressor	E0570
nebulizer heater	E1372
needle with syringe	A4206

Continued

Table 2. HCPCS Alphanumeric Index—cont'd

Description	Code
needles	A4215
neonatal transport, ambulance, base rate	A0225
neostigmine methylsulfate (Prostigmin), injection	J2710
neuromuscular stimulator	E0745
nikethamide (Coramine), injection	J3490
nitrogen mustard, injection	J9230
noncovered procedure	A9270
nonprescription drugs	A9150
nonprofit transport, nonemergency	A0120
O	
occipital/mandibular support, cervical	L0160
orphenadrine citrate (Norflex), injection	L2360
orthoses, thoracic-lumbar-sacral (scoliosis)	L1200
orthotic, knee	L1830
ostomy supplies	A4421
oxacillin sodium (Bactocill), injection	J2410
oxymorphone HCl (Numorphan), injection	J2700
oxytetracycline, injection	J2460
oxytocin (Pitocin), injection	J2590
P	
pacemaker monitor, includes audible/visible check systems	E0610
pacemaker monitor, includes digital/visible check systems	E0615
pad for water circulating heat unit	E0249
pail or pan for use with commode chair	E0167
papaverine HCl, injection	J2440
paraffin	A4265
paraffin bath unit	E0235
paste, conductive	A4558
pelvic belt/harness/boot	E0944
penicillin G benzathine (Bicillin L-A), injection	J0560
penicillin G potassium (Pfizerpen), injection	J2540
penicillin procaine, aqueous, injection	J2510
pentazocine HCl (Talwin), injection	J3070
percussor	E0480
peritoneal straps	L0980
peroxide	A4244
perphenazine (Trilafon), injection	J3310
phenobarbital, injection	J2560
phenobarbital sodium, injection	J2515
phentolamine mesylate (Regitine), injection	J2760
phenylephrine HCl (Neo-Synephrine), injection	J2370
phenytoin sodium (Dilantin), injection	J1165
phototherapy, light	E0202
plasma, single donor, fresh frozen, each unit	P9017
platelet concentrate, each unit	P9019
platelet-rich plasma, each unit	P9020
portable hemodialyzer system	E1635
postural drainage board	E0606
pralidoxime chloride (Protopam Chloride), injection	J2730
prednisolone acetate, injection	J2650
pressure alarm, dialysis	E1540
procainamide HCl (Pronestyl), injection	J2690
prochlorperazine (Compazine), injection	J0780

Table 2. HCPCS Alphanumeric Index—cont'd

Description	Code
progesterone, injection	J2675
prolotherapy	M0076
promazine HCl (Sparine), injection	J2950
promethazine HCl (Phenergan), injection	J2550
propiomazine (Largon), injection	J1930
propranolol HCl (Inderal), injection	J1800
prostheses, above elbow, endoskeletal	L6500
prostheses, below elbow, endoskeletal	L6400
prostheses, hemipelvectomy	L5280
prostheses, intercapsular thoracic, endoskeletal	L6570
prostheses, lower extremity, NOC	L5999
prosthetic services, NOC	L8499
protamine sulfate, injection	J2720
protector, heel or elbow	E0191
Q	
Quad cane	E0105
R	
rack/stand, oxygen	E1355
reciprocating peritoneal dialysis system	E1630
red blood cells, each unit	P9021
regulator, oxygen	E1353
reserpine (Sandril), injection	J2820
restraints, any type	E0710
reverse osmosis water purification, ESRD	E1610
Rh_O(D) immune globulin, injection	J2790
rims, hand (wheelchair)	E0967
Ringer's injection	J7120
rings, ostomy	A4404
S	
safety equipment	E0700
safety visit, wheelchair	E0980
seat attachment, walker	E0156
seat insert, wheelchair	E0992
sensitivity study	P7001
serum clotting time tube	A4771
shunt accessories, for dialysis	A4740
sitz bath, portable	E0160
skin bond or cement, ostomy	A4364
sling, patient lift	E0621
slings	A4565
social worker, nonemergency transport	A0160
sodium succinate, injection	J1720
sorbent cartridges, ESRD	E1636
spectinomycin dihydrochloride (Trobicin), injection	J3320
sphygmomanometer with cuff and stethoscope	A4660
spinal orthosis, NOC	L1499
splint	A4570
splint, hallux-valgus, night, dynamic	L3100
stand/rack, oxygen	E1355
streptokinase-streptodornase, injection	J2995
streptomycin, injection	J3000
streptozocin, injection	J9320

Continued

Table 2. HCPCS Alphanumeric Index—cont'd

Description	Code
succinylcholine chloride (Anectine), injection	J0330
suction pump, portable	E0600
supplies for self-administered injections	A4211
surgical stockings, above-knee length	A4490
surgical supplies, miscellaneous	A4649
surgical trays	A4550
swabs, povidone-iodine (Betadine) or iodine	A4247
syringe	A4213
T	
taxi, nonemergency transportation	A0100
terbutaline sulfate, 0.5 mg, injection	J3105
testosterone cypionate (Depo-Testosterone), injection	J1070
testosterone cypionate and estradiol cypionate (Depo-Testadiol), injection	J1060
testosterone propionate, injection	J3150
testosterone suspension, injection	J3140
tetanus immune human globulin (Homo-Tet), injection	J1670
tetracycline, injection	J0120
tetracycline HCl (Achromycin), injection	J0120
theophylline and mersalyl (Salyrgan), injection	J2810
thiethylperazine maleate (Torecan), injection	J3280
thiotepa (triethylenethiophosphoramide), injection	J9340
thymol turbidity, blood	P2033
thyrotropin (TSH), exogenous, up to 10 IU, injection	J3240
tobramycin sulfate (Nebcin), injection	J3260
toilet rail	E0243
toilet seat, raised	E0244
tolazoline HCl (Priscoline), injection	J2670
tolls, nonemergency transport	A0170
traction device, gravity-assisted	E0941
traction equipment, overdoor	E0860
travel hemodialyzer system	E1635
trays, surgical	A4550
triflupromazine HCl (Vesprin), injection	J3400
trimethaphan camsylate (Arfonad)	J0400
trimethobenzamide HCl (Tigan), injection	J3250
U	
unclassified drugs (contraceptives)	J3490
underarm crutches, wood	E0112
unipuncture control system, dialysis	E1580
urea (Ureaphil), injection	J3350
urinary drainage bag	A4357
urinary leg bag	A4358
urine control strips or tablets	A4250
urine sensitivity study	P7001
V	
vancomycin HCl (Vancocin), injection	J3370
vaporizer	E0605
vascular catheters	A4300
venous pressure clamps, dialysis	A4918
ventilator, volume	E0450
vest, safety, wheelchair	E0980

Table 2. HCPCS Alphanumeric Index—cont'd

Description	Code
vinblastine sulfate, injection	J9360
vinblastine sulfate (Velban), injection	J9360
vitamin B12, injection	J3420
vitamin K, injection	J3430
volume ventilator, stationary or portable	E0450
W	
walker, wheeled, without seat	E0141
walker attachments, platform	E0154
warfarin sodium (Coumadin), injection—unclassified	J3490
washed red blood cells, each unit	P9022
water softening system, ESRD	E1625
wearable artificial kidney (WAK), each	E1632
wheelchair, wide, heavy duty with detachable arms and leg rests	E1092
Y	
youth wheelchair	E1091